Diagnostic Transmission Electron Microscopy of Human Tumors

IDEALIZED ANIMAL CELL

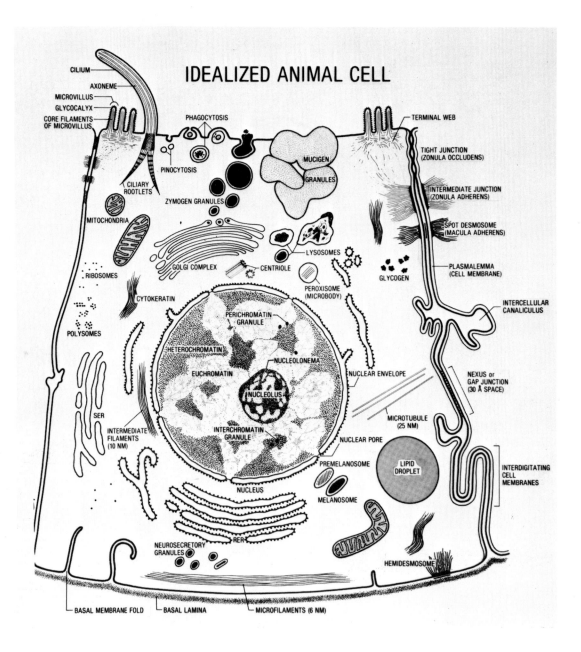

Diagnostic Transmission Electron Microscopy of Human Tumors

The Interpretation of Submicroscopic Structures in Human Neoplastic Cells

ROBERT A. ERLANDSON, Ph.D.

Attending Electron Microscopist
Department of Pathology, Memorial Hospital
for Cancer and Allied Diseases, Memorial
Sloan-Kettering Cancer Center

Assistant Professor of Pathology
Cornell University Medical College

New York City, New York

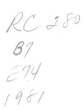 MASSON Publishing USA, Inc.

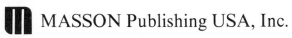 New York • Paris • Barcelona • Milan • Mexico City • Rio de Janeiro

Library of Congress Cataloging in Publication Data

Erlandson, Robert A.

    Diagnostic transmission electron microscopy of
human tumors.

    (Masson monographs in diagnostic pathology; 3)
    Bibliography: p.
    Includes index.
    1. Tumors—Diagnosis. 2. Diagnosis, Electron
microscopic. I. Title. II. Series. [DNLM:
1. Microscopy, Electron. 2. Neoplasms—Diagnosis.
3. Neoplasms—Ultrastructure. W1 MA9309S v. 3 / QZ
241 E69d]
RC280.B7E74   616.99′207582   81-11717
ISBN 0-89352-138-8   AACR2

ISBN 0-89352-138-8
Library of Congress Catalog Card Number: 81-11717
Printed in the United States of America

Masson Monographs in Diagnostic Pathology

Series Editor: Stephen S. Sternberg, M.D.

1. *Tumors and Proliferation of Adipose Tissue:*
   A Clinicopathologic Approach

   By Philip W. Allen (1981)

2. *Diagnostic Immunohistochemistry*

   Edited by Ronald A. DeLellis (1981)

3. *Diagnostic Transmission Electron Microscopy*
   of Human Tumors

   By Robert A. Erlandson (1981)

4. *Meningiomas: Biology, Pathology,*
   and Differential Diagnosis

   By John J. Kepes (1981)

Foreword

Very few physicians appreciate the difficulties of the surgical pathologist. Faced with the cruelties of cancer they cannot be faulted for exerting tremendous pressure on the bench pathologist. The latter, blessed only with the practical experiences of his teachers and rather crude accessory tools such as special stains, must often make educated guesses as to the nature of his material. Surgical pathology, after all, is mostly art and relatively little science. What excitement there was 25 years ago when it appeared that a new tool—the electron microscope—was available to unlock the secrets of tumor diagnosis! Surely, cancers would reveal new organelles, inclusions, or membrane changes to make diagnosis a sure thing. We all know that these expectations were not specifically realized. As a matter of fact, in some quarters electron microscopy of tumors is hardly felt to be worth the price of the microscope. Yet, in a handful of laboratories throughout the world, dedicated workers have built up a powerful body of literature about the ultrastructure of cancers. Rather than finding structures unique to cancer cells, these scientists have succeeded in showing that tumors may be diagnosed on the basis of the presence and arrangements of specific morphologic elements.

Robert A. Erlandson was trained as a biologist with formal education in medical pathology. He is one of the few electron microscopist pathologists to have devoted himself almost entirely to the study of the ultrastructure of tumors. His experience as the electron microscopist for our laboratory as well as his profound knowledge of the literature on this subject makes him a formidable figure in his chosen area. His patience with students and amateurs in the field is well known and his helpful attitude a source of comfort to our surgical pathology staff. The meticulous technique he requires of his technicians and the fantastically clear and relevant photographs he turns out are remarkable.

When Dr. Erlandson first spoke to me about his plans for this monograph, he said that he didn't want to repeat the Atlas or "blown up light microscopic" approach to the problem that several other authors have used but, rather, to examine tumors by reviewing ultramicroscopic structures that are of diagnostic significance. I think that if the reader will slowly and carefully read the text and study the many fine illustrations, he will have taken a first-rate course in the electron microscopy of tumors.

PHILIP H. LIEBERMAN, M.D.
Chief, Surgical Pathology Service
Memorial Hospital for Cancer and Allied Diseases
New York, New York

Preface

Over the past 15 years a large number of papers pertaining to ultrastructural aspects of human tumors have been published. Many of these reports are flawed, either because too few cases were examined, so that they do not reflect the variegated fine structure of a particular nosologic entity, or because the findings were misinterpreted because of lack of cytologic expertise. Nevertheless, information of theoretical, diagnostic, and histogenetic significance has been compiled. Data from original studies, reviews, and a recent book have shown that transmission electron microscopy (TEM) is a valuable adjunct to tumor diagnosis when light microscopic evaluation is equivocal, because neoplasms often retain enough fine structural features of their normal cellular counterparts to establish an accurate diagnosis. The use of TEM is complementary to routine surgical pathology procedures and frequently is definitive when the pathologist has narrowed the diagnostic possibilities in a particular case to a few entities.

The purpose of this monograph is to provide pathologists and other scientists interested in the ultrastructure of human tumors with concise up-to-date information and illustrations covering the diagnostic significance of nuclear and cytoplasmic structures and cell membrane specializations. If the pathologist is able to use such information in a meaningful analysis of diagnostic problems and to evaluate scientific papers accurately, this author will feel that his efforts have been rewarded. The comments made in the monograph are based on the author's electron microscopic examination of more than 3500 human tumors collected over a period of 11 years in the pathology department of Memorial Hospital for Cancer and Allied Diseases, New York City, and on a critical review of the literature.

The monograph is organized differently than most treatises on this subject in that morphology and function of a particular cellular structure are discussed before an illustrated commentary is presented on how the presence of or alteration of this structure may contribute to the diagnosis of a human tumor. For example, one can first read about various types of normal cell junctions, then inquire as to their appearance in a particular sarcoma, e.g., synovial sarcoma. One can also look up diagnostic ultrastructural features of a particular entity or of a broad category of neoplasms, e.g., adenocarcinomas, by consulting the alphabetic listing (Appendix C) of a selected number of human neoplasms keyed to the text. Thus the reader can look up both a particular cell structure and tumor.

The text consists of six chapters and three appendices. Chapter 1 describes procedures for evaluating human tumors and ends with a listing of current reviews and books covering the ultrastructure of human neoplasms. Chapters 2–5 cover the normal morphology, function(s), and appearance in tumors (diagnostic significance) of nuclear, cytoplasmic, cell surface, and selected stromal constituents. Because most structures of diagnostic significance are found in the cytoplasm, organelles, inclusions, and fibers are discussed in greater detail. Only a brief description of the morphology and functions of most cellular constituents is given.

Nevertheless, detailed up-to-date descriptions of neurosecretory-type granules, melanin, intercellular junctions, and especially intracytoplasmic fibers are included, incorporating recent discoveries by cell biologists. The design of the monograph based on particular cell structures also provides for more detailed discussion of a particular category of tumors. For example, the subject of melanin formation (in the inclusions section) logically leads to a discussion of melanocytic nevi and malignant melanomas. Chapter 6 presents 10 cases, illustrating how ultrastructural studies contribute to the evaluation of human tumors; these are followed by a brief summary of the contributions and limitations of this technique based on the author's personal experience. Appendices A–C include preparatory techniques used in our laboratory (Appendix A), the recognition of artifacts (Appendix B), and an alphabetic listing of a selected number of human tumors and their diagnostic ultrastructural features keyed to the main text (Appendix C).

This monograph is not intended to be an encyclopedic compilation of neoplasms and is certainly not intended to substitute for original reports and appropriate textbooks of cytology and pathology. The reader should consult a recent pathology textbook for histologic descriptions of most of the neoplasms described in the monograph. In view of the voluminous literature covering the ultrastructure of human tumors, only selected recent reviews and pertinent references are listed.

ROBERT A. ERLANDSON

Acknowledgments

I wish to express my sincere appreciation to Philip H. Lieberman, M.D., Attending Pathologist and Chief of Surgical Pathology Service, Memorial Hospital for Cancer and Allied Diseases, and Professor of Pathology, Cornell University Medical School, New York City, for his advice and counsel during the preparation of this monograph. I am also indebted to my erstwhile colleague, Bernard Tandler, Ph.D., Professor of Oral Biology and Medicine, School of Dentistry, Case Western Reserve University, Cleveland, for his valued advice and criticism concerning the cell biology content of this manuscript. I would also like to gratefully acknowledge my departmental and surgical colleagues for providing the specimens of human tumors used in the preparation of this book.

My special thanks to Miss Ann Baren and Mrs. Myrna Moy for collecting, processing, and skillfully sectioning and staining the tissues. I am especially indebted to Mr. Roy Keppie for his superb job of printing all the light and electron micrographs from less-than-perfect negatives. Mr. David R. Purnell of the Biomedical Communications Department prepared the line drawing of the idealized animal cell (frontispiece) from my rough sketch.

Miss Barbara Lyngholm did an excellent job of typing the numerous handwritten drafts and researching the case reports. Mrs. Kathryn Clements and Ms. Lisa R. Block skillfully typed the final manuscript.

Finally, I wish to express my gratitude to Fredrick H. Shipkey, M.D., my former boss, for giving me the first opportunity to study the ultrastructure of human neoplasms and for allowing me to reproduce Figure 18 (text Fig. 3-75) from his excellent paper on crystalline inclusions in alveolar softpart sarcomas.

Contents

CHAPTER 1.

Procedure for Evaluating Human Tumors 1

Neoplasms Submitted for Diagnostic TEM at Memorial
  Hospital for Cancer and Allied Diseases 4

CHAPTER 2.

The Nucleus 7

  Nuclear Configurations 7
    Lymphomas 10

  Nucleolus 17

  Nuclear Inclusions 18

CHAPTER 3.

The Cytoplasm 21

  Organelles 21

    Mitochondria 21
      In Cells Synthesizing Steroid Hormones 21
      Mitochondrial Inclusions 23
      Oncocytes 23

    Endoplasmic Reticulum and Ribosomes 26
      Rough Endoplasmic Reticulum 29
      Ribosomes and Polysomes 33
      Smooth Endoplasmic Reticulum 33

    Annulate Lamellae 33

    Golgi Apparatus 35

    Lysosomes 35
      Granular Cell Tumors 38

    Organelle Complexes 41

  Inclusions 42

    Secretory Granules 44
      Mucigen 44
      Zymogen 44
      Neurosecretory-Type Granules (Apudomas) 47

    Glycogen and Lipid 58

    Crystalline Inclusions 60

    Langerhans Granule (Birbeck body) 63

    Lamellar Inclusion Body 65

    Weibel-Palade Body—Vascular Tumors 66

    Melanin 71
      Melanocytic Nevi 72
      Malignant Melanoma 74

  Intracytoplasmic Fibers 77

    Microtubules 77

    Microtrabecular System 78

Contents

Microfilaments—Myofilaments 78
Rhabdomyosarcoma 79
Smooth Muscle Tumors 82
Intermediate Filaments 85
Epidermoid (Squamous-Cell) Carcinoma 87
In Mesenchymal Tumors 89
Hybrid Contractile Cells 89
Myofibroblast 89
Myoepithelial Cell 90

CHAPTER 4.

The Cell Surface 95
Cell Membrane Specializations 95
Plasmalemmal Configurations 95
Pinocytotic Vesicles 95
Asymmetric Unit Membrane (Urinary Bladder Urothelium) 95
Microvilli 99
Intracellular Lumen—Adenocarcinoma 99
Microvillar Configurations 104
Cilia 106
Cell Junctions 107
Junctional Complex 108
Hemidesmosome and Gap Junction 109
Primitive Cell Junctions 111
In Neoplasms other than Typical Carcinomas and
Sarcomas 111
In Sarcomas 115

CHAPTER 5.

Extracellular Constituents 117
Basal Lamina 117
In Neoplasms 117
Collagen 122

CHAPTER 6.

Contributions of TEM to Tumor Diagnosis 125
Case Reports 125
Summary 156
APPENDICES 157
Appendix A. Materials and Methods 157
Appendix B. Artifacts 160
Appendix C. Ultrastructural Tumor Diagnosis—Quick Reference Table 160
References 169
Index 187

CHAPTER I

Procedure for Evaluating Human Tumors

My own examination of more than 3500 neoplasms in the pathology department of Memorial Hospital for Cancer and Allied Diseases and the large number of publications from other pathology departments have shown that high-resolution transmission electron microscopy (TEM) contributes significantly to the evaluation of tumors in the following areas[157]:

1. General submicroscopic anatomy of specific human neoplasms including modification of, or change in numbers of, organelles, inclusions, intracytoplasmic fibers, the nucleus, and cell surface.
2. Histogenesis (cytogenesis) and classification of tumors. Information on the histogenesis of tumors provided by ultrastructural studies is often useful for improving classification schemes. For example, combined electron microscopical and cell surface marker studies have shown that most non-Hodgkin's lymphomas, including the so-called histiocytic lymphomas, are composed of neoplastic B (more rarely T or null) lymphocytes[211,365,381,439,511]; lymphomas composed of neoplastic histiocytes, excluding cases of malignant histiocytosis (histiocytic medullary reticulosis),[266,362,492] are very rare.
3. Diagnostic TEM (the subject of this monograph).
4. Study of functionally active polypeptide hormone or amine-producing neuroendocrine tumors or "apudomas."
5. Experimental tumor pathology. Evaluation of the effects of chemotherapeutic agents and radiation on specific types of neoplastic cells; opportunistic infections in the immunodepressed cancer patient (e.g., *Pneumocystis carinii*[91]) and the evaluation of human tumors grown in tissue or organ culture or in nude mice.

It should be clear to the reader that categories 1–4 are interdependent in that the ultrastructural features of a particular neoplasm often provide information useful for classifying that tumor, e.g., determining whether it is an apudoma, and therefore making an accurate diagnosis.

The present monograph covers only the diagnostic applicability of cell fine structure with respect to human tumors. An ultrastructural description of all neoplasms, including histogenetic and experimental studies, is beyond the scope of this text.

On the basis of our experience over the past 10 years, the following steps and precautions are recommended before making a diagnosis (issuing a TEM supplementary report) on a problem neoplasm submitted for electron microscopic evaluation.

1. Before examining the properly prepared specimen under the electron microscope (Appendix A), it is mandatory to obtain vital clinical information, examine the gross specimen (if possible) and the paraffin-embedded tissue including appropriate special stains, and localize the neoplastic cells of interest in 1-μm-thick epoxy sections. Panoramic low-magnification survey electron micrographs should be taken in addition to high-magnification micrographs (Fig. 1-1).

2. Beware of artifacts attributable to autolysis or necrosis, or both, which are not always visible by light microscopy. It is important to sample viable areas of the tumor. Where possible, avoid examining tumors subjected to chemotherapy or radiation, surgical specimens more than 1 hr after extirpation, specimens from delayed autopsies, and pieces of tissue taken from paraffin blocks (Appendix B).

3. Transmission electron microscopy should not be used to distinguish between benign and malignant neoplasms, because reliable ultrastructural criteria for malignancy are lacking.

4. Be familiar with the spectrum of ultrastructural appearances of a specific nosologic en-

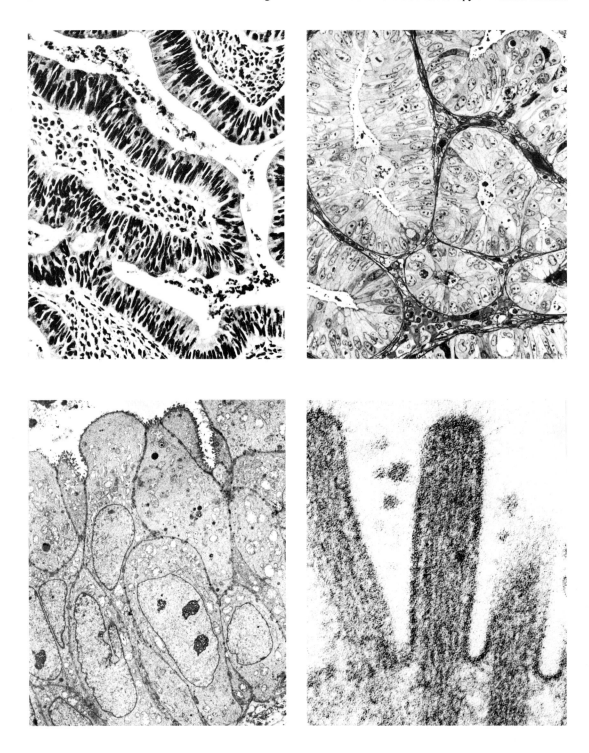

FIGURE 1-1
Adenocarcinoma from the sigmoid colon of a 66-year-old male. Composite illustration comparing H&E stained paraffin-embedded specimen (*upper left*, ×250), toluidine blue stained, epoxy-embedded specimen (*upper right*, ×250), relatively low-magnification electron micrograph (*lower left*, ×2240), and high magnification electron micrograph of a microvillus (*lower right*, ×120,000); note the microfilamentous core extending into the ectoplasm. The magnification and resolution capabilities of TEM should be apparent.

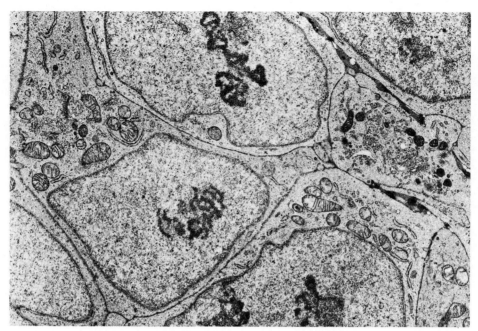

FIGURE 1-2
Undifferentiated malignant ovarian tumor (pelvic mass, 21-year-old female). The neoplasm consists of sheets of polygonal and ovoid cells lacking specific ultrastructural markers. (×7000.)

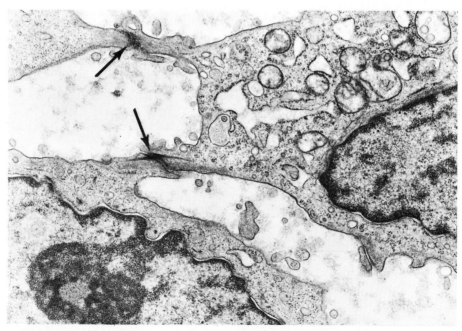

FIGURE 1-3
Spindle cell area of infiltrating duct carcinoma (breast, 60-year-old female). Note that one neoplastic epithelial cell (*right*) is connected to two adjacent cell processes by rudimentary cell junctions (*arrows*). The cells otherwise resemble fibroblasts with a well-developed branching RER. (×16,000.)

tity. Neoplasms of a particular type are like fingerprints—no two are exactly alike. Where possible, it is advisable to have a control file of known cases of specific types of neoplasms, e.g., synovial sarcoma, malignant fibrous histiocytoma, and pulmonary carcinoid tumors. Obtain multiple specimens from a histologically heterogeneous specimen.

5. Identifying a constellation of structures characteristic of the putative cell of origin is often more definitive. For example, ultrastructural features attributed to smooth muscle tumors are parallel bundles of longitudinally oriented actin microfilaments with interspersed fusiform dense bodies, plasmalemmal attachment plaques, numerous surface pinocytotic vesicles, and a well-defined basal lamina (Fig. 3-120). The presence of all these submicroscopic structures makes the diagnosis more certain, because each may be found in other cell types either singly or in combination, e.g., myofilaments of the smooth muscle type are found in myofibroblasts and myoepithelial cells, and pinocytotic vesicles are prominent in endothelial and perineurial cells. The complete, essential characteristics of normal cells, unfortunately, are hardly ever reproduced in tumors derived from them. For a structure to be diagnostic, it must be found in all or a significant number of cases of a particular nosologic entity.

6. Occasional poorly differentiated (anaplastic) tumors are devoid of fine structural features required to establish histogenesis. In some cases it is impossible to determine whether the neoplasm is a carcinoma or sarcoma (Fig. 1-2). It must be emphasized that not all tumors have specific ultrastructural markers that permit them to be recognized (Chapter 6, cases 7–10). No pathologist likes to admit not being able to make a specific, accurate diagnosis. And the surgical pathologist is pressured by the clinician to provide a specific diagnosis so that a therapeutic regimen can be tailored for a particular tumor. Such terms as spindle cell carcinoma or sarcoma, anaplastic tumor, poorly differentiated carcinoma of uncertain histogenesis, and small round cell anaplastic tumor are appropriate, albeit unsatisfactory, when it is impossible to further subclassify the lesion using all available methods. It is my policy not to call a poorly differentiated tumor an amelanotic melanoma just because the clinician or surgical pathologist, or both, suspect it is, if, after painstaking search at high magnification, no premelanosomes can be identified (see discussion of melanoma, p. 74).

7. Tumors derived from controversial hybrid, transitional, or intermediate cells, e.g., the myoepithelial cell, myofibroblast, pericyte, perineurial cell, and facultative fibroblast, with ultrastructural features of two widely divergent types of tissue, are often difficult to interpret, as discussed elsewhere in this volume. Neoplasms derived from blastema or primitive multipotential (pleuripotential) mesenchymal stem cells, and those arising from cells that have migrated from the neural crest, e.g., nephroblastoma (Wilms's tumor),[453,604] pancreatoblastoma,[258] pulmonary blastoma,[198] synovial sarcoma,[411] malignant fibrous histiocytoma,[11,113,195,281,358,591] apudomas (p. 47), also require careful interpretation because of the varied submicroscopic appearance, atavistic features, and multipotentiality of these heterogeneous groups of poorly understood neoplasms. Note any metaplastic changes, e.g., squamous or spindle cell (Fig. 1-3) metaplasia in adenocarcinomas[383] and mesenchymal metaplasia, e.g., cartilage formation, of epithelial cells, e.g., myoepithelial cells (p. 91), or in the connective tissue stroma of neoplasms.

Chapter 6 presents 10 cases that illustrate how the above-listed procedures are applied to the ultrastructural diagnostic evaluation of tumors.

The well-differentiated cell carries the complete genetic information of the individual in a partially repressed state. Derepression of tumor cells, many of which may have an altered genome (aneuploidy, deletions, translocations, and inversions) could lead to unexpected ultrastructural characteristics. The nature of these changes is poorly understood and is beyond the scope of this monograph.

NEOPLASMS SUBMITTED FOR DIAGNOSTIC TEM AT MEMORIAL HOSPITAL FOR CANCER AND ALLIED DISEASES

Examples of neoplasms routinely submitted for ultrastructural evaluation by the electron microscopy laboratory of the pathology department are:

1. All unusual, rare, or interesting tumors, as well as "classic" examples of specific nosologic entities for control files.
2. All undifferentiated (anaplastic) tumors (Chapter 6).
3. Spindle cell sarcomas of questionable histogenesis, e.g., leiomyosarcoma versus malignant nerve sheath tumor. Suspected cases of malignant fibrous histiocytoma, epithelioid sarcoma, or synovial sarcoma.
4. Small, round to oval cell tumors, especially in

TABLE 1-1

EM Differential Diagnosis of Small Round Cell Tumors

	Embryonal Rhabdomyosarcoma	Ewing's Sarcoma	Neuroblastoma	Primitive Neuroectodermal Tumor	Non-Hodgkin's Lymphoma	Small Cell Carcinoma
Nuclear morphology	Often pleomorphic	Round; generally smooth	Round	Round or ovoid	Round, cleaved or convoluted	Round or pleomorphic
Nucleolus	Small or large	Small	Small	Small	Small or large; round	Large; generally round
Cell processes	May form long cell processes	Absent	Dendritic	Dendritic[a]	Absent or filopodia	Inconspicuous
Prominent organelles	Golgi, polysomes, RER	None	None	Variable	Polysomes	Variable; intracellular lumen[a]
Glycogen	May be prominent	Prominent (pools)[a]	Inconspicuous	Rare	Rare	Inconspicuous
Neurosecretory-type granules	Absent	Absent	Present within dendritic processes[a]	Absent	Absent	Present only in apudomas
Intracytoplasmic fibers	Actin and myosin, primitive sarcomeres[a]	Rare	Neurofilaments and microtubules (in cell processes)[a]	Neurofilaments and microtubules (in cell processes)[a]	Rare	Occasional microfilaments and cytokeratin
Intercellular junctions	Inconspicuous, primitive	Rare; primitive	Inconspicuous	Inconspicuous, primitive	Absent[a]	Mature or primitive[a]; junctional complex
Basal lamina	Often conspicuous	Absent	Absent (present in ganglioneuroblastoma)	Absent	Absent[a]	Inconspicuous

[a] Key diagnostic structure.

TABLE 1-2

Ultrastructural Diagnosis of Anterior Mediastinal Tumors

	Thymoma (Epithelial Cell)	Thymic Carcinoid	Non-Hodgkin's Lymphoma	Hodgkin's Disease (Reed-Sternberg Cell)	Seminoma (Germinoma)
Nuclear morphology	Ovoid or cigar shaped. Usually smooth	Round	Round, cleaved, or convoluted	Pleomorphic multilobulated[a]	Round or ovoid
Nucleolus	Small	Small	Small or large, round	Large and round	Prominent nucleolonema[a]
Cell processes	Conspicuous	Inconspicuous	Absent or filopodia	Absent; filopodia, ruffles	Rare
Prominent organelles	Variable	RER; Golgi, polysomes	Polysomes	Polysomes and ribosomes	Variable
Neurosecretory-type granules	Absent	Numerous[a]	Absent	Absent	Absent
Intracytoplasmic fibers	Cytokeratin filaments[a]	Inconspicuous	Rare	Rare	Rare
Intercellular junctions	Desmosomes[a]	Scattered, primitive	Absent[a]	Absent	Inconspicuous
Basal lamina	Inconspicuous (cells closely packed)	Often surrounds cell clusters	Absent[a]	Absent	Rare, incomplete

[a] Key diagnostic structure.

children and adolescents when the clinical and frozen section diagnosis is uncertain. Examples: neuroblastoma, Ewing's sarcoma, embryonal rhabdomyosarcoma, lymphoma (Table 1-1).

5. Anterior mediastinal tumors. Examples: thymoma, non-Hodgkin's lymphoma, germinoma, thymic carcinoid (Table 1-2).

6. Suspected cases of amelanotic melanoma, mesothelioma, non-Hodgkin's lymphoma, oat cell carcinoma, and neuroendocrine tumors (carcinoids—apudomas).

Out of 1030 diagnostic problems examined by TEM (excluding known examples of specific nosologic entities), only 120 tumors lacked sufficient ultrastructural markers to unable us to render an accurate diagnosis.

Selected Reviews and Books—Diagnostic
Electron Microscopy

1. Bauer, W.C., and McGavran, M.H.: Ultrastructure and surgical pathology. In: *Surgical Pathology*, 5th ed. L.V. Ackerman and J. Rosai (eds.). C.V. Mosby, St. Louis, MO, 1974, pp. 7–35.
2. Bonikos, D.S., Bensch, K.G., and Kempson, R.L.: The contribution of electron microscopy to the differential diagnosis of tumors. *Beitr Pathol 158: 417–444, 1976.*
3. Buss, H., and Hollweg, H.G.: Application of scanning electron microscopy to diagnostic pathology. A critical review. In: *Scanning Electron Microscopy/1980/III.* O. Johari and P. P. Becker (eds.). SEM, Chicago, pp. 139–153.
4. Damjanov, I.: *Ultrastructural Pathology of Human Tumors.* Eden Medical Research, St. Albans, VT, 1979, Vol. 1; 1980, Vol. 2. (No photographs.)
5. Erlandson, R.A.: Electron microscopy of human tumors. A short review. *Clin Bull 3: 14–19, 1973.*
6. Ferenczy, A.: Diagnostic electron microscopy in gynecologic pathology. In: *Pathology Annual*, Vol. 14. S.C. Sommers and P.P. Rosen (eds.). Appleton-Century-Crofts, New York, 1979, pp. 353–381.
7. Ghadially, F.N.: *Diagnostic Electron Microscopy of Tumors.* Butterworths, Boston, 1980.
8. Gyorkey, F., Min, K-W., Krisko, I., and Gyorkey, P.: The usefulness of electron microscopy in the diagnosis of human tumors. *Hum Pathol 6: 421–441, 1975.*
9. Mackay, B., and Osborne, B.M.: The contribution of electron microscopy to the diagnosis of tumors. In: *Pathobiology Annual*, Vol. 8. H.I. Ioachim (ed.). Raven Press, New York, 1978, pp. 359–405.
10. Morales, A.R.: Electron microscopy of human tumors. In: *Progress in Surgical Pathology*, Vol. 1. C.M. Fenoglio and M. Wolff (eds.). Masson, New York, 1980, pp. 51–70.
11. Rosai, J., and Rodriguez, H.A.: Application of electron microscopy to the differential diagnosis of tumors. *Am J Clin Pathol 50: 555–562, 1968.*
12. Trump, B.F., and R.T. Jones (eds.): *Diagnostic Electron Microscopy.* John Wiley & Sons, New York, 1978, Vol. 1; 1979, Vol. 2; 1980, Vol. 3.
13. van Haelst, U.J.G.M.: General consideration on electron microscopy of tumors of soft tissues. In: *Progress in Surgical Pathology*, Vol. 2. C.M. Fenoglio and M. Wolff (eds.). Masson, New York, 1980, pp. 225–257.

CHAPTER II

The Nucleus

The nucleus contains the vast bulk of the cellular DNA. It is the source of informational macromolecules (ribosomal, messenger, and transfer RNAs) that control the synthetic activities of the cytoplasm. The nucleus is separated from the cytoplasm by a complex nuclear envelope or membrane. During interphase, nucleocytoplasmic exchange of macromolecules probably occurs via scattered small openings in the nuclear envelope called nuclear pores. The nucleoplasm contains chromatin consisting of DNA and nucleoproteins in clumped or condensed regions, heterochromatin, or in a metabolically active finely dispersed form, euchromatin. During mitosis the chromatin is organized into discrete, easily discernible rodlike chromosomes. In addition to chromatin and the poorly understood perichromatin and interchromatin granules (see Ghadially,[208] p. 25), the nucleus contains one or more prominent spherical bodies called nucleoli, which consist of both, masses of RNA and deoxyribonucleoprotein. Electron micrographs show the nucleolus to be composed of a network of anastomosing strands—the so-called nucleolonema of the light microscopist—and both, granular and nongranular rounded masses (Fig. 2-1).

Electron microscopic studies of human tumors have failed to demonstrate any unique nuclear changes associated with neoplasia. Although pleomorphic nuclei with deep cytoplasmic invaginations, prominent heterochromatin, and enlarged, often multiple, nucleoli (Figs. 2-2 and 2-3) are commonly found in poorly differentiated neoplastic cells, some malignant tumors e.g., neuroblastoma (Fig. 3-53) and Ewing's sarcoma (Fig. 3-70) consist of cells that have a small, smooth-contoured nucleus, finely dispersed chromatin, and a small nucleolus, whereas cells comprising benign neoplasms may have irregularly shaped nuclei with large nucleoli (Fig. 2-4).

The remainder of this chapter discusses some interesting and sometimes diagnostic nuclear configurations (nuclear envelope alterations), the malignant lymphomas, and variations in nucleolar morphology. Nuclear inclusions, although not diagnostically significant, are also briefly covered, as they are found in diverse neoplasms.

NUCLEAR CONFIGURATIONS

I have observed two types of nuclear configurational changes in tumors that are quite rare in non-neoplastic cells: (1) the morphologic manifestations of nuclear envelope plasticity (cytoplasmic invaginations), and (2) abnormal proliferation (nuclear projections, pockets, or blebs).[158]

A relatively common finding in neoplastic cells is the presence of shallow or deep infoldings of the nuclear envelope. Cleaved nuclei have one or two deep invaginations and are prominent in non-Hodgkins lymphomas derived from the cleaved follicular center B lymphocytes[365] (Fig. 2-5) and in granulosa cell tumors of the ovary.[180,206] Cleaved nuclei are also sporadically found in various other benign (Fig. 2-6) and malignant tumors. Convoluted nuclei are characterized by multiple shallow and moderately deep cytoplasmic herniations (Fig. 2-7). They are prominent in non-Hodgkin's lymphomas composed of T lymphocytes (see below). Cerebriform nuclei with multiple deep and shallow nuclear indentations are commonly found in thymus-derived circulating Sézary cells[331,370,371] and in lymphoid cells which comprise the closely related disorder mycosis fungoides[84] (Fig. 2-8). It should be pointed out that scattered foci of cerebriform Sézary-like mononuclear cells are also found in a variety of skin conditions, such as parapsoriasis en plaque,[370] in human umbilical cord blood, and in the blood of healthy persons.[409] Cytogenetic and cytophotometric studies designed to measure the number of chromosomes and DNA content, respectively, of cerebriform nuclei of Sézary cells from four patients with Sézary syndrome demonstrated abnormal DNA values and karyotypes,[369] indicating that marked chromosomal abnormalities may be responsible for the extreme nuclear plasticity of these cells.

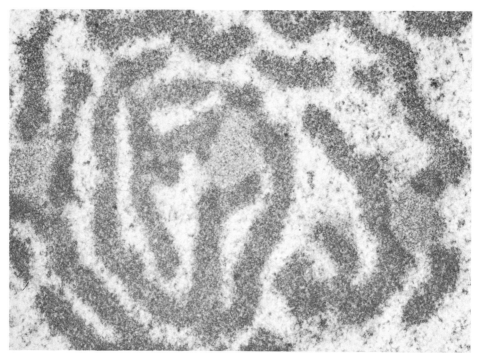

FIGURE 2-1
Epidermoid carcinoma (left upper lobe, lung, 55-year-old female). Ribbon-like nucleolonema and granular rounded masses of nucleolus are illustrated. (×40,000).

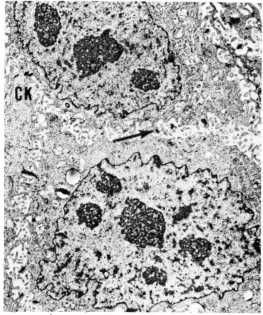

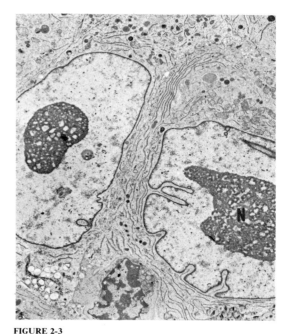

FIGURE 2-2
Squamous carcinoma (tongue, 73-year-old female). The large, pleomorphic nuclei contain multiple nucleoli and evenly dispersed clumped chromatin. Note the microvilluslike surface protrusions, remnants of desmosomes (*arrow*), and cytokeratin filaments (CK). (×31,800).

FIGURE 2-3
Anaplastic lung adenocarcinoma (right upper lobe, 68-year-old male). Two large nuclei are shown. Note the multiple nuclear invaginations and the huge centrally located nucleolus (N). The cytoplasm contains prominent strands of RER and secretory granules and lysosomes of varying size and density. (×3120).

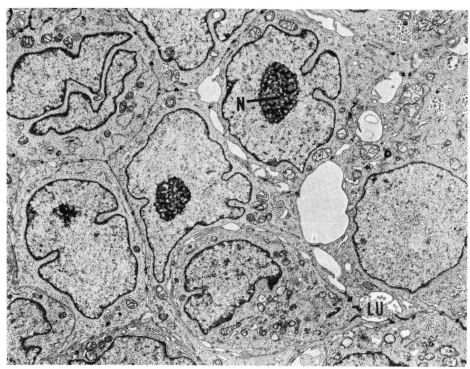

FIGURE 2-4
Cystadenfibroma (ovary, 66-year-old female). Nest of benign neoplastic coelomic epithelial (mesothelial) cells. Note the prominent invaginations of the nuclear envelope and the large nucleolus (N). Lumen (LU). (×4800).

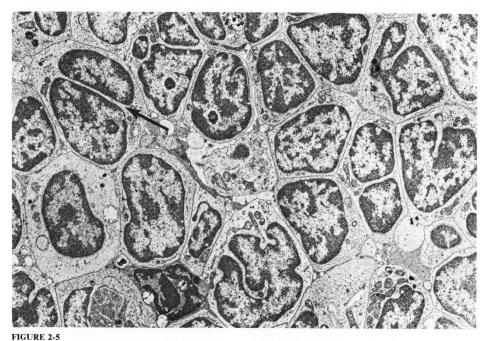

FIGURE 2-5
Malignant lymphoma, poorly differentiated lymphocytic (small cleaved cell type), nodular (axillary lymph node, 59-year-old male). Many of the nuclei exhibit one or two deep infoldings of the nuclear envelope that occasionally appear to bisect the nucleus (*arrow*). (×4800).

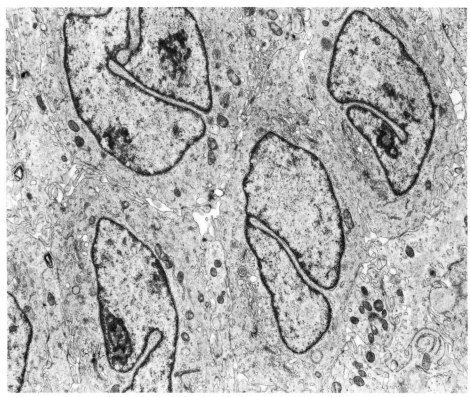

FIGURE 2-6
Benign papilloma (urinary bladder, 67-year-old female). Transitional epithelial cells with prominent deeply cleaved nuclei. (×7600).

The second and less common type of nuclear envelope abnormality consists of an unusual proliferation (excess production) of nuclear membranes resulting in protrusions variously referred to as nuclear projections, blebs, sheets, or pockets (Fig. 2-9).[421,422,544] These structures are formed by apposed extensions of nuclear membranes and either their subjacent fibrous lamina (an approximately 30-nm-thick band of fibrillogranular material of moderate electron density in contact with the inner aspect of the nuclear envelope),[168,396] or heterochromatin. The membranes sometimes arch over to rejoin the main nuclear mass, enclosing a pocket of cytoplasm in the process (Figs. 2-9 and 2-10). In many of the tumor cells, multilobated or satellite nuclei are formed by terminal expansion of the apposed nuclear membranes (Figs. 2-10 and 2-11). Nuclear membrane protrusions are more commonly found in sarcomas, e.g., certain lymphomas and leukemias,[87,118,422] chrondroblastoma,[269,348] and medulloblastoma,[583] as opposed to carcinomas. Satellite nuclei are consistently found in the neoplastic perineurial fibroblasts comprising cases of dermatofibrosar-

coma protuberans (Fig. 2-11), an unusual fibrous skin tumor with a characteristic storiform cell pattern.[10,240] Nuclear protrusions are also found in occasional cases of malignant melanoma.[314] We recently examined a primitive unclassifiable leukemia in a 40-year-old man, the cells of which exhibited both types of nuclear envelope abnormalities in addition to excess production of plasma membranes (Fig. 2-12). Although the precise mechanism for this phenomenon is not known, Ahearn and associates[5] and Shabtai et al.[530] have shown a definite correlation between chromosomal abnormalities and nuclear blebs in several cases of human acute leukemia.

Lymphomas

It is appropriate to discuss briefly the malignant lymphomas, because diagnosis and classification is strongly dependent on the nuclear configuration of the neoplastic lymphocytes composing these tumors.[216,349,365,491,511] Despite intensive light microscopical, ultrastructural, immunologic and cytochemical studies, there is still no universally

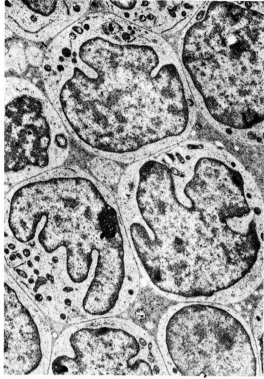

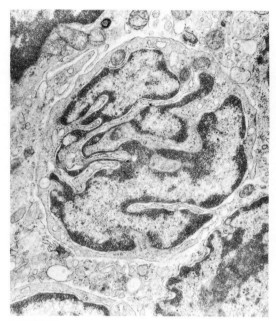

FIGURE 2-8
Mycosis fungoides (skin biopsy, 64-year-old female). Neoplastic lymphoid cell with complexly folded cerebriform nucleus. (×11,200).

FIGURE 2-7
Malignant lymphoma, lymphoblastic type (cervical lymph node, 8-year-old male). Two lymphoid cells showing three cytoplasmic herniations into the nucleus are illustrated. (×6800).

accepted classification of non-Hodgkin's lymphomas.[439] The following discussion of the ultrastructural features of a selected number of malignant lymphomas uses a modified Rappaport classification currently employed at Memorial Hospital for Cancer and Allied Diseases, New York City. Malignant lymphoma, well-differentiated lymphocytic type (synonymous with chronic lymphocytic leukemia) consists of normal-appearing small lymphocytes. True histiocytic lymphomas and plasmacytoid lymphomas are discussed elsewhere in the text. An important diagnostic feature of normal, abnormal, or neoplastic lymphocytes is that they are never joined by cell junctions and do not form an external lamina.

Malignant lymphoma of the poorly differentiated lymphocytic type consists of small or medium-size lymphocytes, or both, with cleaved, noncleaved, or irregularly shaped nuclei presum-

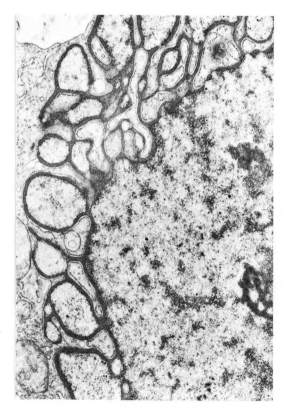

FIGURE 2-9
Metastatic leiomyosarcoma (groin node, 78-year-old female). Portion of nucleus illustrating numerous nuclear membrane protrusions. (×11,200).

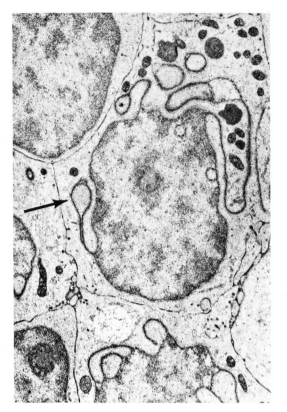

ably derived from the bursal equivalent B lymphocytes (B cells) populating the follicular centers[216,365,511] (Figs. 2-5 and 2-10). Either a follicular (nodular) or diffuse growth pattern may be present. The chromatin is clumped and is usually located adjacent to the nuclear envelope (marginated chromatin). Nucleoli of moderate size are either centrally or peripherally located. The scanty cytoplasm contains only a few organelles. Transformed lymphocytes or immunoblasts, or both (see below), with round nuclei, dispersed chromatin, large nucleoli, and numerous polysomes in an abundant cytoplasm are usually scattered among the cleaved and noncleaved lymphoid tumor cells.

Malignant lymphoma of the lymphoblastic type is composed of distinctive immature lymphoid cells that are indistinguishable from the lymphoblasts and prolymphocytes of acute lymphoblastic leukemia. The patients often have anterior mediastinal masses and involvement of bone marrow and peripheral blood.[74,440,454,511] One type of neo-

FIGURE 2-10
Malignant lymphoma, poorly differentiated lymphocytic (small cleaved cell type), diffuse (groin node, 71-year-old female). Neoplastic B lymphocytes showing nuclear membrane protrusions and a satellite nucleus (*arrow*). (×8400).

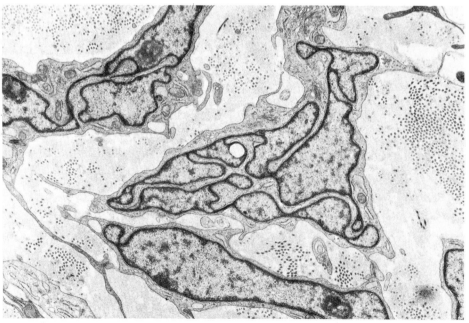

FIGURE 2-11
Dermatofibrosarcoma protuberans (breast, mass, 62-year-old female). Multilobated nuclei in neoplastic perineurial fibroblasts. Cross-sectional collagen fibrils are evident in the stroma. (×9200).

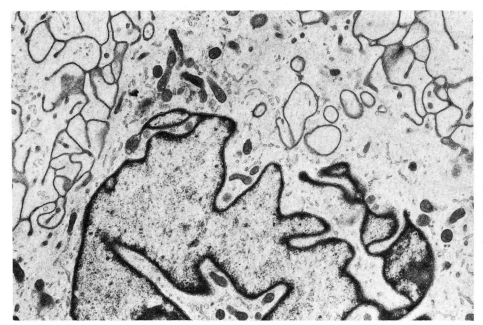

FIGURE 2-12
Primitive unclassifiable leukemia (axillary lymph node, 40-year-old male). Leukemic cell showing pleomorphic nucleus and abnormal cell membrane production. (×10,000).

plastic thymus-derived lymphocyte (T cell) is characterized by convoluted or multisegmented (multilobulated) nuclei, marginated chromatin, and small inconspicuous nucleoli (Fig. 2-7). The cytoplasm contains variable numbers of polysomes and a well-developed Golgi apparatus, e.g., mediastinal lymphomas of childhood and large cell histiocytic lymphomas of T cell type[440,454,511] (Fig. 2-16). Not all lymphoblastic lymphomas are composed of T lymphocytes having prominent nuclear convolutions; many consist of null lymphocytes (cells without surface markers) with uniformly round nuclei or nuclei with one shallow indentation, finely dispersed or marginated chromatin, small nucleoli, and scanty cytoplasm containing few organelles (Fig. 2-13). Nevertheless, convoluted nuclei are occasionally found in null cell lymphomas, and round nuclei in T cell lymphomas (Fig. 2-14). Differentiating T cell from null cell lymphoblastic lymphomas by morphologic methods is not possible. The finely dispersed chromatin (no margination) pattern is highly characteristic of lymphoblasts, wheras the prolymphocytes have occasional foci of heterochromatin and marginated chromatin (Fig. 2-7).[74]

Malignant lymphoma of the histiocytic type—

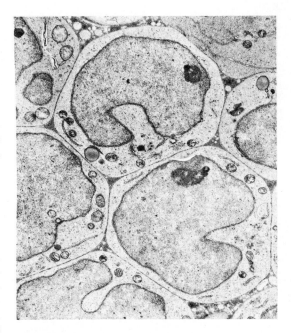

FIGURE 2-13
Malignant lymphoma, lymphoblastic null cell type (cervical lymph node, 8-year-old male). Lymphoblasts with slightly indented nuclei containing finely dispersed chromatin and a small, inconspicuous nucleolus. (×5600).

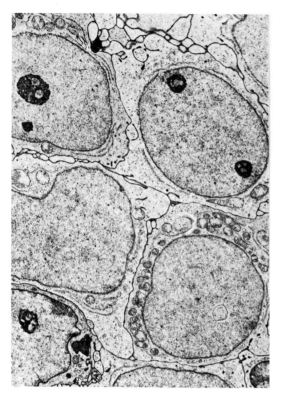

FIGURE 2-14
Malignant lymphoma, lymphoblastic T cell type (cervical lymph node, 46-year-old male). The neoplastic lymphoblasts contain a uniform round nucleus with finely dispersed chromatin and one or two small nucleoli. Ruffling of the cell membrane is evident at the *top right*. (×4000.)

FIGURE 2-15
Malignant lymphoma, histiocytic type, diffuse (submental mass, adult male). Large transformed neoplastic B lymphocytes are illustrated. Note that two of the nuclei are cleaved, nucleoli are large and marginated, and the abundant cytoplasm contains numerous polysomes. (×4700).

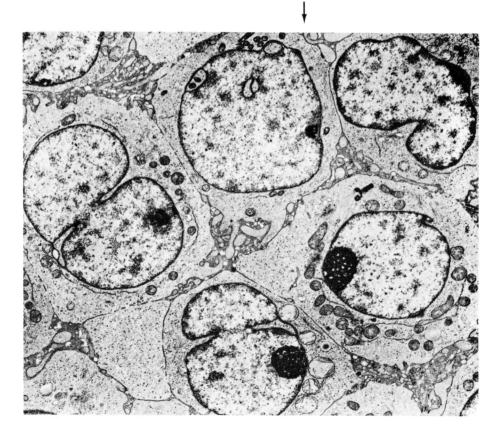

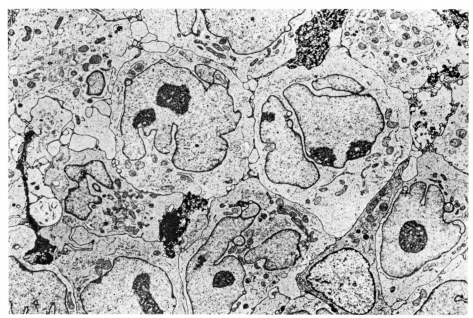

FIGURE 2-16
Malignant lymphoma, T-immunoblastic type, diffuse (groin lymph node, 38-year-old female). Large neoplastic immunoblasts with pleomorphic nuclei containing finely dispersed chromatin and large multiple nucleoli are illustrated. Note the prominent polysomes and scattered segments of RER in the cytoplasm. Remnants of necrotic tumor cells (dark masses) are also evident. (×2800).

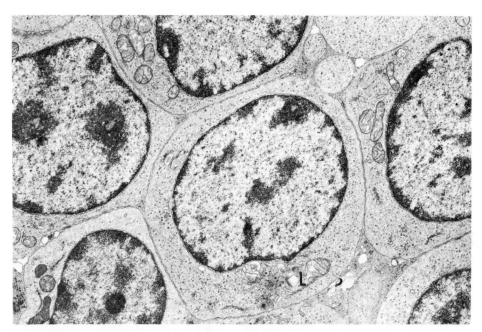

FIGURE 2-17
Malignant lymphoma, undifferentiated, Burkitt-type (cervical lymph node, 5-year-old male). Small lymphoid cells with round nuclei, clumped and marginated chromatin, nucleoli, and numerous cytoplasmic polysomes are illustrated. One of the cells contains two small lipid droplets (L). (×7200).

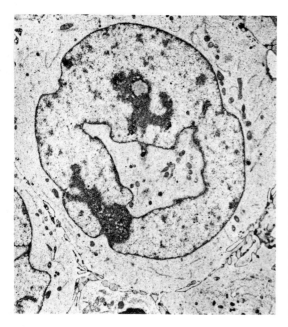

FIGURE 2-18
Hodgkin's disease, mixed cellurlarity type (supraclavicular lymph node, 13-year-old male). Characteristic Reed-Sternberg cell. Because of the plane of sectioning the nucleus is doughnut shaped. Note the two large nucleoli (×3600).

formerly called reticulum cell sarcoma—is recognized as a misnomer. It is a term used to describe a heterogeneous group of neoplasms consisting of large transformed lymphoid cells of B cell, and rarely T cell or null cell origin.[29,211,365,381,476,468,511] In my experience of 60 cases such tumors consist of a wide variety of large lymphoid cells with either noncleaved, cleaved, or convoluted nuclei. The chromatin is usually moderately clumped, and the nucleoli are generally quite large. Polysome rosettes often are abundant in the large noncleaved cells that resemble transformed lymphocytes (Fig. 2-15). Immunoblasts are transformed lymphocytes undergoing plasmacytoid differentiation.[188] The abundant cytoplasm contains fairly numerous long irregular strands of rough endoplasmic reticulum (RER) in addition to large numbers of polysomes. A variant of histiocytic lymphoma consisting of a monomorphic population of immunoblasts is currently called either B-immunoblastic lymphoma[365,439] or immunoblastic lymphosarcoma.[410] We recently studied an unusual case of T cell histiocytic lymphoma (T-immunoblastic type)[512] composed of large pleomorphic lymphoid tumor cells. The nuclei are markedly convoluted, cleaved, and show

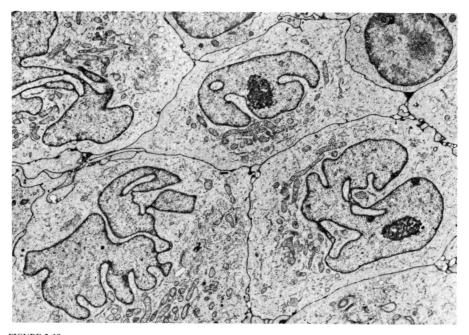

FIGURE 2-19
Hodgkin's disease, nodular sclerosis type (supraclavicular lymph node, 13-year-old female). A cluster of lacunar cells, each containing a large pleomorphic nucleus and prominent cytoplasmic organelles. Note the large size of these cells compared with the small lymphocyte, *upper right corner*. (×4300).

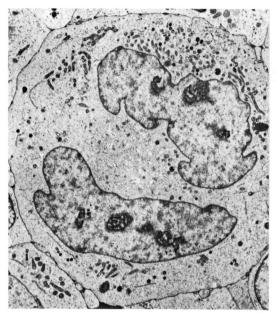

FIGURE 2-20
Hodgkin's disease, mixed cellularity type (celiac axis lymph node, 15-year-old female). Histiocytic variant of Reed-Sternberg cell. Note the abundance of electron-dense lysosomes in the cytoplasm. (×4300).

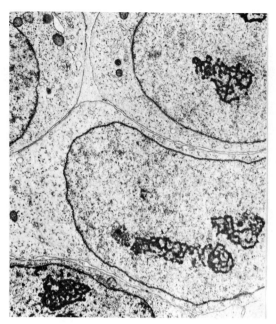

FIGURE 2-21
Seminoma (testicle, 41-year-old male). Twisted nucleolar strands (nucleolonema) are prominent. (×4560).

satellite nuclei. The chromatin pattern is diffuse and large multiple nucleoli are often evident. The cytoplasm contains large numbers of polysomes (Fig. 2-16).

Malignant lymphoma of the undifferentiated type consists of small noncleaved B lymphocytes, supposedly of follicular center origin. One variant is known by the eponym Burkitt's lymphoma.[45] The Burkitt-type undifferentiated lymphoma consists of small lymphoid cells with round nuclei (often with nuclear pockets and one or two small indentations present), some clumped and marginated chromatin, and multiple small nucleoli. The nucleus is surrounded by a thin rim of cytoplasm containing numerous polysomes and, in some cases, scattered lipid droplets (Fig. 2-17).[144,291] Pleomorphism of both the small noncleaved cells and nuclei separates the non-Burkitt type of undifferentiated lymphoma from classic Burkitt's lymphoma[44,365] This latter subtype is not ultrastructurally distinct.

Demonstration of large mononuclear or multinucleate Reed-Sternberg cells in the appropriate background is required for the diagnosis of Hodgkin's disease.[366] The classic Reed-Sternberg cell is a large cell with an abundant cytoplasm containing variable numbers of organelles, scat-

tered small bundles of cytoplasmic fibrils, and numerous ribosomes and polysomes. The nucleus is deeply cleaved, convoluted, or bilobed with a fine chromatin pattern (Fig. 2-18). Each lobe contains a large centrally located nucleolus. In addition to the diagnostic type of Reed-Sternberg cell, there are two variants. The lacunar cell characteristic of the nodular sclerosis type of Hodgkin's disease is larger and contains a prominent multilobulated nucleus[18] (Fig. 2-19). The remaining subtype is a histiocytic variant of the above two cell types. The nucleus is more peripherally located and the cytoplasm contains lipid droplets and lysosomal dense bodies (Fig. 2-20). The lineage of the Reed-Sternberg cell is still disputed, although there is increasing evidence favoring a lymphocytic origin. The different types of Reed-Sternberg cells probably represent stages of a developmental sequence of lymphocytic transformation.[18,27,215]

NUCLEOLUS

Although nucleoli may be large, pleomorphic, multiple, and marginated in neoplastic cells that make up many poorly differentiated tumors (Figs. 2-2 and 2-3), they may be relatively inconspicuous in others, e.g., Ewing's sarcoma, lymphoblastic

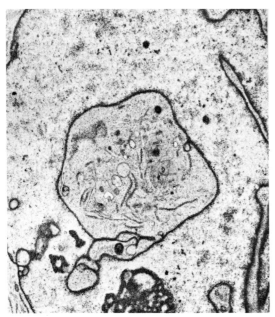

FIGURE 2-22
Adenocarcinoma of lung (right upper lobe, lung, 68-year-old male). Large pseudonuclear inclusion consisting of cytoplasm delineated by nuclear envelope. Other nuclear invaginations are also evident. (×6500).

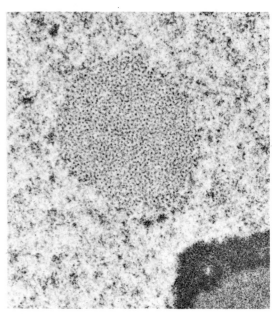

FIGURE 2-24
Recurrent malignant peripheral nerve sheath tumor (chest wall, 79-year-old female). Nuclear body consisting of small granules. Portion of nucleolus is at lower right. (×25,200).

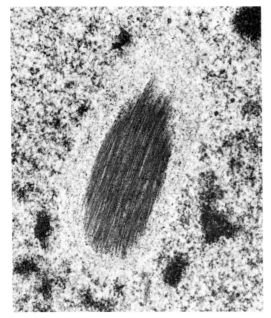

FIGURE 2-23
Infiltrating glioma (cerebrum, 67-year-old male). True nuclear body consisting of closely packed bundles of fibrils surrounded by a more electronlucent halo. (×38,000).

lymphoma, and neuroblastoma (see appropriate sections of text). Enlarged, often marginated, nucleoli are also found in metabolically active nonneoplastic cells,[207] e.g., transformed lymphocytes[599] and regenerating hepatocytes.[47] Such nucleolar changes are indicative of active protein synthesis and of rapid cell proliferation. Nucleolar changes in neoplastic cells, although quite striking in a variety of human tumors, are generally not found consistently in specific nosologic entities, with one exception. Well-developed elongated and twisted nucleolar strands are seen in most, but not all, cell types comprising testicular (Fig. 2-21) and extragonadal seminomas[274,347,391,465,477] and ovarian dysgerminomas.[180] Identification of the rope-like nucleolar pattern is helpful in the differentiated diagnosis of small cell anterior mediastinal tumors, e.g., germ cell tumor versus thymoma, thymic carcinoid, or especially malignant lymphoma (Table 1-2; Appendix C; Chapter 6, case 4; and appropriate sections of the monograph).

NUCLEAR INCLUSIONS

Two types of intranuclear inclusions are occasionally found in individual tumors of diverse histogenesis. The first type is a pseudoinclusion resulting from invaginations of the nuclear envelope

(Fig. 2-22). These inclusions are essentially cross-sectioned areas of cytoplasm separated from the nucleoplasm by the nuclear envelope. The second-type is the true intranuclear inclusion or nuclear body lying within the nucleoplasm. Many different types of true intranuclear inclusions are found in human tumors, the most common of which consist of either parallel bundles of fibrils of varying lengths (Fig. 2-23) or of spherical structures composed of tightly packed clusters of granules (Fig. 2-24) (granular nuclear body) or complexly intertwined fibrils (fibrillar nuclear body). These latter inclusions can be quite small or occupy a large area of nucleoplasm; they are usually not enclosed within a membrane. True intranuclear inclusions are found in both neoplastic and non-neoplastic cells and are associated with cellular hyperactivity, the cause of which may be physiologic (hormonal), drug-induced, viral, or related to specific alterations in the genome of neoplastic cells.[75,135,137,292,549,573,607] I know of no morphologic type of nuclear inclusion that is specific for or found in all cases of a particular neoplasm. In conclusion, intranuclear inclusions are of little if any diagnostic significance with respect to human neoplasms.

CHAPTER III

The Cytoplasm

Ultrastructural features helpful in identifying the cell of origin of a particular tumor are usually found in the cytoplasm, as opposed to the nucleus, of the neoplastic cell. Accordingly, a large portion of this monograph is devoted to cytoplasmic structures. This chapter discusses how the presence, hyperplasia, and/or morphologic alteration of organelles, inclusions, and types of intracytoplasmic fibers can help the pathologist confirm a diagnosis. The demonstration of combinations of cytoplasmic structures related to the physiologic function (e.g., secretion, contraction) of the putative tissue of origin is more significant in this respect. The scope of the monograph does not permit coverage of the multitude of organelle changes induced by drugs, vitamin deficiencies, viral infection, and hormone imbalance.

ORGANELLES

Cytoplasmic organelles are metabolizing structures found in nearly all cells, each characterized by its specific enzyme(s), ultrastructure, and function; they are regarded as the small internal organs of the cell.[59,489] The diagnostic relevance of increased numbers or modifications of specific organelles has been greatly exaggerated in the literature. Many organelle alterations reflect either increased metabolic activity of rapidly dividing cells or anoxic changes.

Some of the basically nonmetabolic intracytoplasmic structures that I have placed in other categories, e.g., inclusions, are often called organelles. For example, the melanosome, the cytoplasmic inclusion formed only in melanocytes, is often called an organelle. Whereas the tyrosinase-containing melanin pigment-producing premelanosome may, with some justification, be regarded as an organelle, mature nonmetabolizing melanosomes are best classified as inclusions. Microtubules are ubiquitous structures found in all cells and are therefore considered an organelle.

I hold that these dynamic structures are part of the complex system of intracellular fibers and should be placed in that category.

Diagnostically significant changes in mitochondria, endoplasmic reticulum and ribosomes, Golgi apparatus, lysosomes, and organelle complexes (close apposition of two types of organelles) are reviewed in this section. Annulate lamellae are also briefly discussed, because a number of recent reports describing the occurrence of these poorly understood transitory organelles in human neoplasms have been published. Peroxisomes (microbodies) and centrioles have no obvious diagnostic relevance to tumor pathology and are not covered.

Mitochondria

Mitochondria are oblong structures consisting of two compartments delineated by membranes, one inside the other. The inner membrane forms distinct crests of fingerlike projections—the cristae—that extend into the mitochondrial matrix. Mitochondria contain a complex system of enzymes that function primarily in trapping the energy liberated by catabolism as adenosine triphosphate (ATP), the process known as oxidative phosphorylation. The mitochondrial matrix also contains matrix granules (depots of divalent cations), DNA, and ribonucleoprotein granules.[575]

Variations in mitochondrial morphology are of limited diagnostic value. Normal-looking mitochondria are seen in most properly prepared viable human tumor cells, whereas swollen, distorted, or pyknotic organelles are frequently seen in anoxic cells. A certain type of mitochondrion must be seen in most tumors of a particular type to be considered diagnostic for that neoplasm.

In cells synthesizing steroid hormones

Mitochondria found in cells producing steroid

21

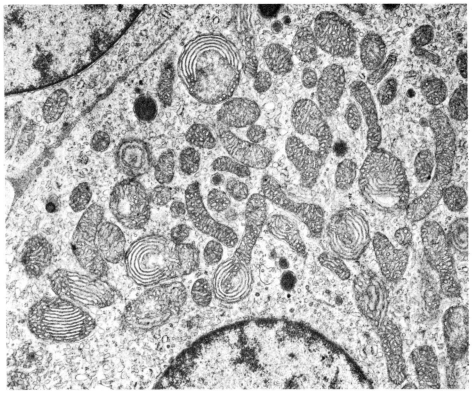

FIGURE 3-1
Adrenocortical adenoma (adrenal gland, 41-year-old male). Portion of neoplastic zona fasciculata cell illustrating mitochondria with tubulovesicular cristae, SER, and electron-dense membrane-bound lysosomes. (×14,700.)

hormones, e.g., in the adrenal gland, ovary, and testis, frequently possess tubulovesicular cristae of the type found in zona fasciculata cells of the adrenal gland (Fig. 3-1).[363,585] These cristae appear as vesicles lying free in the mitochondrial matrix or as concentric closely packed lamellar structures (Fig. 3-2), as opposed to the more common straight, interdigitating lamellar cristae (Fig. 3-8).

Mitochondria containing tubulovesicular cristae are prominent in the large polyhedral cells of the zona fasciculata and in benign and some malignant tumors arising in this zone, e.g., those producing Cushing's syndrome,[208,293,450,585] Leydig (interstitial) cell tumors of the testis (or ovary) that produce androgenic steroids,[39,284,295,550] feminizing or virilizing ovarian sex cord–stromal tumors—especially luteomas,[205,270,323,374] and some rare ovarian Sertoli cell tumors,[238] also consist of cells containing mitochondria with tubulovesicular cristae. Tumors derived from the cells of the zona glomerulosa, e.g., adrenal adenomata secreting excessive amounts of aldosterone (Conn's syndrome), contain mitochondria with the more common lamellar cristae (so-called sarcotubular cristae),[164,208,288,585] whereas those originating from the zona reticularis, e.g., androgen-producing (virilizing) adenomas and cardinomas, and black adenomata[7,208,585,616] possess mitochondria of both types, including intermediate forms. Cells comprising black adenomas are distinguished by abundant cytoplasmic liposfuscin (see p. 37, Fig. 3-31). A rare feminizing adrenocortical carcinoma obtained from a 29-year-old man, however, consisted of cells having large numbers of mitochondria, most of which had only lamellar cristae.[420] Some of the mitochondria also contained electron-dense inclusions. Large or so-called giant mitochondria are also found in cells of benign adenomas (Cushing's syndrome) and in many carcinomas.[585] Unfortunately, many malignant or nonfunctioning tumors, or both, derived from the above organs do not contain mitochondria with tubulovesicular cristae or other organelles com-

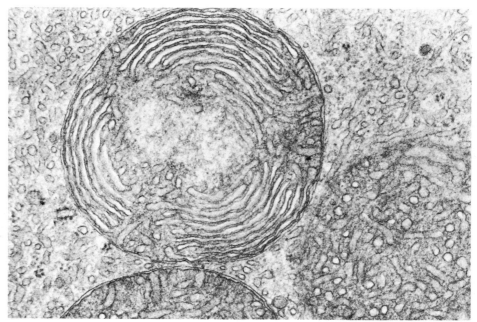

FIGURE 3-2
Higher-magnification micrograph of cytoplasm of cell illustrated in Figure 3-1. Note the concentric and vesicular appearance of the cristae and the anastomosing tubules of the SER. (×37,800.)

monly found in steroid secreting cells (see p. 33)—are often those that pose diagnostic difficulties.

Mitochondrial inclusions

Mitochondrial inclusions of various types are found in diverse tumors and likewise are of little diagnostic significance. These may be amorphous or electron-dense (Fig. 3-3) rodlike helical structures (actually modified cristae) running parallel to the long axis of the mitochondrion[528] (Fig. 3-4), or they may be pseudocrystalline or crystalline.[257,390] Pseudocrystalline (paracrystalline) inclusions are commonly found in hepatocytes in cases of focal nodular hyperplasia and benign hepatomas arising in women taking oral contraceptives[30,296] (Fig. 3-5). These latter inclusions are also found in occasional normal hepatocyte mitochondria[642] and are common nonspecific concomitants of cellular injury.

Oncocytes

Perhaps the most interesting mitochondropathy is the accumulation of large numbers of mitochondria in oncocytes and in neoplasms composed

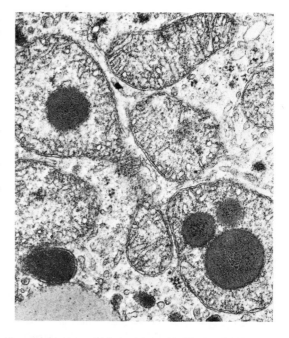

FIGURE 3-3
Adenomatous hyperplasia (adrenal cortex, 34-year-old female with Cushing's syndrome). Focus of mitochondria with tubulovesicular cristae, two of which contain amorphous electron-dense inclusions. (×30,000.)

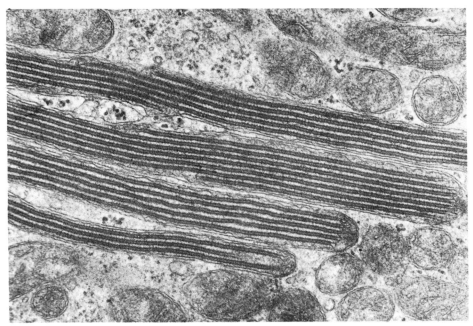

FIGURE 3-4
Oxyphilic parathyroid adenoma (parathyroid gland, 24-year-old female). Mitochondria with long, parallel helical cristae. These modified cristae may be mistaken for a mitochondrial inclusion. (×43,200.)

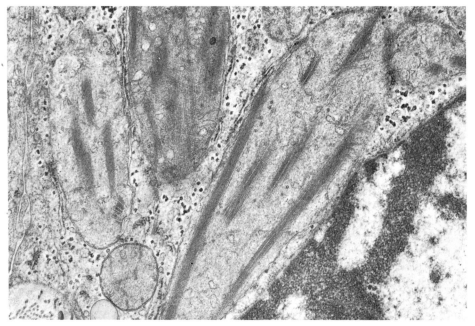

FIGURE 3-5
Focal nodular hyperplasia (liver, 34-year-old female who had taken oral contraceptives for 9 years). Large mitochondria containing paracrystalline inclusions consisting of parallel arrays of fibrils. Electron-dense irregularly shaped small glycogen particles are also evident in the cytoplasm. (×20,000.)

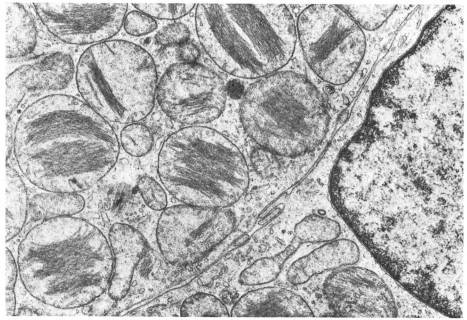

FIGURE 3-6
Oncocytoma (parotid gland, 63-year-old male). Portion of two oncocytes showing closely packed mitochondria with lamelliform cristae. (×16,200.)

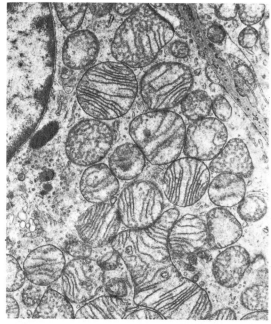

FIGURE 3-7
Granular cell carcinoma (kidney, 18-year-old male). The cytoplasm is occupied by numerous mitochondria of normal morphology. (×10,800.)

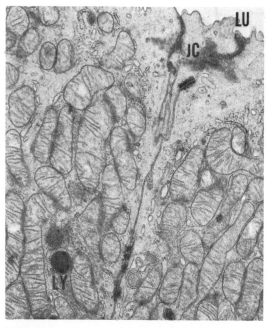

FIGURE 3-8
Warthin's tumor (parotid gland, 40-year-old male). Portions of the apical cytoplasm of two oncocytic epithelial cells lining a papillae. Note that the mitochondria lack the densely packed lamelliform cristae that are present in other areas of the tumor. Junctional complex (JC), lumen (LU), and lysosome (LY). (×12,600.)

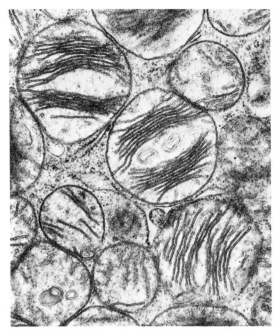

FIGURE 3-9
Hürthle cell tumor (thyroid gland, 34-year-old male). Portion of senescent oncocyte illustrating closely packed mitochondria, many of which have aggregated cristae. (×24,000.)

of these cells (oncocytomas). Oncocytes are large epithelial cells with an extremely acidophilic and granular cytoplasm.[235] Tandler and associates[576] have defined two classes of oncocytes: (1) cells containing pleomorphic mitochondria with elongated densely packed lamelliform cristae (Fig. 3-6) lacking intramitochondrial dense granules, but sometimes containing inclusions of various kinds; and (2) oncocytic cells containing large numbers of closely apposed mitochondria of normal morphology that also lack intramitochondrial dense granules (Fig. 3-7). The latter type of mitochondrion is probably the precursor of the first, as both are usually found in either the same or different oncocytic cell(s) comprising a particular tumor (see below) (Fig. 3-8). Mitochondria with densely packed lamelliform cristae are prominent in so-called senescent or condensed oncocytes, where they occupy virtually the entire cytoplasmic matrix (Fig. 3-9). Cells that contain this type of mitochondrion are easy to label as oncocytes, whereas those that possess only the normal variety require closer scrutiny. Large numbers of this latter type of mitochondrion in close contact with each other must be observed in order for the cell to merit the appellation of oncocyte.

Oncocytes are found in a variety of normal and pathologic tissues including neoplasms, e.g., sali-

vary glands, parathyroid glands, pancreas, and Hashimoto's thyroiditis. The following human tumors are composed of oncocytes: (1) oncocytoma of the parotid gland[279,569,576] (Fig. 3-6), (2) Warthin's tumor[578] (Fig. 3-8), (3) Hürthle (more correctly Askanazy) cell tumors of the thyroid gland[174,615] (Fig. 3-9), (4) benign renal oncocytoma[109,308,650] and some granular cell carcinomas of the kidney (Fig. 3-7), (5) oncocytic adenoma of the pituitary gland,[38,165,324,337] and (6) individual cases of certain other neoplasms such as many oxyphilic parathyroid adenomas,[402,445] some cases of fibroadenoma of the breast,[24] and bronchial oncocytoma.[171,516]

Ultrastructural studies are often necessary to confirm the nature of marked cytoplasmic granularity and eosinophilia, which may be attributable to abundant mitochondria (oncocytes), but also could be attributable to large numbers of lysosomes (granular cell tumors, p. 38). I have seen intense cytoplasmic eosinophilia in a thyroid lesion erroneously called a Hürthle cell adenoma until electron microscopic (EM) studies showed that it consisted of cells with prominent dilated cisternae of RER (Fig. 3-10). The granular intracisternal proteinaceous precipitate accounted for the unusual cytoplasmic eosinophilia of this oncocytoid hyperplastic lesion.

It is important to remember that cells in many different types of neoplasms may contain numerous mitochondria. They are not oncocytes unless the strict criteria described above are met. The significance of the oncocytic transformation is unknown, but it may represent a compensatory hyperplasia and hypertrophy of biochemically defective organelles.[576]

Endoplasmic Reticulum and Ribosomes

This section discusses the diagnostic relevance of a well-developed membrane-bound cavitary system, e.g., endoplasmic reticulum (ER) and the presence of numerous 12- to 15-nm ribonucleoprotein particles (ribosomes). The order of presentation is as follows: (1) ribosome-studded cisternae—the rough (granular) endoplasmic reticulum (RER)—especially well developed in cells actively engaged in protein synthesis; (2) single ribosomes and clusters of these particles called polysomes (also termed polyribosomes) lying free in the cytoplasmic matrix; and (3) the anastomosing tubules of the smooth surface endoplasmic reticulum (SER), which functions primarily in the

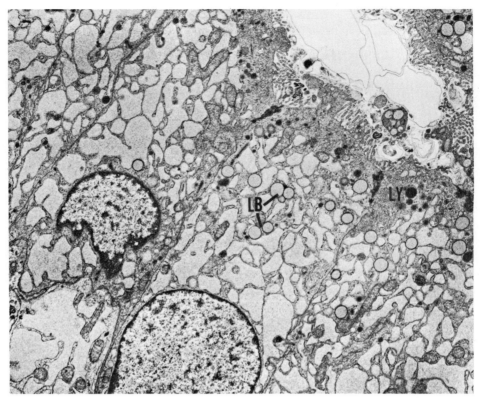

FIGURE 3-10
Oncocytoid adenomatous hyperplasia (thyroid gland, 21-year-old male). The cytoplasmic eosinophilia of the hyperplastic follicular epithelial cells is attributable to numerous dilated RER cisternae containing a granular proteinaceous substance. Lipid bodies (LB), lysosomes (LY). (×6240.)

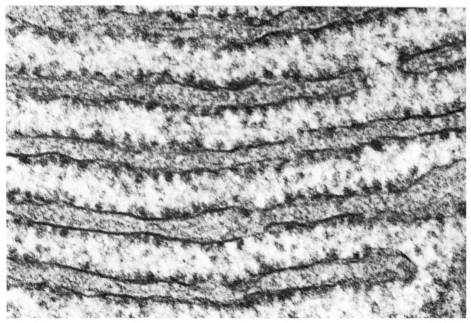

FIGURE 3-11
Anaplastic tumor (lung metastases, 50-year-old female). Stacked cisternae of the RER studded with ribosomes on the outer surface of their limiting membranes. (×104,000.)

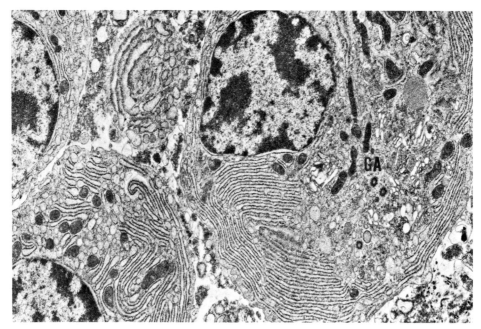

FIGURE 3-12
Plasmacytoma (humerus, 84-year-old male). Neoplastic plasma cells. The peripherally located nuclei exhibit prominent marginated clumps of chromatin. The cytoplasm contains a well-developed Golgi apparatus (GA) and curvilinear stacked RER cisternae. (×8400.)

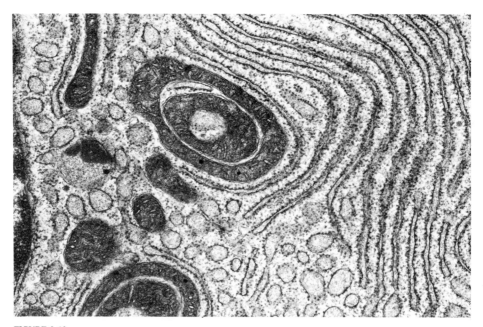

FIGURE 3-13
Plasma cell myeloma (clavicle, 64-year-old female). Portion of cytoplasm showing profiles of RER (some are seen in cross section) and two unusual circular mitochondrial configuration in which one mitochondrion is located inside the other. (×24,000.)

biosynthesis of glycogen, steroid hormones and cholesterol, in lipid metabolism, and in the detoxification of many lipid-soluble drugs, such as phenobarbital. It should be pointed out that there is structural and functional continuity between the endoplasmic reticulum, ribosomes, and other organelles (e.g., Golgi apparatus, lysosomes).

Rough endoplasmic reticulum

The cytoplasm of nearly all cells, especially those producing proteins for export, contains a more or less continuous network of membrane-bound cisternae studded with ribosomes, or RER (Fig. 3-11). Although RER is found in virtually all neoplastic cells, it varies in amount. Rough endoplasmic reticulum in the form of stacked or branching configurations is conspicuous in a number of different tumors. Elongated curvilinear stacked RER cisternae are prominent in certain tumors whose histogenic precursors secrete abundant protein, e.g., plasma cell tumors (plasmacytoma, multiple myeloma)[28,385,543] (Figs. 3-12 and 3-13), acinic cell carcinomas of the parotid gland,[161] the rare acinar cell tumors of the pancreas,[93] and in lymphomas composed of plasma-

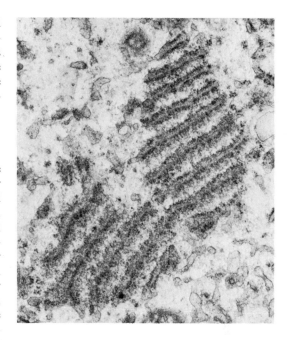

FIGURE 3-14
Adrenocortical carcinoma (adrenal gland, 2-year-old female). Portion of cytoplasm showing two stacks of short RER cisternae. (×20,000.)

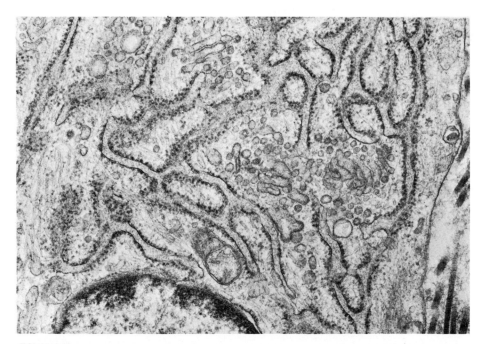

FIGURE 3-15
Low-grade fibrosarcoma (popliteal fossa, 17-year-old male). Juxtanuclear cytoplasm of neoplastic fibroblast showing branching cisternae of RER and clusters of small Golgi vesicles. (×32,400.)

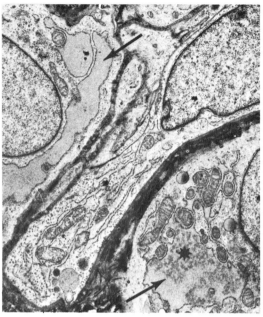

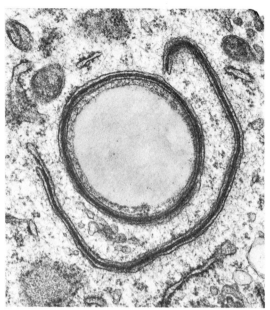

FIGURE 3-16
Malignant fibrous xanthoma (chest wall, 22-year-old female). Portions of fibrous and xanthomatous cells illustrating prominent dilated cisternae of RER (*arrows*). Note the more electron-dense precipitate in one of the cisternae (asterisk). The cells are surrounded by collagen fibrils. (×6400.)

FIGURE 3-18
Liposarcoma (thigh, 44-year-old female). Two paired cisternae of RER, one of which encloses a lipid droplet, are illustrated. Note that only a few ribosomes remain on the outer membranes. (×33,600.)

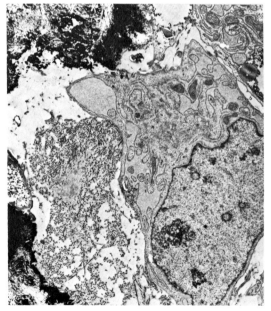

FIGURE 3-17
Osteogenic sarcoma (humerus, 11-year-old female). Neoplastic osteoblast (a fibrocytic cell) containing prominent dilated cisternae of RER. The surrounding matrix consists of osteoid (a type of collagen) and calcified osteoid (*black areas*). (×3840.)

cytoid cells.[89,410] Short stacked segments of RER are found in adrenocortical carcinomas[585] (Fig. 3-14) and in hepatocellular carcinomas.[231,257] Branching cisternae of RER are a feature of neoplasms composed of fibroblasts or fibroblastlike cells, e.g., fibrosarcoma (Fig. 3-15), malignant fibrous xanthoma (Fig. 3-16), myofibroblast tumors (see p. 90), and osteoid-producing neoplasms[22,210,481,483,524,558,559] (Fig. 3-17). The cisternae may be dilated and contain a finely granular proteinaceous precipitate in many of the above-mentioned tumors (Figs. 3-16 and 3-17). Whorl-like configurations of RER are nonspecific.

A number of other interesting modifications of RER have also been noted. Intricately intertwined or complex undulating cisternae of RER have been found in a variety of hematopoietic neoplasms.[611] Paired cisternae, consisting of two back-to-back cisternae of RER separated by an electron-dense layer, are occasionally found in a variety of human tumors[237] (Fig. 3-18).

As a general rule, less-differentiated tumors have a poorly developed RER. This holds true for most of the intracytoplasmic structures discussed in this text.

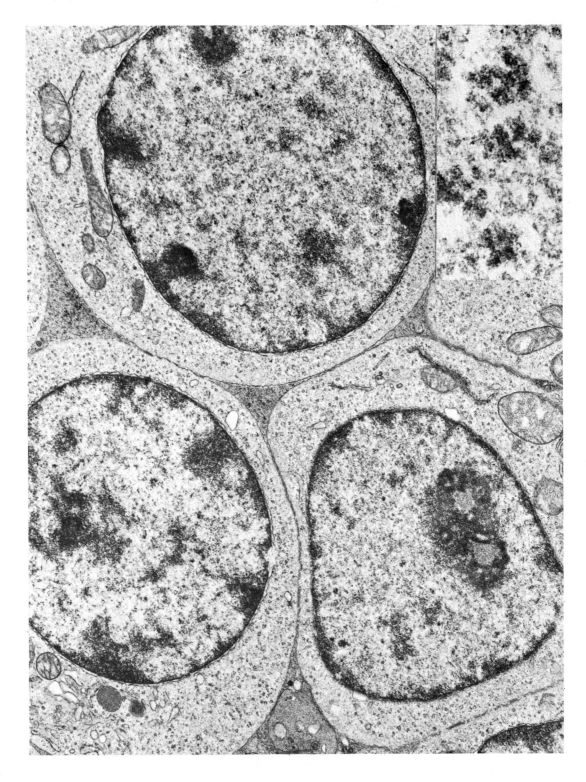

FIGURE 3-19
Malignant lymphoma, undifferentiated Burkitt's type (cervical lymph node, 5-year-old male). Note the clusters of ribosomes (polysomes) in the cytoplasm of the small noncleaved neoplastic B lymphocytes (×12,400). *Inset*, high-magnification micrograph of polysomes. (×140,000.)

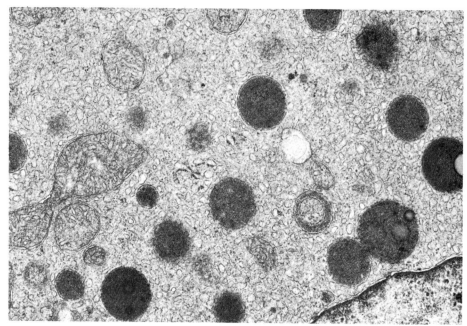

FIGURE 3-20
Interstitial (Leydig) cell tumor (testis, 17-year-old male). Note the complex anastamosing SER tubules, mitochondria with tubulovesicular cristae, and membrane-bound lysosomes with a heterogeneous electron-dense content. (×21,000.)

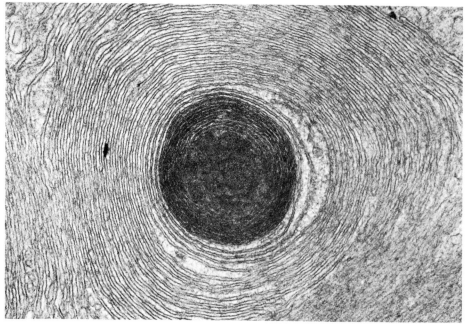

FIGURE 3-21
Membranous whorl with electron-dense core from the same neoplasm shown in Figure 3-20. (×42,000.)

Ribosomes and polysomes

Ribosomes—both free and associated with the RER—are the sites at which protein synthesis takes place in the cytoplasm. I have observed large numbers of both individual ribosomes and polysomes (Fig. 3-19) in non-Hodgkin's lymphomas composed of neoplastic cells that resemble transformed lymphocytes (Fig. 2-14) or immunoblasts.[188,410] Many rapidly growing immature neoplastic cells engaging in the active production of proteins for endogenous use contain numerous free polysomes.[207,208]

Smooth endoplasmic reticulum

The cells comprising neoplasms that elaborate steroid hormones usually contain well-developed smooth (agranular) endoplasmic reticulum in addition to other organelles and inclusions, e.g., mitochondria with tubulovesicular cristae, lysosomes, and lipid, usually found in these hormonally active cells (Fig. 3-1, 3-2, and 3-20). Membranous whorls consisting of concentric flattened cisternae of SER are also found in some of these tumors, particularly interstitial (Leydig) cell tumor of the testis (Fig. 3-21).[39,395,550] and pituitary adenomas.[325]

The following ovarian sex cord–stromal tumors often have hormonal activity (feminizing or virilizing) and are usually composed of cells with a prominent SER in addition to the other organelles and inclusions associated with the elaboration of steroid hormones: (1) granulosa–theca cell tumor,[180,374] (2) Sertoli-Leydig cell tumor,[238,284,302] (3) hilus cell tumor,[407] luteoma of pregnancy,[205] (4) lipid (lipoid) cell tumors[270] (the origin of which is unknown), and (5) a rare virilizing tumor with adrenocortical hormonal activity.[323]

Adenomas of the adrenal cortex[7,164,208,293,585] and occasional adrenocortical carcinomas (glucocorticoids and mineralocorticoids)[616] (p. 22); benign hepatomas[204,296] and well-differentiated hepatocellular carcinomas,[372,449] and Sertoli cell adenomas of the testis[1] also consist of cells with a well-developed SER in addition to other cytoplasmic structures characteristic of the cell of origin, e.g., glycogen in neoplastic hepatocytes.

Annulate Lamellae

Annulate lamellae consist of parallel arrays of cisternae interrupted at regular intervals by pores (small annuli) with diaphragms[305] (Fig. 3-22). The

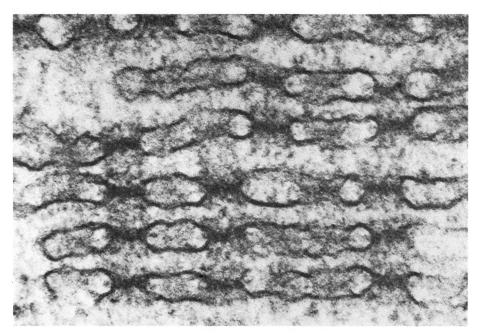

FIGURE 3-22
Pulmonary blastoma (lung, 64-year-old male). Portion of cytoplasm of primitive respiratory epithelial cell illustrating parallel arrays of annulate lamellae consisting of ellipsoidal smooth-walled cisternae joined by membranous pores or annuli. Note the fibrillogranular material associated with the annuli. (×132,000.)

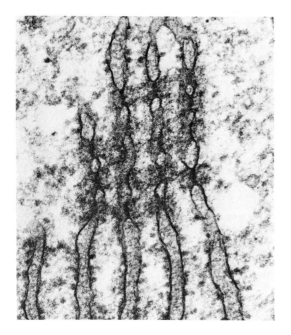

FIGURE 3-23
Anaplastic carcinoma (cervical lymph node, 62-year-old female). Annulate lamellae continuous at both ends with RER. (×64,000.)

lamellar cisternae, which resemble a segment of nuclear envelope, are often continuous at their ends with RER (Fig. 3-23) and are frequently located near the Golgi apparatus. Although these structures are probably derived from the nuclear envelope and may represent a developmental stage in the formation of RER, the precise origin and function of annulate lamellae have not been firmly established.[568]

Annulate lamellae are particularly prominent in oocytes, spermatids, and Sertoli cells and have been found in a variety of human neoplasms, particularly carcinomas.[568] This unusual organelle is occasionally prominent in parathyroid adenomas composed of chief cells[16,70,115,153] and in immature neoplastic germ cells.[136,180,256,316] I have seen numerous cisternae of annulate lamellae, often associated with mitochondria or whorl-like configurations of ER, in one out of 16 parathyroid adenomas (Fig. 3-24), in a pulmonary blastoma (Fig. 3-22), and sporadically in other tumors of diverse histogenesis. Watanabe et al.[631] reported the presence of these structures in lymphocytic cells in four cases of diffuse histiocytic lymphoma. In my experience, annulate lamellae are more commonly found in carcinomas, as opposed to

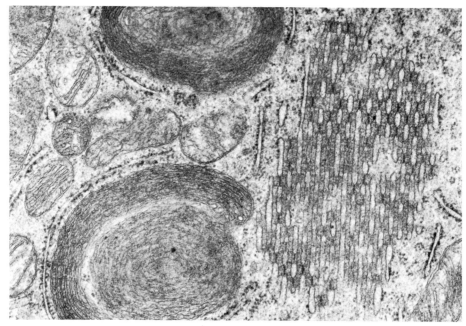

FIGURE 3-24
Parathyroid adenoma composed of chief cells (parathyroid gland, 54-year-old female). Portion of cytoplasm illustrating annulate lamellae and ellipsoidal and crescentic mitochondria partially enveloped by a RER cistern. (×34,200.)

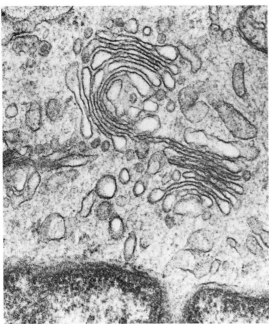

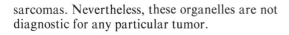

FIGURE 3-25
Spindle cell malignant tumor (axillary lymph node, 79-year-old female). Saccular and vesicular components of two Golgi apparati are illustrated. *Bottom*, a portion of the nucleus. (×56,000.)

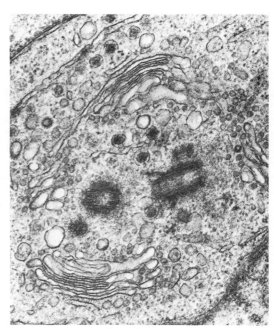

FIGURE 3-26
Merkel cell carcinoma (axillary lymph node, 68-year-old male). Perinuclear Golgi region of cell. Note the closely packed parallel smooth-surfaced Golgi cisternae, the Golgi vesicles, the paired centrioles, and the 100-nm dense-core endosecretory granules that are probably packaged on GERL membranes. (×34,000.)

sarcomas. Nevertheless, these organelles are not diagnostic for any particular tumor.

Golgi Apparatus

The Golgi apparatus or complex consists of flattened saccules or cisternae, often slightly curved and arranged in parallel array, numerous small 30- to 80-nm vesicles, and larger vacuoles (Fig. 3-25). The inner surface (trans aspect) is called the forming face, whereas the outer surface (cis aspect) is referred to as the maturing face.[59,149] The primary function of the Golgi apparatus in secretory (glandular) cells is the accumulation and concentration of proteinaceous secretory products synthesized on ribosomes.[273] The Golgi apparatus is capable of synthesizing complex carbohydrates and coupling them to proteins (glycoproteins). Melanosome formation (p. 71) is also associated with the RER and Golgi apparatus.[276] This organelle is usually well developed in secretory cells as well as in the more differentiated tumors derived from them.

Between the nucleus and the innermost Golgi saccules lies a region of SER with a complex specialized structure. This hydrolase-rich region,

continuous with the RER and referred to as GERL (Golgi-Endoplasmic Reticulum-Lysosome), forms lysosomes, and in some endocrine cells possibly forms neurosecretory granules[446] (Fig. 3-26). Techniques for identifying acid phosphatase activity are necessary for visualizing GERL and primary lysosomes (see below).

The Golgi apparatus may be well developed, hypertrophied, dilated, or distorted in many normal, abnormal, or neoplastic cells that are not obviously secretory (Fig. 3-25). It is not a diagnostically significant organelle.

Lysosomes

Primary lysosomes are small (0.25-0.5 μm), membrane-limited bodies of variable electron density that contain various acid hydrolases (Figs. 3-27 and 3-28). They are found in nearly all types of cells. Lysosomes participate in the intracellular digestion of cytoplasmic structures (autophagy) or material taken into the cell by the process of phagocytosis, or endocytosis (heterophagy). Fusion of the primary lysosome with these substances of intra- or extracellular origin results in the forma-

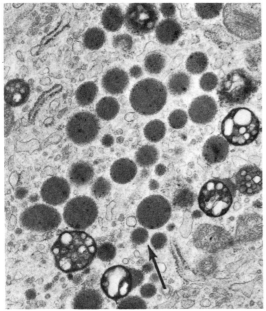

FIGURE 3-27
Hürthle cell adenoma (thyroid gland, 59-year-old female). Portion of cytoplasm containing secondary and possibly some more homogeneous primary lysosomes (*arrow*). (×18,400.)

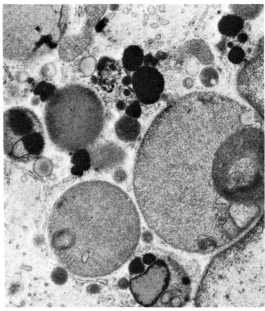

FIGURE 3-29
Thymoma (hilar mass, 63-year-old male). Portion of cytoplasm of thymic epithelial cells showing a cluster of pleomorphic secondary lysosomes. The contents of the phagosomes are of variable morphology and electron density (×14,400.)

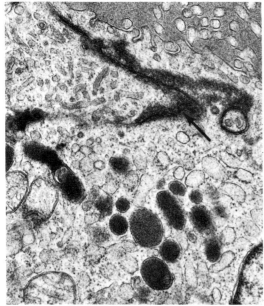

FIGURE 3-28
Low-grade follicular carcinoma (thyroid gland, 59-year-old female). Juxtaluminal cytoplasm of neoplastic follicular epithelial cell (the lumen, *top*) illustrating what are most likely primary lysosomes. The dense material (*arrow*) is a tangential section of a tight and intermediate cell junction. Moderately electron-dense colloid is present in the lumen. (×22,400.)

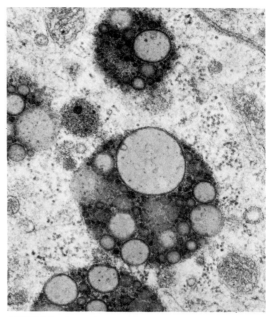

FIGURE 3-30
Parathyroid adenoma (parathyroid gland, 63-year-old female). Portion of cytoplasm of a neoplastic clear cell (appearance due to abundant cytoplasmic glycogen) containing lipofuscin granules. Note the lipid bodies in the matrix of the granules. (×32,200.)

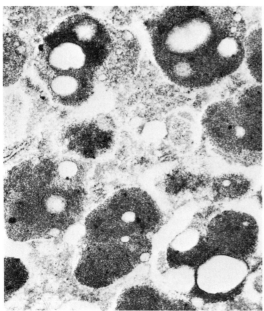

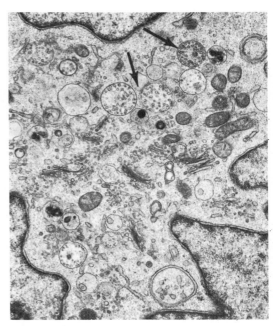

FIGURE 3-31
Black adenoma (adrenal gland, 86-year-old female). Portion of cytoplasm containing numerous lipofuscin granules. The tissue was obtained from a paraffin block. (×21,600.)

FIGURE 3-32
True histiocytic lymphoma (cervical lymph node, 28-year-old male). Indented Golgi region of neoplastic histiocyte illustrating multivesicular bodies (*arrows*). These lysosomal organelles consist of numerous small vesicles within a membranous sac. (×11,200.)

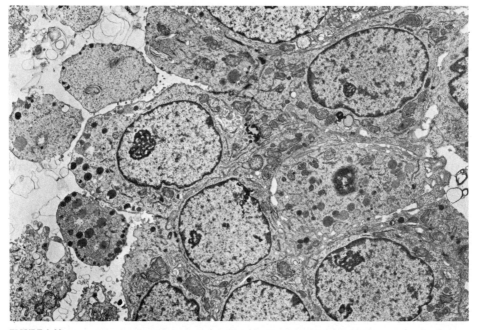

FIGURE 3-33
Carcinoma *in situ* (prostate gland, 43-year-old male). Low magnification micrograph of a nest of neoplastic prostatic epithelial cells. Note the numerous cytoplasmic lysosomes of variable size and density. (×4000.)

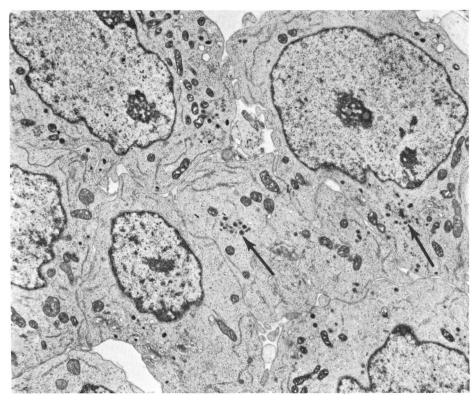

FIGURE 3-34
Myelomonocytic leukemia (axillary lymph node, 60-year-old male). Isolated granules and clusters of lysosomal organelles (*arrows*) are present in the cytoplasm of the leukemic cells. (×5280.)

tion of pleomorphic structures of variable electron density called secondary lysosomes. The latter include phagosomes (Fig. 3-29), residual bodies (sometimes called telolysosomes), lipofuscin pigment (Figs. 3-30 and 3-31), and presumably the multivesicular body[59] (Fig. 3-32). Collections of lysosomes are often mistaken for secretory granules. For example, in microfollicular thyroid carcinomas it is frequently difficult to distinguish small lysosomes from neurosecretory-type granules found in medullary carcinoma.[614]

Pleomorphic secondary lysosomes are particularly abundant in epithelial cells of the normal, hyperplastic, and neoplastic thyroid[61,300] (Figs. 3-27 and 3-28) and prostate[76,231,388] (Fig. 3-33) glands. Hydrolysis of thyroglobulin (stored in colloid) to release thyroxine takes place in the lysosomes of the thyroid follicular cells.[59] The demonstration of numerous lysosomes in a metastatic tumor in the proper clinicopathologic setting is suggestive of, but not necessarily diagnostic for, a primary carcinoma of the thyroid or prostate gland. I have also found lysosomes to be prominent in interstitial cell tumors of the testis, myelocytic

and monocytic leukemias (Figs. 3-34 and 3-35), true histiocytic lymphomas (Fig. 3-32), cases of malignant histiocytosis (Fig. 3-36), and the ganglion cells found in ganglioneuroblastomas.[649]

Granular cell tumors

Granular cell tumors (so-called granular cell myoblastomas),[98,286,413,547,548,610,635] granular cell ameloblastomas,[441,577] granular cell ameloblastic fibromas,[639] and granular cell tumors of infants (congenital epulis)[294] are characterized histologically by clusters of plump cells having acidophilic granular cytoplasm. Electron microscopic studies (see above references) have demonstrated that the cytoplasmic granularity is caused by the presence of large numbers of autophagosomes, residual bodies, and ceroid-lipofuscin inclusions (Fig. 3-37). Angulate bodies, large ovoid membrane-limited structures containing numerous "microtubules" (Fig. 3-38), are found in undifferentiated fibroblastlike cells at the periphery of the nests of tumor cells and also in occasional granular cells. The significance of these peculiar structures is not

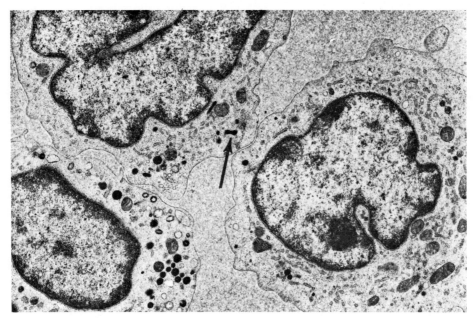

FIGURE 3-35
Acute myelomonocytic leukemia (peripheral blood, 27-year-old male). Portion of three neoplastic myelomonocytic cells from buffy coat specimen illustrating round electron-dense primary granules and dumbbell-shaped tertiary granules (*arrow*). (×8400.)

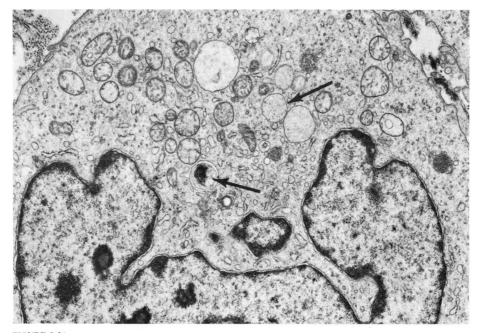

FIGURE 3-36
Malignant histiocytosis (supraclavicular lymph node, 17-year-old male). Portion of neoplastic histiocyte
showing bean-shaped nucleus and lysosomal structures of variable density (*arrows*) located primarily in
the Golgi region of the cell. (×9200.)

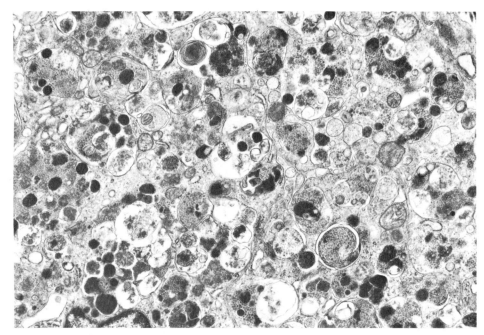

FIGURE 3-37
Granular cell tumor (thigh, 42-year-old female). Large numbers of various types of secondary lysosomes are present in the cytoplasm of the cells comprising these tumors of unknown histogenesis. (×12,000.)

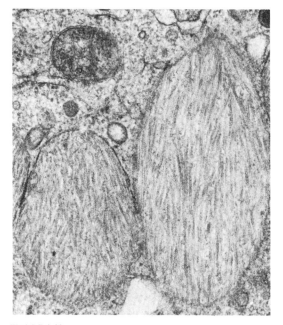

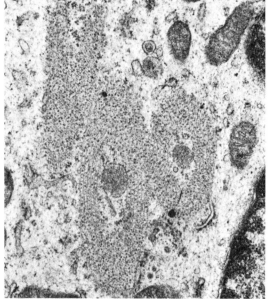

FIGURE 3-38
Granular cell tumor (knee, 52-year-old female). Two membrane-limited angulate bodies containing numerous microtubules are shown. (×45,000.)

FIGURE 3-39
Hairy cell leukemia (peripheral blood, 55-year-old male). Three linear ribosome–lamella complexes are illustrated. Two of these structures enclose a portion of cytoplasm. (×21,000.)

known. Although a Schwann cell origin is favored by many investigators,[98,208,286,548,610,635] these tumors may arise in other cell types.[111]

The above-mentioned granular cell tumors are remarkable neoplasms of uncertain histogenesis with a unique metabolism that causes acceleration of autophagocytosis with an increased accumulation of secondary lysosomes mostly in the form of residual bodies and ceroid-lipofuscin pigment. These tumors can usually be readily diagnosed by light microscopy combined with acid phosphatase staining procedures.

Organelle Complexes

Elaborate structural complexes of various kinds between two different types of organelles (or an organelle and an inclusion) are occasionally seen in neoplastic as well as nonneoplastic cells. Most of these structures are fortuitous findings of little or no diagnostic specificity.

Intracytoplasmic ribosome–lamella complexes,[654] arranged linearly or concentrically (Figs. 3-39 and 3-40), are found in some cases of chronic

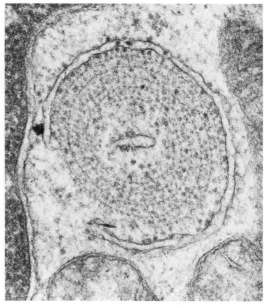

FIGURE 3-40
Concentric ribosome–lamella complex partially enclosed by a RER cistern from same specimen illustrated in Figure 3-39. (×64,000.)

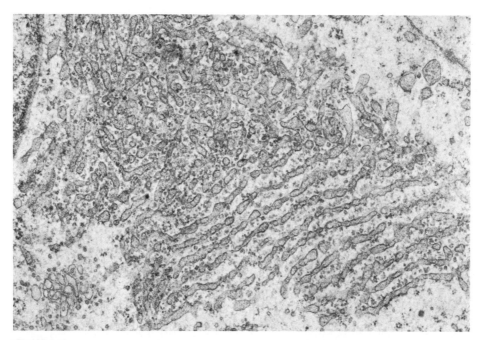

FIGURE 3-41
Papillary intraductal and infiltrating duct carcinoma (breast, 59-year-old female). So-called glycogen body consisting of complex labyrinths and linear arrays of smooth-membraned cisternae and glycogen particles. (×21,600.)

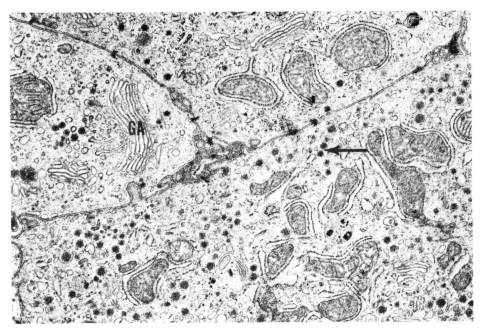

FIGURE 3-42
Medullary carcinoma (thyroid gland, 70-year-old female). Portion of cytoplasm of three neoplastic thyroid epithelial cells joined by small desmosomes. Note the Golgi apparatuses (GA), 220 nm endosecretory granules (*arrow*), and individual cisternae of RER wrapped around the mitochondria. (×9200.)

lymphocytic leukemia, lymphosarcoma cell leukemia, and monoblastic leukemia[28,85,557]–they are particularly prominent (found in 50% of patients) in the lymphomonocytoid cells (the cells frequently express markers of both B lymphocytes and monocytes) comprising hairy cell leukemia, so named because of the prominent long surface microvilli.[85,290] They consist of alternating layers of ribosomelike granules and lamellae composed of double tubule structures.[501] Ribosome–lamella complexes have also been observed in occasional nonhematopoietic neoplasms, e.g., paragangliomas,[435] and an adrenocortical adenoma.[262]

I have seen complex labyrinths and linear arrays of smooth-membraned cisternae intricately associated with glycogen particles (glycogen body) in neoplastic epithelial cells comprising a case of papillary and infiltrating duct carcinoma of the female breast (Fig. 3-41).

Another interesting organelle complex consists of individual cisternae of RER wrapped around a mitochondrion. I have found significant numbers of these nonspecific structures in a medullary carcinoma of the thyroid gland (Fig. 3-42), in a parathyroid adenoma derived from chief cells, and in a pleomorphic adenoma of the submandibular gland.

Structurally ordered complexes of mitochondria and RER are quite striking in the cytoplasm of the physaliferous and stellate cells comprising human chordomas, a tumor that arises from remnants of the embryonic notochord. In these complexes, single mitochondria alternate with single cisternae of RER, with each organelle separated from its neighbor by an interval of constant width (Fig. 3-43). They are found in most but not all cases of chordoma, and their significance is unknown.[162] Thiele and associates[596] reported a similar complex in a parathyroid adenoma of the chief cell type.

It must be emphasized that except for the ribosome–lamella structures (it can be argued that the lamellae is not a true organelle) observed in many cases of hairy cell leukemia and the mitochondria–RER complexes found in most chordomas, organelle complexes are incidental findings of no known diagnostic significance.

INCLUSIONS

Cytoplasmic inclusions are considered to be nonmetabolizing accumulations of the products of cell metabolism, normal or abnormal, such as secretory granules, glycogen, lipid droplets, pigments, and crystals.[59] In contrast to organelles, inclusions are dispensable and often temporary constituents of the cytoplasm. (Many cell biologists, however, regard inclusions to be just as essential to the

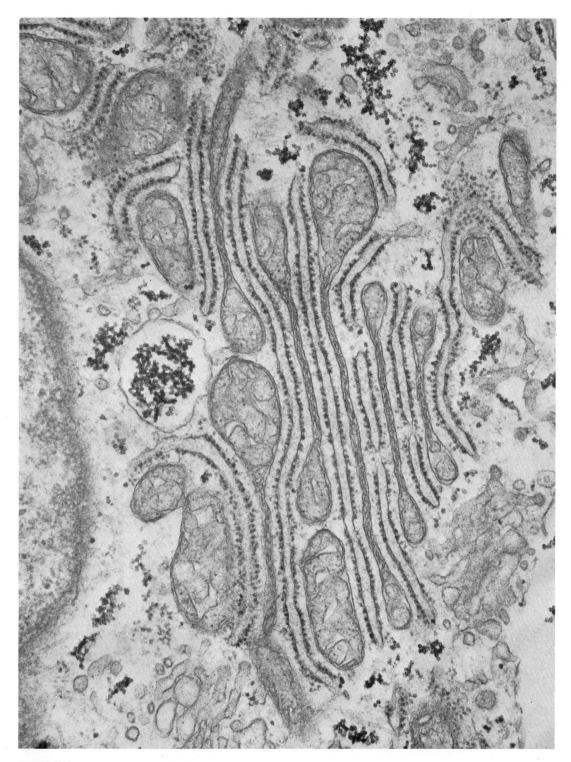

FIGURE 3-43
Chordoma (sacrum, 60-year-old female). Typical mitochondria-RER complex in vacuolated physaliferous cell. Note that the mitochondria are attenuated in their central regions and bulbous at their ends. Small clusters of glycogen particles, some in vacuoles, are also evident. (×56,500.) (Reproduced, with permission, from Erlandson et al. Ultrastructure of human chordoma. Cancer Res 28:2115–2125, 1968).

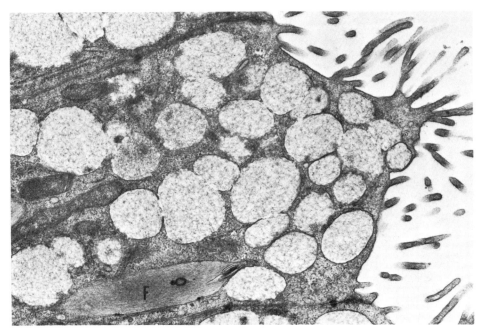

FIGURE 3-44
Endocervical mucosa (endocervix from 31-year-old female with clear cell carcinoma of the cervix). Apical
(luminal) portion of mucin-producing endocervical columnar epithelial cell. Note the reticulated structure
of the mucigen granules, fusion of granules, and elongated fibrillary body (F). (×16,800.)

function(s) of cells in which they occur as are organelles.) This section discusses the problems encountered in identifying the various types of secretory granules and other inclusions found in human tumors, as well as the diagnostic significance of these structures.

Secretory Granules

Three categories of secretory granules—mucigen, zymogen, and neuroendocrine—are found in adenocarcinomas and neuroendocrine tumors. The first two types (exocrine) are expelled into either alveoli, ducts, or body surfaces (e.g., bronchial lumen). Neurosecretory-type (neuroendocrine or endosecretory) granules are liberated into the connective tissue stroma either by exocytosis (fusion of granule membrane with plasmalemma) or by transmembrane effusion (diffusion with no membrane disruption),[509] and either act locally or diffuse into adjacent capillaries for systematic distribution. It should be understood, however, that the normal modes of extrusion are not always evident in neoplastic tissue.

Mucigen

The most commonly encountered protein-containing secretory granules found in human neo-

plasms, especially adenocarcinomas, are mucigen (mucin) granules. Classic membrane-limited mucigen granules, as found in goblet cells, range from 0.7 to 1.8 μm in diameter, and are often fused to each other (an artifact of fixation) (Fig. 3-44). Most mucigen granules have a reticulated electron-lucent substructure of variable density and on occasion contain an opaque spherule (Fig. 3-45). Structureless or homogeneous more electron-dense granules are also commonly found in mucin-secreting neoplastic cells (Fig. 3-46); the latter granule type may be mistaken for a zymogen granule. Elongated fibrillary bodies are also occasionally seen (Fig. 3-44).

As immature or atypical mucigen granules vary in size, shape, and density in many mucin-producing neoplastic cells, histochemical stains are required for their identification.[430] For example, the immature small (200 nm), membrane-limited, electron-dense mucigen (?) granules located in the apical cytoplasm of neoplastic colonic epithelial cells (Fig. 3-47) are indistinguishable by morphology from neurosecretory-type granules.[252] Only the classic mucigen granules can be identified with certainty by fine structural examination.

Zymogen

Zymogen (serous) granules are another class of

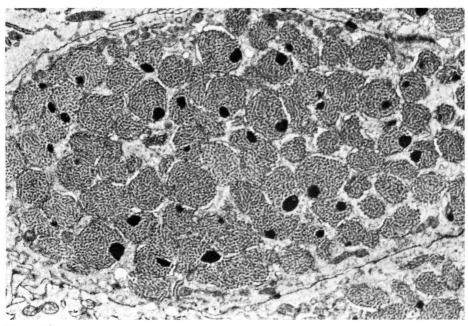

FIGURE 3-45
Mucin-producing adenocarcinoma (stomach, 36-year-old male). Portion of apical cytoplasm of neoplastic goblet cell showing marginated electron-opaque spherule in many of the mucigen granules. (×7360.)

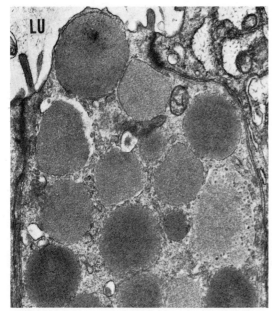

FIGURE 3-46
Well-differentiated duct cell adenocarcinoma (pancreas, 72-year-old female). More electron-dense homogeneous mucigen granules in subluminal cytoplasm of neoplastic goblet cell. Lumen (LU). (×15,600.)

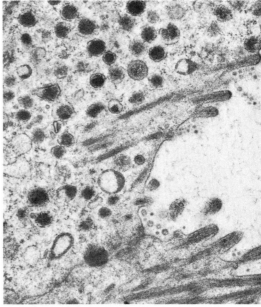

FIGURE 3-47
Adenocarcinoma (sigmoid colon, 66-year-old male). Immature 200-nm mucigen granules (?) that are morphologically indistinguishable from neurosecretory-type granules located in subluminal cytoplasm of neoplastic epithelial cell. (×21,600.)

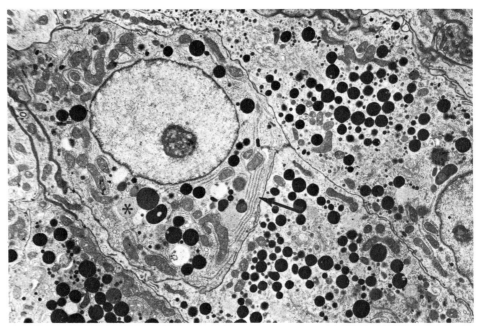

FIGURE 3-48
Well-differentiated acinic cell carcinoma (parotid gland, 16-year-old female). Portion of four neoplastic acinar cells. Note the variable size of the electron-dense zymogen granules. Partially extracted granules (*asterisk*), RER (*arrow*). (×5400.)

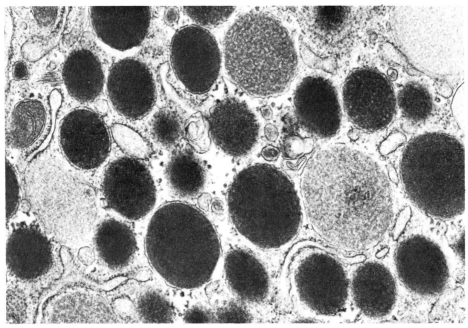

FIGURE 3-49
Acinar cell carcinoma (pancreas, 64-year-old male). The tumor consisted primarily of cysts of variable size lined by one or two layers of well-differentiated acinar cells. Portion of cytoplasm showing typical membrane-limited electron-dense zymogen granules and low-density variants that resemble mucigen granules. (×25,000.)

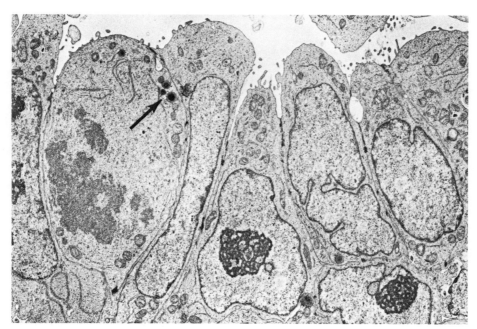

FIGURE 3-50
Papillary serous cystadenocarcinoma (ovary, 52-year-old female). Note the absence of zymogen or serous granules in the neoplastic surface mesothelial cells. Peculiar lipid droplets (*arrow*) are present in the mitotic cell. (×5000.)

protein-containing secretory granule found in the apical cytoplasm of acinar cells of certain exocrine glands (e.g., gastric chief cells, pancreatic acinar cells, serous acinar cells of salivary glands, and small glands scattered throughout the upper respiratory tract). Paneth cells,[606] which occur only in small groups in the lower portion of the intestinal crypts of Lieberkuhn, also contain zymogen granules. Strictly speaking, zymogen refers to a proenzyme-containing granule such as trypsinogen, whereas serous granules contain the enzyme in its final form, e.g., amylase.

Zymogen granules are membrane-limited spherical structures measuring 0.5–1.5 μm in diameter (Fig. 3-48). The homogeneous granular matrix is quite electron dense when well preserved, and in certain cases may contain an even denser spherule. Swollen, partially extracted, poorly preserved zymogen granules of low electron density are virtually indistinguishable from mucigen granules (Fig. 3-49). Cells containing zymogen granules are prominent in acinic cell carcinomas of the parotid gland[161,297,541] (Fig. 3-48), pancreatic acinar cell tumors[88,93] (Fig. 3-49), pancreatoblastoma,[258] an infantile type of pancreatic carcinoma, and in rare acinar cell carcinomas arising in the larynx[129] and lung.[172] Neoplastic Paneth cells with osmiophilic zymogen granules containing lysozyme (a marker for Paneth cells)

and mucosubstances are occasionally found in gastrointestinal (GI) tract neoplasms.[246]

It is worthwhile to note at this point that the designation serous tumor does not necessarily mean that the cells comprising the neoplasm produce zymogen granules. Ovarian serous cystadenomas, derived from the surface mesothelial covering, contain nonciliated neoplastic cells with scattered small mucigen, rather than serous granules in their apical portions.[178,311] In my experience, apical secretory granules of any kind are rarely found in either benign or malignant ovarian serous cystadenomas (Fig. 3-50). It cannot be overemphasized that extreme caution must be used in interpreting the nature of secretory granules by morphology alone.

Neurosecretory-type granules (apudomas)

Perhaps the most interesting and controversial class of secretory granules are the relatively small membrane-encased dense core or neurosecretory-type granules that contain amines or polypeptide hormones. Found in a variety of neuroendocrine tumors, these granules range in size from 80 to 600 nm and are generally spherical (Fig. 3-51), although oblong and pleomorphic varieties have also been described (Fig. 3-52). Bloodworth et al.[58] prefer the term endosecretory granules for

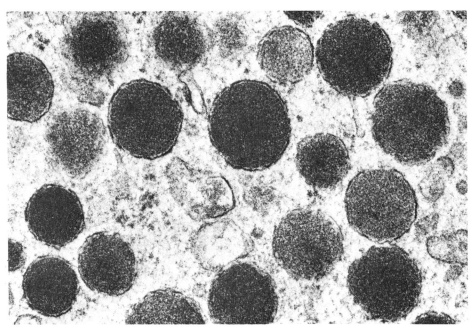

FIGURE 3-51
Metastatic islet cell carcinoma (liver, 54-year-old female). Portion of cytoplasm showing relatively large (average diameter, 350 nm) spherical membrane-limited dense-core neurosecretory-type or endosecretory granules. (×41,400.)

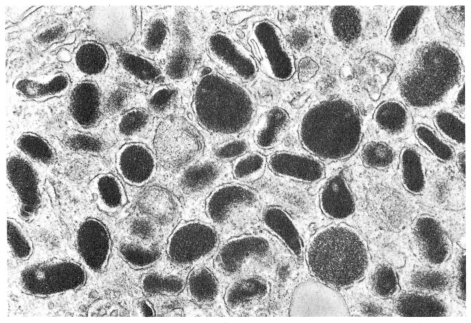

FIGURE 3-52
Carcinoid tumor (ileum, 52-year-old female). Spherical and 180 × 400-nm average diameter pleomorphic endosecretory granules characteristically found in midgut carcinoid tumors are illustrated. (×40,000.)

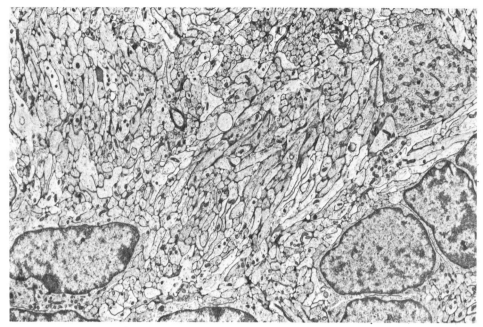

FIGURE 3-53
Neuroblastoma (perirenal lymph node, 8-year-old female). Portion of metastatic tumor in lymph node showing neuroblast cell bodies and profusion of neuritic processes. (×4320.)

those found in tumors that are not part of the nervous system.

Pearse's APUD (Amine Precursor Uptake Decarboxylation) concept[459] of a widely dispersed system of endocrine cells presumed to be of neural crest origin that helps explain the histochemical and ultrastructural similarities of a variety of endocrine cells and tumors derived from them—apudomas or neuroendocrinomas—has gained rapid acceptance,[103,110,223,460,461] although of the 40 original members, only six (thyroid C cells, carotid body type 1 cell, chromaffin cells of the adrenal medulla and sympathetic nervous system, urogenital tract enterochromaffin (EC) or E cells, and the melanoblast) are of proved neural crest origin. Pearse and Polak[462] now suggest that all APUD cells are derived from neuroendocrine-programmed cells originating in the embryonic ectoblast.

Not all apudomas are of neural crest, placodal, ectodermal, or ectoblastic origin. For example, the origin of islet cells is disputed[20,339,475]—intermediate stages between typical centroacinar or ductular cells and neoplastic endocrine cells have been described.[357,510] Adenocarcinoid tumors consisting of amphicrine cells[522] that contain both mucigen and neurosecretory granules within the

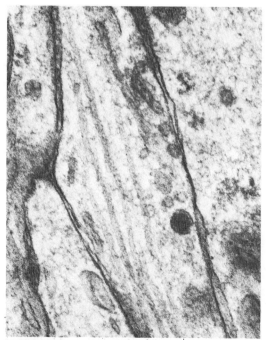

FIGURE 3-54
Neuroblastoma (cf. Fig. 3-53). Portion of four neuritic processes one of which contains characteristic neurotubules (actually microtubules) and a neurosecretory granule measuring 86 nm in diameter. (×72,000.)

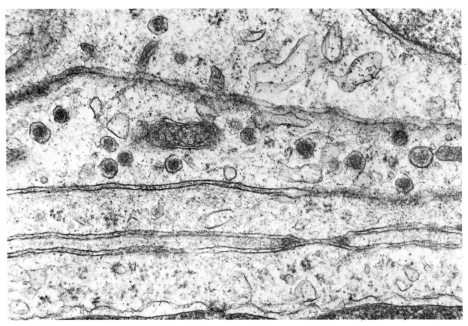

FIGURE 3-55
Esthesioneuroblastoma (antrum, 33-year-old male). Neuroblast cell processes, one of which contains numerous
110-nm neurosecretory granules. (×45,000.)

same cells have also been reported.[2,122] Evidence
for the endodermal origin of digestive, respiratory,
and pancreatic neuroendocrine cells is reviewed by
Sidhu.[539] Although the APUD concept has certain
flaws, it still offers the best explanation for the
multitude of widely dispersed neuroendocrine
neoplasms with similar biochemical, histochemical, and ultrastructural features.

Examples of tumors containing neurosecretory-type granules and possibly arising from
APUD cells include the following:

1. The large group of carcinoid tumors[110,212,463]
   (see below).
2. Neuroblastomas[376,497,590,651] (Figs. 3-53 and
   3-54) and esthesioneuroblastomas arising
   from the olfactory placode[107,595] (Fig. 3-
   55).
3. Medullary thyroid carcinomas[245] (Fig. 3-
   42).
4. Pheochromocytomas[83,377,584] (Fig. 3-61).
5. Paragangliomas[106,203,230,259,333,334] (Fig. 3-
   56).
6. Rare Merkel cell tumors of the
   skin[141,538,540,580] wherein the granules are
   usually located just beneath the plasmalemma
   (Chapter 6, case 5).
7. Pituitary adenomas (Table 3-1)—only the
   granule morphology of the five cell types
   comprising the anterior pituitary gland as

determined by electron microscopic immunocytochemical methods is listed in Table
3-1.[58] Cell features and granule morphology
are usually significantly altered in pituitary
adenomas, e.g., multiple hormone production
and stem cell tumors, so that ultrastructural
criteria useful for identifying cell types and
hormones in the normal pituitary gland
are often not applicable to tumor
cells.[23,97,165,260,261,325,327,351,493,520,521,523,582]

8. Tumors arising from pancreatic islet cells and
   adjacent duodenal wall (see below). Except for
   the beta cell, the other cell types found in the
   normal islet are also found in the GI
   tract[58,73,86,96,131,229,287,429,552] (Table 3-2).
   According to Pearse and Polak,[462] gastroenteropancreatic (GEP) cells are derived from
   "neuroendocrine programmed cells of ectoblastic origin," and not from the neural crest.
9. Pulmonary tumorlets.[479]
10. Oat cell carcinoma, a highly malignant variant
    of bronchial carcinoid tumor.[186,224,244,401] In
    our experience, not all oat cell carcinomas
    arising in the lung are composed of cells con-
    taining neurosecretory-type granules; ex-
    cluding small cell squamous carcinomas,[112,378]
    about one-third are probably anaplastic
    bronchial basal cell tumors. So-called oat cell
    carcinomas have also been described in other
    organs.[394,432,499,587,593] The term oat cell is

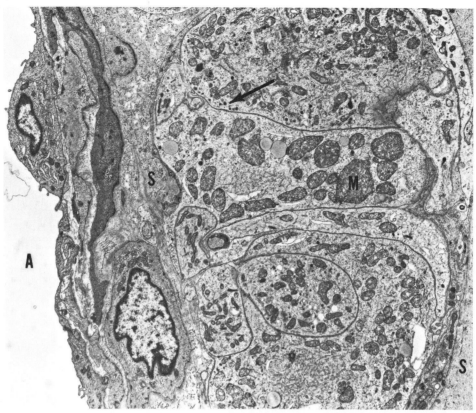

FIGURE 3-56
Carotid body tumor (carotid body, 72-year-old male). Portion of carotid body tumor showing a nest of neoplastic chief cell processes. Note the dense-core granules (*arrow*), megamitochondria (M), arteriole (A), and stroma (S). (×5040.)

descriptive. These tumors are not apudomas unless scattered clusters of neurosecretory-type granules are demonstrated by electron microscopy (Chapter 6, case 6).

Carcinoid tumors are a heterogeneous group of hormonally active or inactive neoplasms most of which occur in the GI tract. They are composed of either solid nests of uniform small cells (insular pattern) or, less commonly, of bands, ribbons, or trabeculae of tumor cells. These neoplasms can be divided into three groups[463,529,641]:

1. *Foregut carcinoids* (bronchus, thymus, stomach, upper duodenum, pancreas, and liver). The main secretory product is 5-hydroxytryptophan (5-HTP). The endosecretory granules are small (average diameter, approximately 150 nm) and

TABLE 3-1

Secretory Granule Morphology—Cells of the Anterior Pituitary[58]

Cell Type	Hormone	Secretory Granule Ultrastructure		
		Diameter (nm)	Shape	Core Density	Halo
Corticotroph	Adrenocorticotropic (ACTH)	300–350	Spherical	Variable	None
Gonadotroph	Follicle-stimulating (FSH)	250–300	Spherical	Dense	None
		400–450	Spherical	Variable	None
	Luteinizing (LH) or Interstitial-cell-stimulating (ICSH)	250–300	Spherical	Dense	None
Lactotroph	Prolactin (PRL)	500–600	Spherical	Dense	None
Somatotroph	Growth (GH)	350–450	Spherical	Dense	None
Thyrotroph	Thyroid-stimulating (TSH)	50–150	Spherical	Dense	Variable

TABLE 3-2

Classification of Cells Comprising the Gastroenteropancreatic Endocrine System[a]

Cell Type	Location	Secretory Granule Morphology (EM)				Postulated Polypeptide Hormone	Tumor Syndrome
		Diameter (nm)	Shape	Core	Halo		
Alpha (A)	Pancreas, stomach	200–400	Round	Black	Gray	Glucagon	Glucagonoma (? Diabetes)
Beta (B)	Pancreas	250–350	Round or oblong	Para-crystalline	Clear	Insulin	Insulinoma (hypoglycemia)
Delta (D)	Pancreas, duodenum, and jejunum	200–450	Round	Gray to black	None	Somatostatin	Somatostinoma (Steatorrhea, Achlorhydria, Diabetes mellitus)
Pancreatic Polypeptide (PP)	Pancreas	150–170	Round	Black	Narrow clear	Pancreatic Polypeptide	
Gastrin (G)	Pyloric antrum and duodenum	200–400	Round	Variable density	None	Gastrin	Gastrinomas (Zollinger-Ellison syndrome)
Enterochromaffin (EC) (Kultschitzky cell)	Stomach through rectum	200–600	Round pleomorphic (in midgut)	Gray to black	Variable	Motilin, Substance P, Amines 5-HTP and 5-HT	Carcinoid syndrome
D₁	Pancreas, stomach, upper duodenum	140–190	Round	Variable density	None	VIP, GIP, or HPP[b]	?Verner-Morrison syndrome
Intermediate (I)	Lower jejunum and ileum	240–280	Round	Black	None	Cholecystokinin-Pancreomyzin	
Large (L)	Small and large intestines	260–400	Round	Black	None	Enteroglucagon (Glicentin)	
Secretin (S)	Primarily duodenum and jejunum	100–200	Round or oblong	Black	Narrow clear	Secretin	

[a] Not all the 15 identified types of the 1977 Lausanne classification[552] are listed. The data were obtained from various sources.
[b] *Abbreviations:* VIP = Vasoactive intestinal polypeptide; GIP = gastric inhibitory polypeptide; HPP = human pancreatic polypeptide.

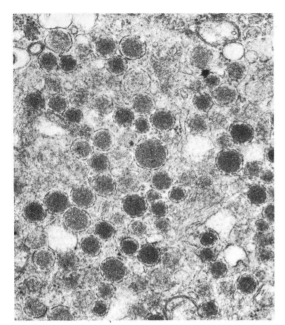

FIGURE 3-57
Carcinoid tumor (within a rectal polyp, 43-year-old female).
Cluster of endosecretory granules ranging from 170 to 350 nm
in diameter. (×31,000.)

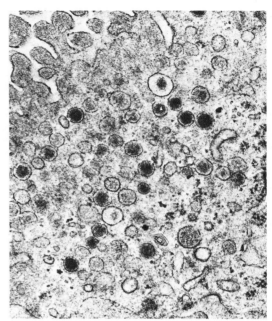

FIGURE 3-58
Carcinoid tumor (left upper lobe, lung, 51-year-old female).
Apical cytoplasm of neoplastic Kulkschitzky cell. Note the
small (140-nm average diameter) endosecretory granules.
(×32,000.)

uniformly round. Foregut carcinoids are argyrophil positive (stain with metallic silver after
addition of exogenous reducing agent) and argentaffin negative (do not reduce ammoniacal
silver nitrate).

2. *Midgut carcinoids* (lower duodenum, jejunum,
   ileum, appendix, and right hemicolon). Insular
   growth pattern. The main secretory product is
   5-hydroxytryptamine (5-HT) also known as
   serotonin. The secretory granules are large and.
   pleomorphic (see below) and are argentaffin
   positive and argyrophil negative.

3. *Hindgut carcinoids* (left hemicolon, anus, and
   rectum). Trabecular growth pattern. No known
   secretory product (the main product is
   biochemically inactive). The endosecretory
   granules are large and round (average diameter, 190 nm) (Fig. 3-57) and are basically both
   argentaffin and argyrophil negative.

In addition to the organs above-listed, carcinoid
tumors have also been found in the esophagus,[587]
ovary,[56,480,529] testicle,[571] uterine cervix,[395]
breast,[132] and kidney,[555] middle ear,[434] and will
undoubtedly be reported in other organs of the
body. Ultrastructural identification and characterization of endosecretory granules is often essential for the diagnosis of carcinoid tumors, but
it is of little value for establishing the site of origin

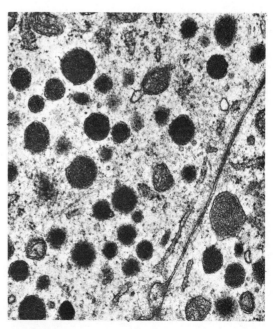

FIGURE 3-59
Carcinoid tumor (left upper lobe lung, 65-year-old female). The
neoplastic Kultschitzky cells in this tumor contain a population
of large (280-nm) endosecretory granules in addition to the
140-nm granules (cf. Fig. 3-58). (×32,000.)

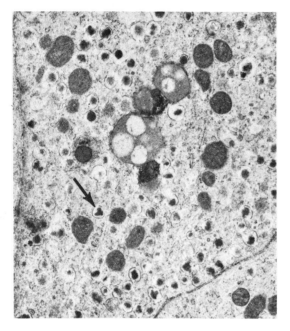

FIGURE 3-60
Insulinoma (pancreas, 60-year-old male with hypoglycemia).
Portion of cytoplasm of neoplastic beta cell showing endosecretory granules with crystalline core (*arrow*) mixed with
granules with an amorphous electron-dense core. It is difficult
to see the core periodicity in the vast majority of cases.
(×12,800.)

of metastatic neoplasms because of overlapping
granule morphology (exceptions are given below).
For example, Serratoni and Robboy[529] could not
distinguish foregut and hindgut carcinoids on the
basis of granule morphology alone.

Contrary to popular belief, electron microscopy
alone is of limited value in determining the pro-
totypical cell or type of polypeptide hormone or
amine produced by apudomas. Many recent
studies show that granular size varies considerably
within the same cell or in individual tumors of the
same type, e.g., carcinoid tumors arising within the
lung[95,232] (Figs. 3-58 and 3-59). In many instances,
it is also very difficult to relate a given apudoma
with confidence to its presumed precursor
cell.[58,126,229,361,463] For example, Creutzfeldt et
al.[127] showed that the ultrastructural appearance
of the endosecretory granules in 10 gastrinomas in
patients with Zollinger-Ellison syndrome was not
uniform and that multiple hormone production
was frequent.

The demonstration of neuro- or endosecretory
granules in a lesion using standard procedures,
including electron microscopy, does not necessarily
mean that the patients will exhibit symptoms of
excess hormone or amine production. The granules
in many cases contain only prohormones, which
are unable to convert to active hormones.[110,630]

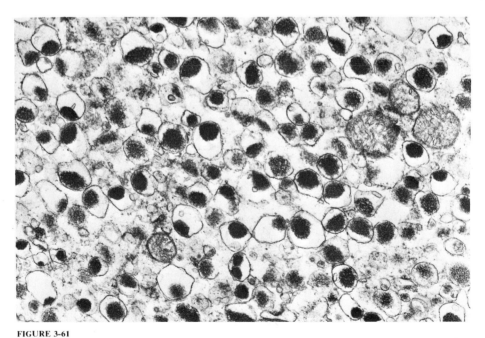

FIGURE 3-61
Pheochromocytoma (adrenal gland, 66-year-old female with paroxysmal hypertension). Portion of cytoplasm
of large epithelioid medullary chromaffin cell. Note the eccentrically positioned dense core of the norepi-
nephrine-containing granules. (×17,600.)

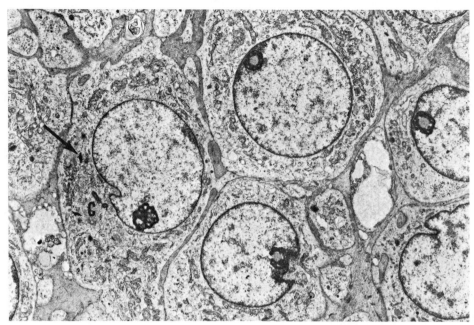

FIGURE 3-62
Juxtaglomerular cell tumor (kidney, 14-year-old female with hypertension). Clusters of polygonal and round juxtaglomerular cells in a dense fibrillogranular stroma. Note the renin granules (*arrow*). Centrioles (C). (×6720.)

The secretion of various endocrine substances (ectopic or multiple hormone production) by apudomas and tumors composed of a mixture of endocrine cell types is also not uncommon.[94,127,223,395,451] For example, secretion of more than one hormone is a recognized feature of islet cell tumors.[58,72,73,126]

There are certain neuroendocrinomas, however, in which the neurosecretory granule morphology can be more confidently identified with a specific kind of APUD cell or a neuroendocrine cell type preponderant in a given organ. Insulinomas, derived from pancreatic beta cells, contain endosecretory granules with a distinctive crystalline core[79,128] (Fig. 3-60). Poorly differentiated functioning insulinomas, however, have been described that are composed principally of cells without crystalline granules intermingled with cells containing only a few immature beta granules.[73,570] A distinctive feature of the neurosecretory granules in most extraadrenal pheochromocytomas is the eccentrically positioned dense-core characteristic of norepinephrine (NE)-containing granules[83,208,377,584] (Fig. 3-61). Renin-secreting juxtaglomerular cell neoplasms (a rare kidney tumor) (Fig. 3-62) that induce hypertension, contain

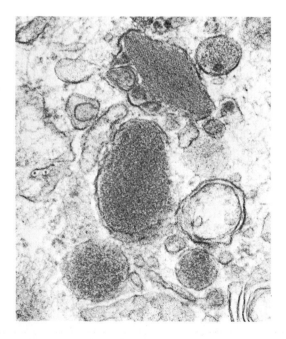

FIGURE 3-63
Juxtaglomerular cell tumor (cf. Fig. 3-62). Rounded granules with a granular electron-dense content and a rhomboid protogranule with a crystalline core. (×66,000.)

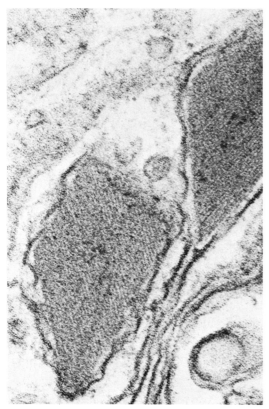

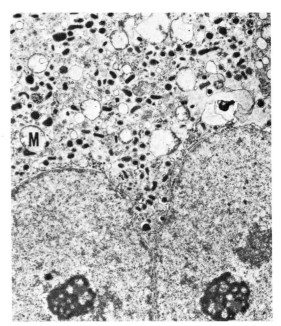

FIGURE 3-65
Carcinoid tumor (ovary, 70-year-old female). Portion of bi-nucleate cell containing both spherical and pleomorphic granules. The mitochondria (M) are dilated due to delayed fixation. (×8800.)

FIGURE 3-64
Detail of crystalline core of two protogranules. Note the periodicity of the crystalline lattice. (×111,000.)

pleomorphic mature granules and highly characteristic rhomboid protogranules[31,427,464] (Figs. 3-62 and 3-63). Many of the rhomboid granules have a periodic crystalline core (Fig. 3-64).

Neoplasms consisting of cells that contain both spherical and oblong (also called pleomorphic) granules are much less common than are those with only spherical granules. So-called pleomorphic granules (180 × 400 nm; see Fig. 3-52) have been found in midgut carcinoids presumably arising from the EC cell also known as the Kultschitzky-Masson cell,[55,58,377] in ovarian carcinoids[529] (Fig. 3-65), in a testicular carcinoid tumor,[571] and in a carcinoid tumor of the pancreas.[457] Except for some beta granules, all the endosecretory granules found in islet cell tumors are spherical (Fig. 3-51). I have found pleomorphic granules in only carcinoid tumors, arising in the ileum, appendix, ovary, and pancreas. Therefore, the demonstration of pleomorphic granules in a metastatic tumor suggests a limited number of possible primary sites. In our laboratory, a small carcinoid tumor in the ileum was located after pleomorphic granules were found in metastatic tumor cells in a cervical lymph node (Fig. 3-66).

Alveolar soft part sarcomas,[353] soft tissue tumors of undetermined histogenesis with a distinctive organoid appearance, often consist of large polyhedral cells that contain a biphasic population of cytoplasmic secretory granules. The larger (average diameter, 430 nm) membrane-limited inclusions resemble small mucigen granules, whereas the smaller (86–200 nm) electron dense inclusions correspond to neurosecretory-type granules (Fig. 3-67). Although it has been proposed that these tumors arise from paraganglia,[609,636] this contention is disputed, because specific stains for these granules (Grimelius, argentaffin, etc.) are negative, the histology is different, and paragangliomas do not arise within skeletal muscle.[151,617] This is a perfect example of how the ultramicroscopic appearance of a secretory granule can be misleading. Distinction between small primary (or possibly secondary) lysosomes and neurosecretory-type granules can be difficult or impossible in tumors consisting of cells containing only scattered small dense-core granules.[251]

Although electron microscopy is helpful in establishing the secretory nature (exocrine or endocrine) of a primary or a metastatic tumor, it often fails to provide information sufficient to

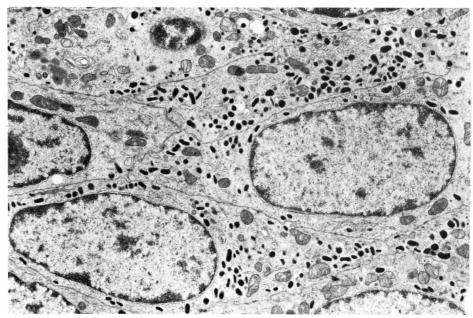

FIGURE 3-66
Metastatic carcinoid tumor (Lower jugular lymph node, 52-year-old female). The presence of pleomorphic granules in the spindle-shaped tumor cells suggested a possible primary tumor in the midgut. Exploratory laparotomy revealed a small primary carcinoid tumor in the ileum. (×7200.)

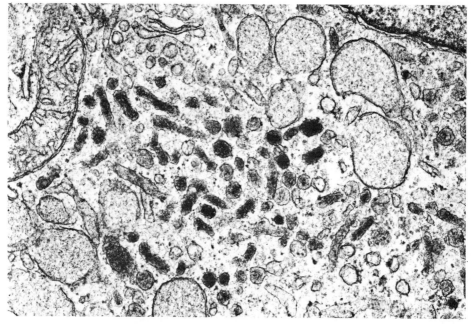

FIGURE 3-67
Alveolar soft part sarcoma (paraaortic lymph node, 24-year-old male). Large (430-nm) mucigenlike granules and smaller (86–200-nm) electron-dense neurosecretory-type granules are illustrated. The true nature of both of these granule types is not known. (×34,000.)

determine its precise histogenesis or the chemical composition of the secretory granules. To improve diagnostic accuracy, ultrastructural observations should always be correlated with clinical and histologic findings including special stains and immunocytochemical investigations for specific types or classes of secretory granules. Immunologic techniques (e.g., immunoperoxidase reaction) at the ultrastructural level for a specific polypeptide hormone and/or assay for hormone activity of extracted tissue samples is often necessary to determine what specific hormone(s) is/are contained in the granules found in neoplastic cells. Unfortunately, these techniques are generally not as widely available as is electron microscopy.

Glycogen and Lipid

Glycogen particles and lipid droplets are found in a wide variety of tumors and are of limited diagnostic significance. But the presence of these inclusions is often helpful in determining the site of origin or histogenesis of certain anaplastic, metastatic, or primary small cell tumors.

Animal cells can store carbohydrates in the form of glycogen. The appearance of glycogen in electron micrographs depends on the method of tissue preparation. Well-fixed glycogen exists in two particulate forms: (1) beta glycogen, irregularly shaped 15–30-nm single particles; and (2) alpha glycogen, rosettelike aggregates that are particularly prominent in hepatocytes (Fig. 3-68). Unfortunately, both collidine-buffered fixatives and uranyl acetate pretreatment almost invariably extract and distort glycogen particles (Figs. 3-69 to 71). Lipid droplets appear as gray-to-black amorphous spherical structures of varying size in properly prepared tissue (Fig. 3-68). They are usually not bounded by a membrane. Even after extensive extraction or deformation, both structures are generally easily recognized in thin sections.

Glycogen and lipid are quite prominent in metastatic clear cell carcinomas of renal origin[156,567] (Fig. 3-69). The presence of pools of cytoplasmic glycogen particles in otherwise undifferentiated small round cell tumors of bone or, more rarely, soft tissues, is diagnostic for Ewing's sarcoma of bone[360,380] (Fig. 3-70) or extraskeletal Ewing's sarcoma[382,640] (Fig. 3-71), respectively, as glycogen is rarely found in lymphomas.[381] It is important to confirm the absence of ultrastructural features characteristic of other small round cell tumors[211,318,381,651] (Table 1-1). A case of neuroblastoma with clinical and histopathologic features of Ewing's sarcoma was found, upon ultra-

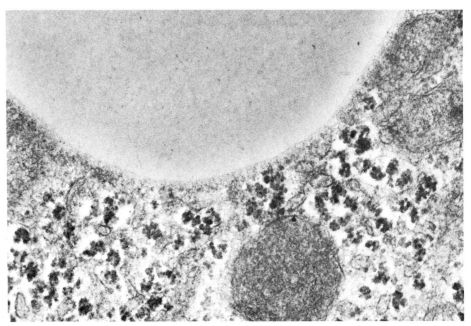

FIGURE 3-68
Focal nodular hyperplasia (liver, 51-year-old female). Portion of hepatocyte cytoplasm containing numerous rosettelike aggregates of alpha glycogen particles. Note that the structureless lipid droplet (*top*) is not surrounded by a membrane. (×60,000.)

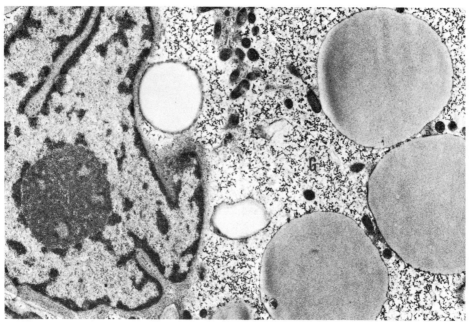

FIGURE 3-69
Metastatic clear cell carcinoma of the kidney (thigh, 80-year-old male). Note the cleaved nucleus with the large central nucleolus, the large lipid droplets, and the coarsely particulate glycogen (G). The round and ellipsoidal dense structures are mitochondria. (×10,400.)

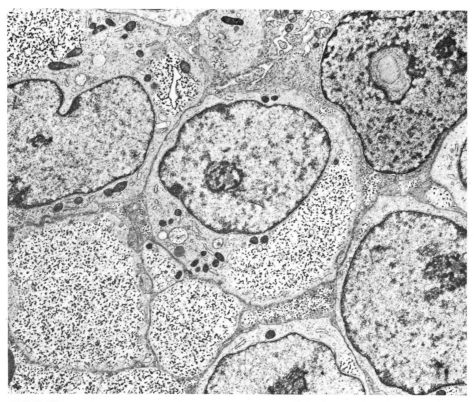

FIGURE 3-70
Ewing's sarcoma (scapula, 16-year-old female). Nests of small round cells containing abundant cytoplasmic glycogen are illustrated. (×6240.)

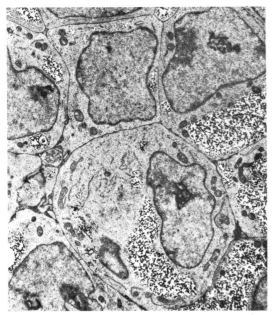

FIGURE 3-71
Extraskeletal Ewing's sarcoma (posterior thigh, 19-year-old male). The findings are identical to that of Ewing's sarcoma of bone. Note the large pools of cytoplasmic glycogen. (×4320.)

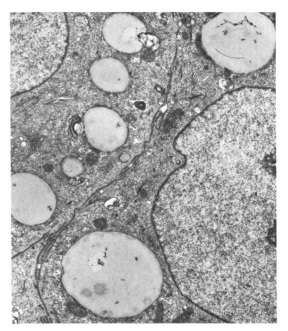

FIGURE 3-72
Sebaceous hyperplasia (nasolabial fold 82-year-old male). Portions of two alveolar epithelial cells from a hyperplastic sebaceous gland. Note the sebum (fat) droplets in the cytoplasm. (×7200.)

structural evaluation, to contain neurosecretory granules in addition to glycogen.[605] Electron microscopy cannot confirm a diagnosis of Ewing's sarcoma unless glycogen is found in the cytoplasm of the neoplastic cells.

Cytoplasmic glycogen is also particularly abundant in the following neoplasms: (1) benign hepatic adenomas,[204,296] (2) clear cell carcinoma of the female reproductive tract[142,182,513] (any tumor arising from müllerian epithelium has the potential to produce vast amounts of glycogen), (3) chondrosarcoma,[159] (4) parathyroid adenomas composed of chief cells with abundant clear cytoplasm,[102,326] and (5) the rare benign clear cell tumor of the lung (Sugar tumor).[40,255] The latter is a unique tumor of unknown histogenesis in which the glycogen is both free and membrane bound, as in glycogen storage diseases.

The diagnostic value of the presence of lipid droplets or vacuoles (Figs. 3-68, 3-69, and 3-72) is limited to possibly confirming a diagnosis of poorly differentiated liposarcoma[66,173,307] and differentiating an ovarian thecoma from a fibroma; theca cells are atypically plump and lipid-laden.[17,180] Lipid (lipoid) cell ovarian neoplasms composed of cells resembling luteinized ovarian stromal cells and Leydig cells or hilus cells[270] contain prominent lipid in addition to other cyto-

plasmic organelles and inclusions associated with steroid hormone synthesis (see p. 33).

Certain histiocytic tumors, i.e., atypical fibroxanthomas[12,33] (Fig. 3-73) and benign and malignant fibrous histiocytomas[11,113,195,281,358,591] also characteristically contain lipid droplets in addition to lysosomes. These latter tumors are a morphologically heterogeneous group. They vary from purely histiocytic neoplasms (malignant histiocytoma), to those consisting of both fibroblasts and histiocytes (classical malignant fibrous histiocytoma), to almost purely fibroblastic tumors (pleomorphic fibrosarcoma).[415] The origin of the so-called tissue histiocyte is unclear. It may represent the morphologic state of a mesenchymal cell rather than a particular cell type.[591]

Crystalline Inclusions

Crystalline or pseudocrystalline inclusions are occasionally found within the cisternae of the RER, in the mitochondrial matrix, or in the cytosol. These inclusions are usually the products of deranged protein synthesis.

Leydig (interstitial) cells of the testis and hilus cells from the ovary contain characteristic crystals of Reinke (Fig. 3-74). In electron micrographs, the

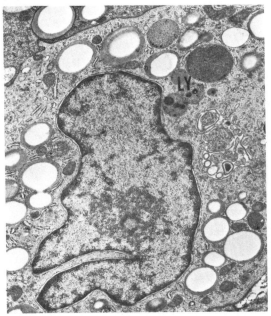

FIGURE 3-73
Atypical fibroxanthoma (intracutaneous nodule, upper arm, 65-year-old female). Histiocyte containing numerous partially extracted lipid droplets. Secondary lysosomes (LY). (×9600.)

FIGURE 3-74
Normal Leydig cell (testicle from a 17-year-old male with a Leydig cell tumor). The Reinke crystal consists of parallel arrays of beaded filaments. The dense granules are artifacts of precipitated osmium tetroxide. (×64,000.)

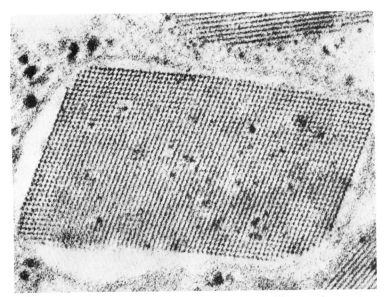

FIGURE 3-75
Alvelolar soft part sarcoma (lung metastasis from thigh primary, 44-year-old female). Cross section of atypical crystal (*center*). The dense lines consist of irregularly outlined points arranged along two axis that intersect at an angle of 75°. Portions of two crystals with a periodic pattern of 10 nm are also evident (×136,000). (Reproduced, with permission, from Shipkey et al. Ultrastructure of alveolar soft part sarcoma. Cancer 17: 821–830, 1964).

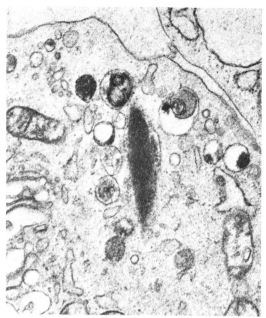

FIGURE 3-76
Granulocytic sarcoma (cervical lymph node, 17-year-old male). Elongated, finely granular electron-dense Auer body with pointed ends in neoplastic granulocyte. (×23,200.)

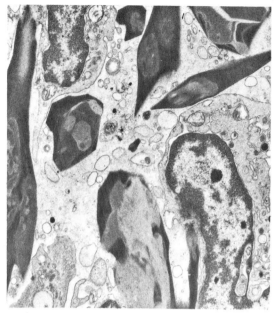

FIGURE 3-78
Seven large extracellular Charcot–Leyden crystals are illustrated (cf. Fig. 3-76). Note the density variation in the core of the crystals. (×9000.)

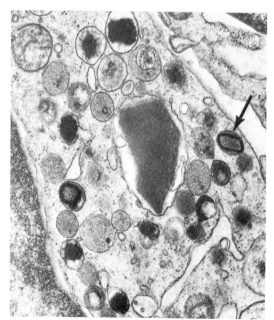

FIGURE 3-77
Small Charcot–Leyden crystal in neoplastic eosinophilic myelocyte (cf. Fig. 3-76). Note the rectangular amorphous crystalloid bar (*arrow*) in some of the secondary granules. (×23,200.)

crystals resemble a hexagonal prism of variable size, consisting of highly ordered 5-nm-thick filaments.[437] The chemical composition and function of these crystals is not firmly established. Reinke crystals or their precursor forms are considered pathognomonic for the identification of ovarian hilus cells.[182,407] Although these crystals are found in testicular Leydig cells[169] (Fig. 3-74) and possibly in spindle-shaped cells located in periendothelial spaces in the human adrenal cortex,[379] they are rarely found in tumors derived from these cells.[39,46,182] Likewise, Charcot-Böttcher crystalloids characteristic of Sertoli cells, were never observed in Sertoli cell tumors of the ovary or testis[238] until recently.[589] These so-called crystalloids actually consist of closely packed electron-dense longitudinal arrays of fibrils lacking a geometric crystalline lattice.

Rectangular crystalloids delineated by a single-unit membrane are found in the cytoplasm of the basal pyramidal cells of Warthin's tumor.[579] They appear to form within structures that resemble microbodies.

Membrane-bound rhomboid proteinaceous crystals and spicules of varying size are found in the cytoplasm of the peculiar epithelioid cells comprising alveolar soft part sarcoma[151,537,609] (Fig. 3-75). Identification of these crystals may be of diagnostic value in the differentiation of tumors with organoid or alveolar patterns. Crystalline inclusions, however, are found in only about one-third of cases,[353] and were not present in the last six cases I examined.

Certain fairly distinctive crystalline inclusions are found in neoplastic granulocytes. Auer bodies are intracytoplasmic needlelike crystalline inclusions (Fig. 3-76) encountered most commonly in acute promyelocytic leukemia and in occasional cases of acute myeloid and myelomonocytic leukemia.[28,80,214,533] They are probably derived from the electron-dense, round, azurophilic or primary granules (secondary or specific granules are more electron lucent and tertiary granules are dumbbell-shaped and electron-dense),[525] because both inclusions generally display strong peroxidase activity. Charcot-Leyden crystals of varying forms are easily recognized by light microscopy because of their large size (Figs. 3-77 and 3-78). They are found in both degenerating normal and occasional neoplastic eosinophils,[21,25,152] and are thought to be derived from degraded or recombined crystalloids originating from the distinctive eosinophil granule.[414] Demonstration of these peculiar crystals is helpful in establishing eosinophilic lineage, although it is doubtful that they are present in immature neoplastic eosinophils.

A number of reports have documented the presence of rectangular proteinaceous crystals within dilated cisternae of the RER in rare cases of chronic lymphocytic leukemia (CLL) and in some non-Hodgkin's lymphomas. These crystals are usually, but not always[336] distinguishable from the needlelike Auer bodies encountered in occasional promyelocytic leukemia cells. In most cases they consist of precipitated immunoglobulin M (IgM) lambda chains. For example, crystalline (also fibrillar or granulofilamentous) structures were reported in 13 of 61 patients with CLL,[557] and IgM lambda crystals have been described in three cases of immunocytoma, a lymphoma of low-grade malignancy.[179] It must be emphasized that demonstration of most types of crystalline inclusions is of very limited diagnostic significance.

Langerhans Granule (Birbeck Body)

Langerhans granules or Birbeck bodies, originally observed in the Langerhans cells of the epider-

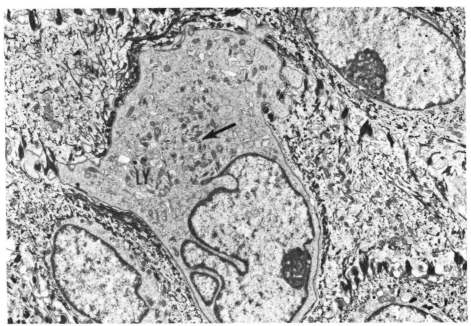

FIGURE 3-79
Langerhans cells (skin, flank, 22-year-old male. From skin biopsy taken 20 days post-bone marrow transplant for aplastic anemia). Langerhans cell surrounded by keratinocytes. Numerous Birbeck bodies (*arrow*, use hand lens) and lysosomes (LY) are evident in the cytoplasm. Note the cytoplasmic invaginations into the nucleus. (×5280.)

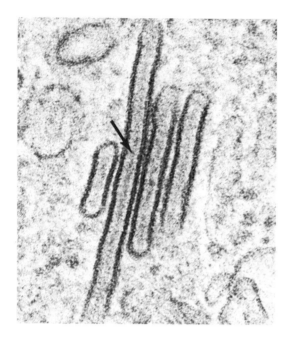

FIGURE 3-80
Langerhans cell (normal skin biopsy, 48-year-old male). The zipperlike periodic core (*arrow*) is evident in portions of the Birbeck bodies. (×168,000.)

mis,[53] (Fig. 3-79) are distinct rod-shaped membranous structures having a zipperlike periodic core[496] (Fig. 3-80). They are often continuous with the plasmalemma and are probably derived from this membrane. Langerhans granules are characteristically present in the cytoplasm of the histiocytic cells comprising eosinophilic granuloma[34,134,425,444] (Langerhans cell granulomatosis).[355] Langerhans cells are occasionally evident in normal lymph nodes and some lymphomatous nodes,[622] in many cutaneous diseases,[12,482,534] and in numerous other organs and diseases (Shelly and Juhlin).[534]

Pale-staining monocytic cells in cases of so-called Letterer-Siwe disease,[92,531] the most malignant entity of histiocytosis-X or Hand-Schuller-Christian disease, also contain these granules. Lieberman and associates[354] have convincingly shown that the latter two terms are inappropriate and confusing, whereas Letterer-Siwe disease is a clinical term used to characterize various malignant histiocytic lymphomas and occasional infectious processes. We have found the presence of these distinctive inclusions to be helpful in confirming a diagnosis of Langerhans cell granulomatosis (eosinophilic granuloma) (Fig. 3-81).

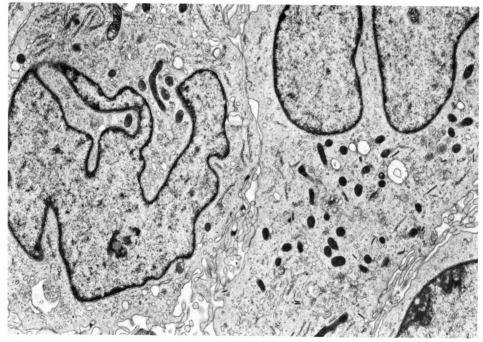

FIGURE 3-81
Eosinophilic granuloma (cervical lymph node, 23-year-old female). Two Langerhans cells, one with a cleaved nucleus (*right*) and one with a convoluted nucleus (*left*) are shown. Birbeck bodies (use hand lens) are scattered throughout the cytoplasm of the cell (*right*). (×8000.)

Recent studies suggest that these granules might play a role in immune responses.[285,565]

Lamellar Inclusion Body

Type 2 alveolar pneumocytes or granular pneumocytes have characteristic intracytoplasmic lamellar inclusion bodies composed of concentrically arranged or straight and parallel electron-dense membranes (Figs. 3-82 to 3-84) that superficially resemble lipoprotein or phospholipid myelin figures. These structures are the major source of surfactant, a material rich in dipalmityl lecithin.[26] Diagnosis of alveolar cell carcinoma is facilitated by demonstration of type 2 alveolar pneumocyte

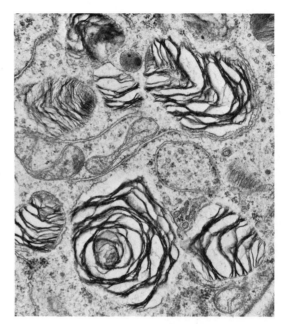

FIGURE 3-82 →
Bronchiolar carcinoma, Clara cell type (right lower lobe lung, 71-year-old male). Portion of cytoplasm of normal granular pneumocyte illustrating characteristic lamellar inclusion bodies. (×19,200.)

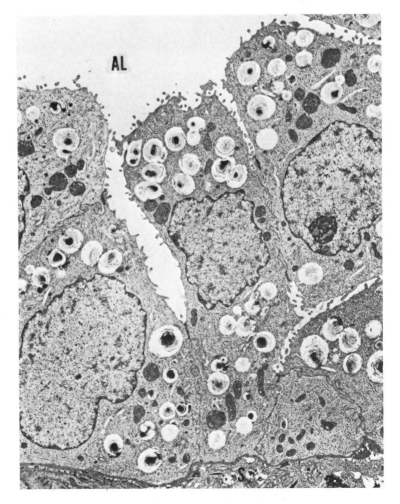

FIGURE 3-83
Pleomorphic adenocarcinoma (right lower lobe lung, 45-year-old male). Hyperplastic columnar granular pneumocytes adjacent to the tumor. Note the stubby surface microvilli and lamellar inclusion bodies. Alveolus (AL), stroma (S). (×4800.)

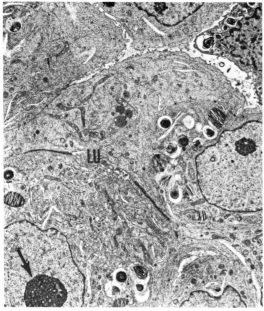

FIGURE 3-84
Pleomorphic adenocarcinoma (right lower lobe lung, 59-year-old female). Portion of a cluster of neoplastic granular pneumocytes. Note the lamellar inclusion bodies, large nucleolus (*arrow*), and lumen (LU). (×3600.)

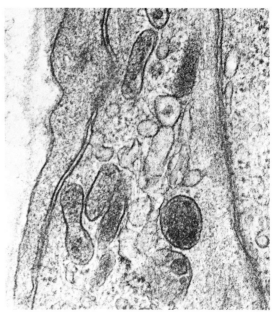

FIGURE 3-86
Myxoma (cheek, 32-year-old male). Assorted rod- and dumbbell-shaped Weibel-Palade bodies in endothelial cell cytoplasm. Note that most of these peculiar inclusions lack a striated core. (×52,000.)

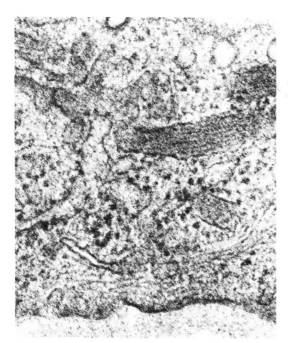

FIGURE 3-85
Childhood sarcoma of undetermined histogenesis (left external oblique muscle, 16-year-old male). Portion of normal endothelial cell cytoplasm containing three Weibel-Palade bodies, note the striated substructure. (×78,000.)

inclusion bodies.[69] Recent investigative studies in our laboratory and in others have shown that most so-called bronchioloalveolar carcinomas[356] consist of neoplastic cells showing bronchiolar cell differentiation (e.g., cuboidal Clara cells with apical electron-dense secretory granules) and should be called bronchiolar carcinomas.[69,160,228,328] Neoplastic granular pneumocytes must be distinguished from hyperplastic type 2 cells (Fig. 3-83), which are present in most of these neoplasms. I have found neoplastic type 2 cells to be a component of occasional bronchiolar and peripheral lung adenocarcinomas. They are recognizable by their pleomorphism and intimate association with other neoplastic cell types (Fig. 3-84).

Weibel-Palade Body—Vascular Tumors

Weibel and Palade[632] originally described a peculiar rod-shaped body with a longitudinally oriented electron-dense striated or tubular core (Figs. 3-85 and 3-86) in arterial endothelial cells. This unusual inclusion is believed to be a specific ultrastructural marker for endothelial cells[329] and for neoplasms of vascular (endothelial cell) origin, e.g., sclerosing hemangioma.[100,299] The function of the Weibel-Palade body, which superficially resembles a lysosome, is unknown.

In addition to Weibel-Palade bodies, normal endothelial cells are characterized by the following features: (1) long, thin bipolar cell processes that may form marginal folds (fingerlike attenuated terminal cell processes that project into the lumen) (Fig. 4-9); (2) a basal lamina; (3) numerous pinocytotic vesicles on both apical and basal plasma membranes; and (4) tight junctions (p. 108). The ultrastructural diagnosis of vasoformative tumors derived from endothelial cells requires the demonstration of cells with most of the above-mentioned features.[100,176,299,500,561,594]

Benign endothelial cell tumors [e.g., hemangioma (Fig. 3-87) and hemangiomatosis (Fig. 3-88)] often consist of flattened cells lining slitlike vascular channels. Most ultrastructural markers (including Weibel-Palade bodies) of the prototypic endothelial cell are usually identifiable. Angiosarcomas show more pronounced cellular pleomorphism (Fig. 3-89), and the formation of tumor capillaries is often required for diagnosis. Hemangioendothelial sarcomas (hemangioendotheliomas) of bone[561] characteristically consist of plump neoplastic endothelial cells that project into a vascular lumen (Fig. 3-90). The cytoplasm

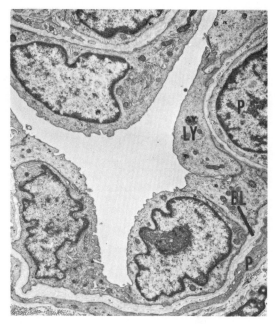

FIGURE 3-87
Hemangioma (skin, back, 8-year-old male). Portion of benign neoplastic arteriole. The bulbous endothelial cells are separated from a single layer of pericytes (P) by a reduplicated thin basal lamina (BL). Only lysosomes (LY) (no Weibel-Palade bodies) are visible at this magnification. (×5250.)

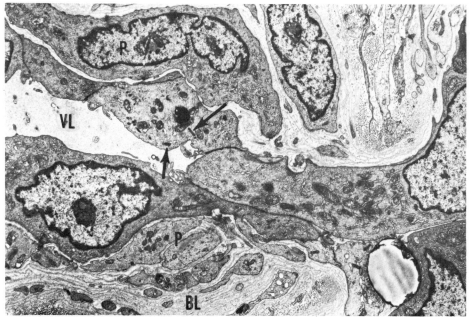

FIGURE 3-88
Benign hemangiomatosis (subcutaneous tissues, anterior chest wall, 39-year-old female). The specimen consisted of a diffuse proliferation of blood vessels of varying sizes in subcutaneous tissue. Note the flattened endothelial cells lining the vessel wall. Vascular lumen (VL), pericytes (P), reduplicated basal lamina (BL), and Weibel-Palade bodies (*arrows*). (×4320.)

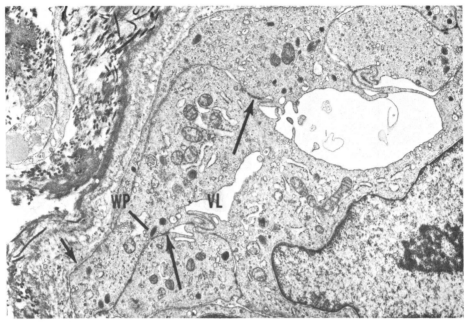

FIGURE 3-89
Pleomorphic angiosarcoma (anterior chest wall, 38-year-old male). Portion of vascular channel lined by large pleomorphic neoplastic endothelial cells containing both lysosomes and Weibel-Palade bodies (WP). The neoplastic endothelial cells are separated from the collagen stroma by a thin basal lamina (*short arrow*). Abortive vascular lumen (VL), cell junctions (*long arrows*). (×10,400.)

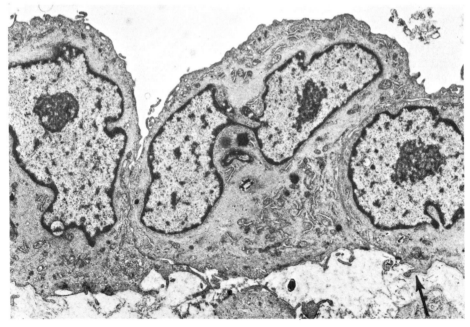

FIGURE 3-90
Hemangioendothelioma (ilium, 33-year-old male). Portion of a vascular channel. The plump neoplastic endothelial cells comprising this malignant tumor contain pleomorphic nuclei and perinuclear bundles of intermediate filaments (organelle-free areas), and bulge into the lumen. Note the remnants of basal lamina (*arrow*). The round electron-dense structures in the cytoplasm are lysosomes. (×5760.)

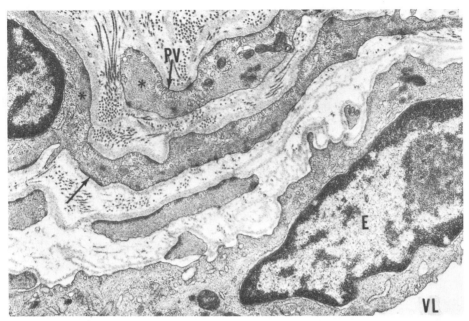

FIGURE 3-91
Neurofibroma (skin, anterior knee, 15-year-old female). Vascular channel surrounded by numerous pericytes showing smooth muscle cell differentiation. Note the surface pinocytotic vesicles (PV), attachment plaques (*arrow*), and microfilaments (asterisk). The pericytes are enveloped by a frayed basal lamina. Endothelial cell (E), vascular space or lumen (VL). (×13,200.)

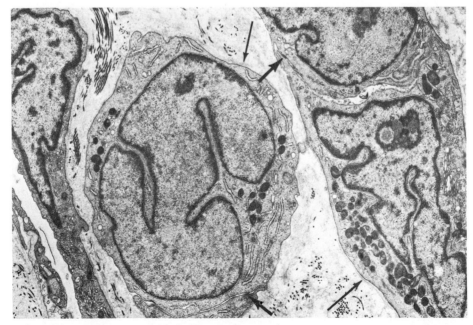

FIGURE 3-92
Metastatic hemangiopericytoma (paravertebral mass, 46-year-old female). Portions of four neoplastic pericytes joined by a primitive cell junction (*short arrows*) and partially invested by basal lamina (*long arrows*). A normal vessel is seen at *left*. (×8000.)

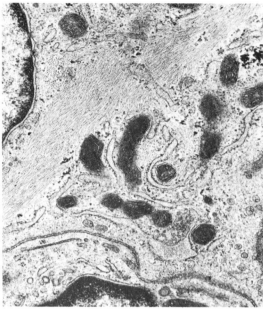

FIGURE 3-93
Metastatic hemangiopericytoma (ilium, 54-year-old male). Bundles of nonspecific 10-nm intermediate filaments are present in the cytoplasm of one of the cells. (×20,000.)

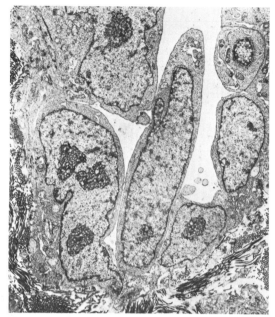

FIGURE 3-94
Postmastectomy lymphangiosarcoma (upper arm, 70-year-old female). Vascular channel lined by highly atypical endothelial cells one of which contains three large nucleoli. The neoplastic endothelial cells are not separated from the stromal collagen fibrils by a basal lamina. (×3430.)

contains large numbers of intermediate filaments (Fig. 3-131) and scattered lysosomes. Weibel-Palade bodies, if present, are helpful in confirming a diagnosis of a tumor of endothelial cell genesis. In my experience, however, they are absent in most vascular tumors, an observation that has been corroborated by numerous other studies.[176,500,561,594,600]

The pericyte, a mesenchymal cell having multipotential capabilities, intimately surrounds most endothelial cells. These peripheral cells are usually enveloped by basal lamina, display surface pinocytotic vesicles, and contain variable amounts of longitudinally oriented microfilaments and dense plasmalemmal attachment plaques (Fig. 3-91). Rhodin[488] postulated that the pericyte is the primitive mesenchymal cell that is the precursor of vascular smooth muscle.

Vascular neoplasms composed of elongated oval cells proliferating around numerous capillaries and believed to be derived from pericytes, are appropriately called hemangiopericytomas. Various fine structural studies of hemangiopericytomas, although supporting pericytic cytogenesis, have also demonstrated the multidirectional differentiation of these transitional cells into fibroblasts, phagocytic cells, possibly endothelial cells, and especially leiomyocytes.[35,150,233,426,472,487] Having examined six cases, it is my impression that these tumors

cannot be reliably diagnosed by electron microscopy because (1) there are no specific ultrastructural markers, and (2) most are composed of poorly differentiated mesenchymal cells (Figs. 3-92 and 3-93).

Some other poorly understood vascular tumors are worthy of brief mention. Postmastectomy lymphangiosarcoma (Stewart-Treves syndrome) is an uncommon malignant tumor that occurs in an edematous upper extremity following radical mastectomy for mammary carcinoma. Electron microscopic studies have failed to demonstrate conclusively an origin in lymphatic capillaries.[146,227,303,408,542,623] I have examined one convincing case that arose in the edematous right arm of a postmastectomy patient. Figure 3-94 illustrates the absence of a basal lamina[344] in this case. Kaposi's sarcoma, a tumor consisting of a variable mixture of vasoformative elements and spindle cells,[78,350,428] and the so-called cerebellar hemangioblastoma,[108,553] are most likely derived from multiple cell types of vascular lineage, e.g., endothelial cells and pericytes. In conclusion, demonstration of vascular channels lined by cells with endothelial cell markers is generally required for the ultrastructural diagnosis of vascular neo-

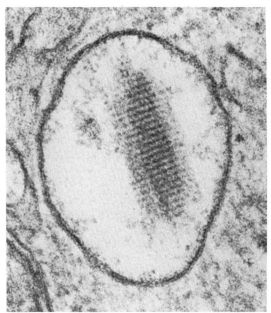

FIGURE 3-95
Malignant melanoma (left side of scalp, 50-year-old male). Stage II premelanosome consisting of a striated inclusion within a vesicle. (×168,000.)

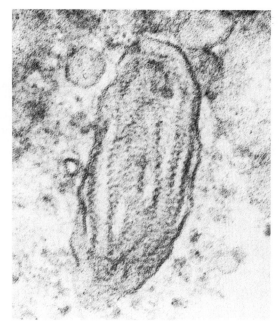

FIGURE 3-96
Balloon cell malignant melanoma (anterior chest wall, 65-year-old male). Stage II premelanosome containing a pleated-coil inclusion. (×120,000.)

plasms. The endothelial cells are not neoplastic in hemangiopericytoma.

Melanin

Perhaps the most significant pigment to the diagnostic electron microscopist is cutaneous (neural crest) melanin, as ultrastructural evidence of the synthesis of this inclusion in poorly differentiated neoplastic cells conclusively establishes the diagnosis of malignant melanoma. Melanocytes, dendritic melanin-producing cells, are derived from the neural crest.[638] They occur primarily as isolated cells in the basal epidermis, although they are also present in the mucous membranes, the pigmented epithelium of the retina and uveal tract, and the pia arachnoid.

Black-brown eumelanin, the major type of melanin in humans, consists of polymerized indole-5,6-quinone. This compound is synthesized from dopaquinone intermediates, with tyrosinase as the major catalytic enzyme.[276,277,474] Melanin formation actually begins with the synthesis of tyrosinase on ribosomes. The tyrosinase is then transported to small vesicles via the RER and Golgi apparatus (Jimbow, refs. 276, 277). Four morphologic stages of melanosome development are recognized.[52,187] The nonspecific small vesicles described above, also called stage I premelano-

somes, subsequently enlarge and elongate into stage II premelanosomes recognized by their characteristic striated (Fig. 3-95) or pleated-coil inclusions (Fig. 3-96). (Stage II and III premelanosomes and stage IV melanosomes are illustrated using neoplastic melanocytes.) Stage III premelanosomes show deposits of melanin pigment (Fig. 3-97), and the uniformly electron-dense fully melaninized structures are called the mature or stage IV melanosomes (Fig. 3-98).

Two classes of tumors composed of neoplastic melanocytes, i.e., the benign melanocytic nevi and the malignant melanomas, are described below. (Melanin is also found in other tumors of neuroectodermal origin; see p. 77.) Electron microscopy is often essential to diagnosing amelanotic malignant melanomas because histochemical stains for melanin (Masson-Fontana's silver nitrate or the DOPA reaction) can give false-positive or negative-results, and the tyrosinase reactions are nonspecific.[243,377]

A second form of melanin, so-called neuromelanin, found in neurons of the substantia nigra, locus ceruleus of the midbrain, various ganglia, and certain pigmented tumors (e.g., pigmented neuroblastoma) is not discussed here. Neuromelanin is a waste product of catecholamine metabolism (a lipofuscin-type secondary lysosome) not asso-

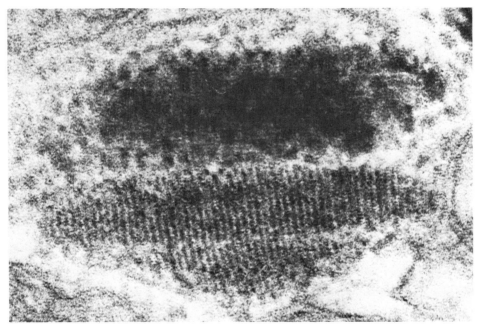

FIGURE 3-97
Malignant melanoma (buccal mucosa, 67-year-old male). Advanced stage III premelanosome (*top*) with abundant deposits of melanin pigment overlying a striated stage II premelanosome. (×216,000.)

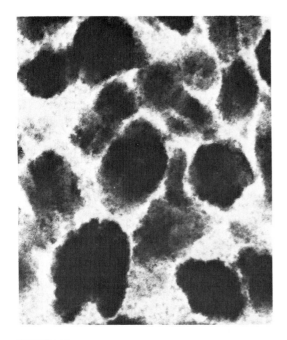

FIGURE 3-98
Blue nevus (skin, lower leg, 55-year-old male). Fully melanized mature stage IV melanosomes in cytoplasm of nevus cell. (×80,000.)

ciated with premelanosomes (see Mullins, ref. 431).

Melanocytic nevi

Melanocytic nevi are congenital or acquired benign neoplasms consisting of pigmented or nonpigmented melanocytes (nevus cells) and, in some entities, of neural elements.[48,133,419] Dermal melanocytes are seen in skin biopsies, and nevus cells are probably transformed melanocytes.[48] Melanocytic nevi may begin as intraepidermal junctional nevi. The cells then migrate into the dermis, forming a compound nevus when found in both the epidermis and dermis, and eventually forming an intradermal nevus when they are no longer present in the basal epidermis.

Nevus cells are uniformly round or occasionally spindle-shaped and are usually arranged in nests within the basal epidermis or dermis, or both. Nevus cells are characterized by the following ultrastructural features:

1. Spherical or indented nuclei containing finely dispersed chromatin (euchromatin) and a medium-size nucleolus.

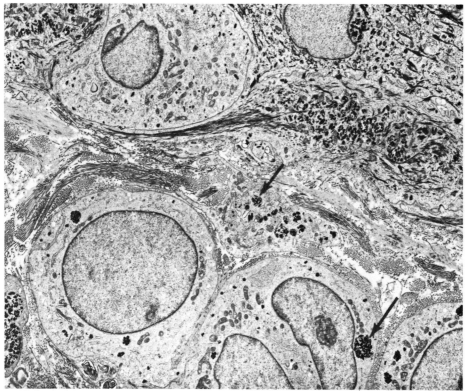

FIGURE 3-99
Compound nevus with prominent junctional component (lower abdomen, 27-year-old female). Nevus cells in upper dermis (one is also in basal epidermis). The nevus cells are round, and the nuclei contain finely dispersed chromatin. Melanosomes occur both singly and in clusters (*arrows*). The keratinocytes are joined by numerous desmosomes and contain prominent curvilinear bundles of cytokeratin filaments. (×4560.)

2. Variable numbers of both polymorphic and normal melanosomes in different stages of development occurring singly or in clusters, with some cells (and nevi) containing no premelanosomes or melanosomes.

3. Inconspicuous organelles, except for occasional clusters of mitochondria and abundant ribosomes.

4. Prominent bundles of intermediate-size cytoplasmic filaments (see p. 85) in approximately one-quarter of the neoplasms.

5. Scattered foci of microvilli and rare primitive cell junctions.

6. Occasional cells partially invested by external lamina (Figs. 3-99 to 3-101).[51,133,418,419,436]

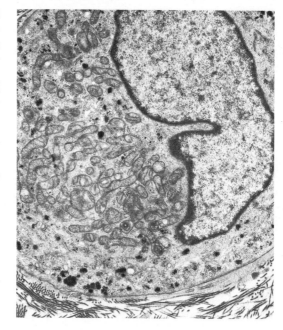

FIGURE 3-100
Pigmented compound nevus (back, 27-year-old female). Portion of nevus cell located in mid dermis. Note the abundant mitochrondria and the pigmented melanosomes. (×7800.)

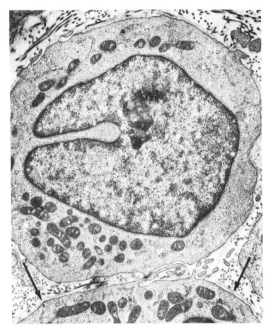

FIGURE 3-101
Compound nevus (lower abdomen, 35-year-old female). Two unpigmented dermal nevus cells joined by a primitive cell junction. The lower cell is partially invested by external lamina (*arrows*). (×7000.)

Giant spherical melanosomes are a consistent feature of pigmented nevus cells comprising nevus spilus and of the epidermal melanocytes found in the *cafe-au-lait* spots of neurofibromatosis.[278,317] These macromelanosomes, which can measure up to 5 μm or more in diameter, are the result of deranged melanosome synthesis.

Blue nevi consist of spindle-shaped cells having long cytoplasmic processes separated by dense bundles of collagen fibrils (Fig. 3-102). The histogenesis of these intradermal nevi, including the cellular and rare malignant variants, is controversial, because neuroid configurations are often identified.[248,406] Bhawan et al.[51] favor origin from an undifferentiated cell of neural crest origin capable of both melanocytic and neural differentiation.

I have recently examined two cases of this entity. Large numbers of mature stage IV melanosomes intermixed with isolated premelanosomes are evident in the cytoplasm of the melanocytic cells (Fig. 3-102). Melanophages, dermal histiocytes that have ingested melanin, are also found in pigmented nevi. It is important to distinguish cells that phagocytize melanin (e.g., melanophages, keratinocytes, and Schwann cells) from melanin-producing cells (melanocytes). The former cells usu-

ally contain clusters of melanosomes within phagosomes (a type of secondary lysosome) (Fig. 3-103), also called compound bodies, whereas the latter cells contain isolated melanosomes in all stages of development (Figs. 3-105 and 3-106).

Malignant melanoma

Most malignant melanomas arise from melanocytes in the basal epidermis of the skin. The cells comprising these tumors are generally quite pleomorphic and often contain more premelanosomes than mature melanosomes. Amelanotic melanomas frequently bear only widely scattered premelanosomes.[49] Ultrastructural demonstration of normal-appearing or recognizable aberrant premelanosomes (Figs. 3-95 to 97, 104 to 106) is often crucial to confirm a diagnosis of amelanotic melanoma.

I have noted three recognizable varieties of premelanosomes in both pigmented and amelanotic melanomas. The most prevalent subtype is the lamellar premelanosome measuring 95–107 × 240–520 nm. These distinctive ellipsoidal, membrane-enclosed structures are easily recognized by their striated core consisting of parallel perpendicularly arranged filaments (Figs. 3-95 and 3-97). In the pigmented melanomas, varying amounts of melanin are deposited on this internal structure (Fig. 3-97). Another much less common aberrant subtype is the helical or spiral premelanosome, consisting of zig-zag coiled filaments (Figs. 3-96, 3-104, and 3-105). Helical premelanosomes are either ellipsoidal or spherical, are often not enclosed in a unit membrane, and are about the same size as lamellar premelanosomes. The last subtype is the granular premelanosome, which is a small, spherical membranous sac containing varying numbers of electron-dense amorphous microgranules (Figs. 3-106 and 3-107) that resemble the vesiculoglobular bodies described by Jimbow and co-workers.[276] The premelanosomes and microgranules are found in both amelanotic and pigmented melanomas. The first two types are variants of stage II and III premelanosomes, whereas the granular premelanosomes resemble stage I premelanosomes with melanin deposits.

A diagnosis of amelanotic malignant melanoma requires ultramicroscopic identification of either the lamellar or spiral premelanosome (Chapter 6, case 3). The presence of only lysosomelike structures having a disorganized internal structure of variable density is not diagnostic. Unfortunately, premelanosomes are frequently sparse and often require a time-consuming search at magnifications

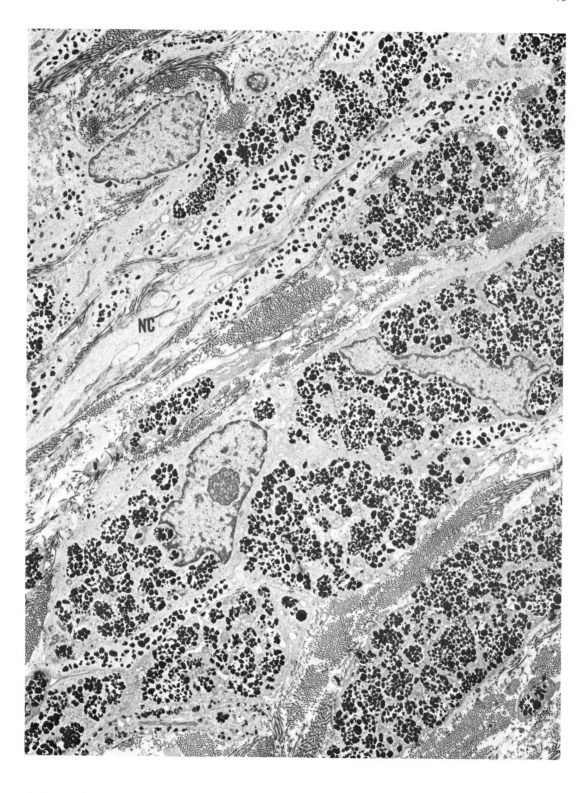

FIGURE 3-102
Blue nevus (cf. Fig. 3-98). Heavily pigmented spindle-shaped cells separated by dense bundles of collagen fibrils. It is difficult to distinguish nevus cells from melanophages in this micrograph. Neuroid configuration (NC). (×6080.)

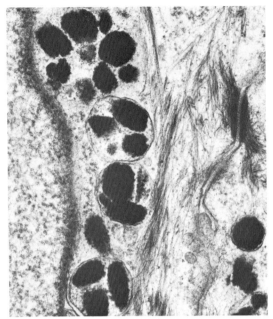

FIGURE 3-103
Pigmented junctional nevus (abdomen, 61-year-old male).
Keratinocytes containing clusters of melanosomes within
membranous sacs (secondary lysosomes) and individual melanosomes in the cytosol. Note the cytokeratin filaments and
the desmosome. (×40,000.)

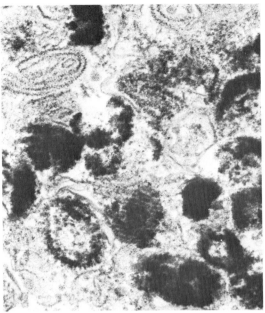

FIGURE 3-105
Superficial spreading malignant melanoma (anterior thigh,
70-year-old female). Portion of cytoplasm of neoplastic mela-
nocyte showing ellipsoidal helical premelanosomes consisting
of zig-zag coiled filaments and aberrant partially and fully
melaninized melanosomes. (×62,000.)

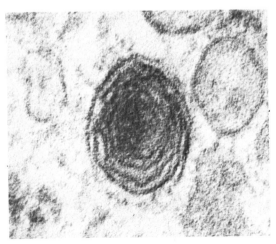

FIGURE 3-104
Amelanotic malignant melanoma (distal urethra, 59-year-old
male; see Chapter 6, case 3). Helical premelanosome. Note the
periodicity of the coiled fibril. (×172,000.)

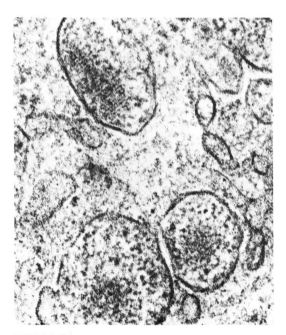

FIGURE 3-106
Malignant melanoma (lower leg, 56-year-old female). An ellipsoidal lamellar or striated premelanosome (*top*) and four
granular premelanosomes are shown. The vesicles contain
varying numbers of microgranules. (×100,000.)

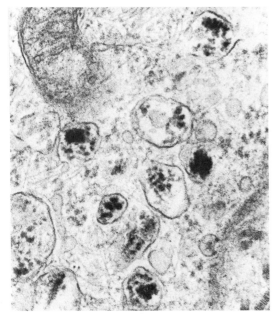

FIGURE 3-107
Cellular blue nevus (upper arm, 32-year-old female). Aberrant granular premelanosomes. The vesicles contain electron-dense pleomorphic melanin granules. (×54,000.)

TABLE 3-3

Intracytoplasmic Fibers—Cytoskeleton

Class	Average Diameter (nm)
1. Microtubules	25
2. Muscle myosin	15
3. Intermediate filaments	10
Cytokeratins (tonofilaments)	
Desmin (muscle cells)	
Glial filaments	
Neurofilaments	
Vimentin (mesenchymal cells)	
4. Microfilaments	6
Actin	
Nonmuscle myosin	
5. Microtrabecular system	3–6
Intracellular scaffolding (high-voltage EM)	

INTRACYTOPLASMIC FIBERS

Probably the most complex and also misunderstood structures in both normal and neoplastic cells are the so-called intracytoplasmic fibers. The protein composition of these fibers is currently the subject of intense investigation by cell biologists. The morphologist, however, has to contend with recognizable sizes and patterns of distribution in the cytoplasm. On the basis of measurements of their average diameter, five major classes of intracytoplasmic fibers have been identified (Table 3-3).

This section describes the major classes of intracytoplasmic fibers, including the heterogeneous protein subtypes. Proper identification of the correct classes of fibers is essential for the differential diagnosis of human neoplasms. As most microfilaments are composed of the contractile protein actin, they are included in the section on myofilaments (see below). Skeletal and smooth muscle tumors, intermediate filaments, and hybrid contractile cells are also discussed.

Microtubules

Microtubules are found in at least some stage of the life cycle of all eukaryotic cells and are easily recognized in well-fixed tissues (Figs. 3-108 and 3-109). They are dynamic tubular structures composed of 13 longitudinally oriented protofilaments composed of globular proteins called alpha- and beta-tubulins. High-molecular-weight microtubule-associated proteins (MAPs) project from their surface.[147,148,495,551,645] Microtubules are essential for cell division (centrioles and spindle

ranging up to 60,000×. I have examined specimens from metastatic amelanotic malignant melanomas derived from pigmented primary tumors that are so poorly differentiated that they only produce essentially empty precursor vesicles derived from the condensing vacuoles of the Golgi apparatus.[68] The three types of premelanosomes or variants thereof (the terminology varies) have also been reported to be present in dysfunctional and neoplastic melanocytes both *in vivo* and in cell cultures.[116,117,133,189,268,315,398,417,418,486,601]

Neoplasms containing the cutaneous (neural crest) type of melanin pigment ultrastructurally associated with the presence of premelanosomes have been described in various sites in the central and peripheral nervous system, e.g., melanotic medulloblastoma,[64] meningeal melanocytoma,[359] and melanotic nerve sheath tumors,[387,405] as well as in other tumors derived from the neural crest division of the neuroectoderm, e.g., malignant melanotic neuroectodermal tumor of infancy[139,442] and spinal melanotic clear cell sarcoma.[456]

To my knowledge, no cytoplasmic inclusions acceptable as a premelanosome have been illustrated in the spindle cells of desmoplastic malignant melanoma.[120] The cells are either dedifferentiated melanocytes with fibroblastic features[613] or fibroblasts—a scirrhous reaction to the melanoma.[332]

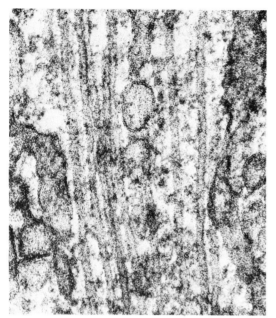

FIGURE 3-108
Microtubules (HeLa cell in telophase, tissue culture). The mitotic spindle consists of microtubules with an average diameter of 25 nm. Longitudinally sectioned. (×30,000.)

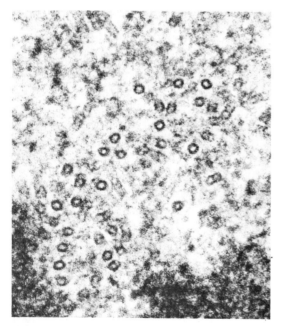

FIGURE 3-109
Microtubules (HeLa cell in metaphase, tissue culture). Cross-sectioned microtubules comprising the spindle. Portions of chromosomes are seen in the *lower portion* of the micrograph. (×35,000.)

apparatus), constitute the axoneme of cilia, are involved in maintaining cell shape, and participate in the movements of organelles and inclusions. Microtubules are particularly prominent in axons, neoplastic Schwann cell processes (e.g., benign solitary schwannomas[163]), and in neuroblast cell processes.[651]

Microtrabecular System

The microtrabecular system consists of an intracellular scaffolding or meshwork of 3–6-nm filaments visualized using high-voltage (1-million-volt) electron microscopes.[646] The filaments comprising this system are ubiquitous and are currently of no diagnostic significance.

Microfilaments—Myofilaments

The contractile protein, actin, is found in both muscle (Fig. 3-110) and nonmuscle cells[340,470] (Fig. 4-20). It has been shown to be the major component of the 6–7-nm microfilaments by means of heavy meromyosin (head fragments of the myosin molecule) binding, which results in the formation of characteristic arrowhead complexes, and by indirect immunofluorescence staining with antiactin antibodies.[340,342]

Although most investigators assume that the majority of 6–7-nm microfilaments in neoplastic cells are composed of actin, myosins with an average diameter of approximately 6 nm have recently been isolated from nonmuscle cells.[3,247,342,470] Therefore, this type of myosin cannot be identified by routine electron microscopy. Localization is achieved using antimyosin antibodies (indirect immunofluorescence). On the basis of the above findings, it should be assumed that both nonmuscle myosin and actin comprise the ectoplasmic microfilament bundles observed in many different types of neoplastic cells.

The last major subtype of myofilament is the 15-nm muscle myosin filament located in the A band of sarcomeres (Fig. 3-110), the cytoplasmic contractile units of skeletal muscle. Similar myosin fibrils are also found in smooth muscle cells.

When compared with their normal counterparts, neoplastic cells generally contain an increased amount of contractile proteins (myofilaments) organized into a microfilamentous apparatus consisting of actin, actinin, myosins, and so forth (demonstrated by immunofluorescent antibody techniques).[199,373]

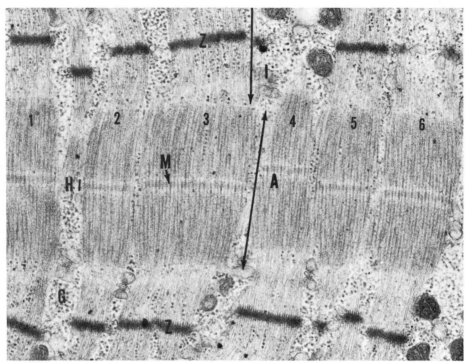

FIGURE 3-110
Normal skeletal muscle (pectoralis major muscle from radical mastectomy specimen). Portion of sarcoplasm showing longitudinal sections of six sarcomeres delineated by Z discs (Z). A band (A), H band (H), M band (M), and incomplete I band (I). Glycogen (G). (×28,000.)

Rhabdomyosarcoma

In skeletal (striated) muscle cells, myofibrils are the smallest contractile units visible under the light microscope. Electron microscopic examination demonstrates that they consist of alternating 7-nm actin myofilaments and 15-nm filaments in parallel arrays arranged in repeating banded contractile units called sarcomeres (Fig. 3-110) delineated by chemically complex Z discs, consisting primarily of alpha-actinin intimately surrounded by the intermediate filament proteins desmin, synemin, and vimentin (see p. 86). Actin filaments extend from the Z discs, constitute the I band, and extend into the adjacent A band, which is composed principally of muscle myosin fibrils. The interaction of actin and muscle myosin filaments during contraction is regulated by the proteins tropomyosin and troponin, whereas desmin and vimentin may be involved in maintaining the lateral registration of myofibrils, thereby producing the characteristic banding pattern of striated muscle.[225,342]

When remnants of sarcomeres or Z disc fragments scattered among parallel alternating 7- and 15-nm filaments are identified in the cytoplasm of poorly differentiated neoplastic cells a diagnosis of rhabdomyosarcoma should be considered[319,377,424,484] (Figs. 3-111 to 3-115); this is the minimum requirement for the electron microscopic diagnosis of rhabdomyosarcoma.

A problem for the electron microscopist is rhabdomyosarcoma of infancy and childhood—alveolar, embryonal, and botryoid rhabdomyosarcoma—as the demonstration of cross-striations by light microscopy is not an absolute requirement for diagnosis.[221] For example, the overall pattern of alveolar rhabdomyosarcoma is epithelial-like, and cells containing recognizable arrays of actin and myosin myofilaments may not be ultrastructurally identified in so-called obvious cases diagnosed by light microscopy. Alveolar rhabdomyosarcoma is most likely a primitive sarcoma consisting of mesenchymal cells found at the stage of somite formation in the embryo.[114] A gradation of maturation from multipotential mesenchymal cells to those with unequivocal features of skeletal muscle is usually evident.[412] When asked to confirm a tentative histologic diagnosis of embryonal or alveolar rhabdomyosarcoma, the electron microscopist should attempt to demonstrate recognizable arrays of actin and myosin (Figs. 3-111 to

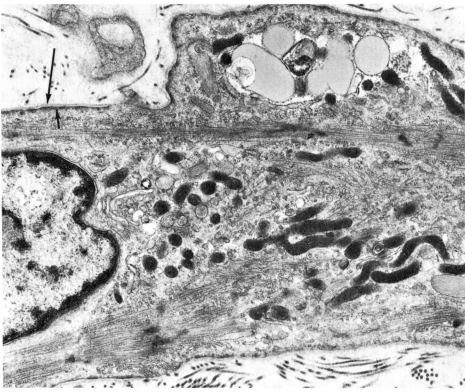

FIGURE 3-111
Metastatic embryonal rhabdomyosarcoma (axilla, 16-year-old male). Portion of a fairly well-differentiated rhabdomyoblast. Note the sarcomere remnants, dense attachment plaques (*short arrow*), and external lamina (*long arrow*). (×14,400.)

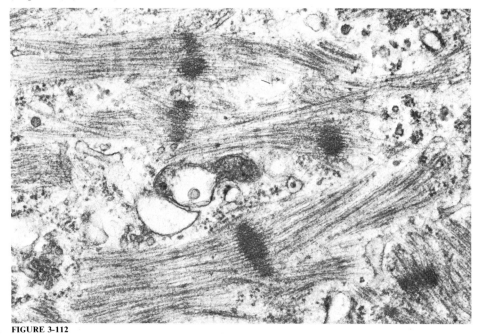

FIGURE 3-112
Heterologous mixed müllerian tumor (uterus, 54-year-old female). The most abundant component was adult-type pleomorphic rhabdomyosarcoma. Portion of rhabdomyoblast cytoplasm showing disorganized remnants of sarcomeres. Note the prominent Z discs. (×38,400.)

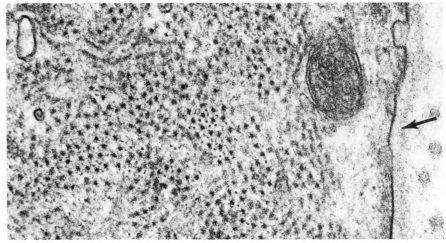

FIGURE 3-113
Metastatic embryonal rhabdomyosarcoma (cf. Fig. 3-111). Cross-sectioned disarrayed sarcomeres. Note the thin actin filaments surrounding the thicker myosin fibrils. External lamina (*arrow*). (×82,000.)

3-113). In cross section, each myosin fibril is surrounded by variable numbers of actin filaments (Fig. 3-113). Evidence of remnants of Z discs (Fig. 3-115) or ribosomes, in single-file arrangement (Fig. 3-114) makes the diagnosis more secure. Use caution, however, as disorganized sarcomeres are frequently found in regenerating skeletal muscle cells (Fig. 3-116).

In summary, fine structural demonstration of recognizable arrays of actin and myosin myofilaments or primitive disorganized sarcomerelike structures is pivotal for a diagnosis of childhood

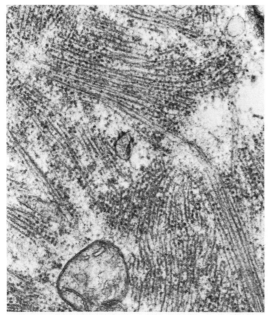

FIGURE 3-114
Botryoid embryonal rhabdomyosarcoma (vagina, 15-month-old female). Disorganized parallel bundles of 14-nm myosin fibrils associated with rows of ribosomes. This is the minimum requirement for the ultrastructural diagnosis of embryonal rhabdomyosarcoma. (×36,000.)

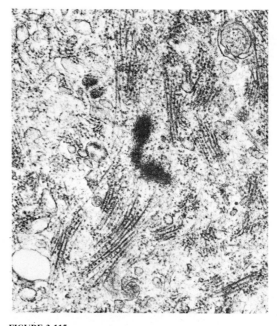

FIGURE 3-115
Pleomorphic rhabdomyosarcoma (scapula, 21-year-old female). Portion of a large, round rhabdomyoblast showing linear arrays of myosin–ribosome complexes and a central focus of Z disc substance. (×30,000.)

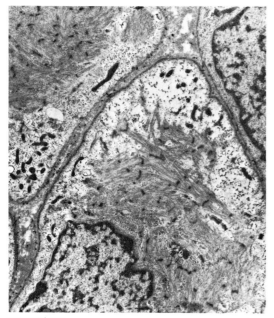

FIGURE 3-116
Pindborg tumor (mandible, 17-year-old male). The odontogenic tumor infiltrated the medial pterygoid muscle. Regenerating myocytes from site of incisional biopsy are illustrated. Note the disorganized sarcomeres in the sarcoplasm. (×6000.)

rhabdomyosarcoma, as small cell sarcomas of undetermined histogenesis may be erroneously called rhabdomyosarcoma[424] (Chapter 6, case 7). It is possible, however, that some of these tumors consist mainly of myoblast precursor cells (primitive mesenchymal cells) containing only abundant ribosomes, a prominent RER, and bundles of 6-nm actin microfilaments or 10-nm intermediate (Z disc-associated) filaments that may precede the formation of myosin fibrils and Z discs.

Neoplastic rhabdomyoblasts are occasionally found to be a component of other neoplasms excluding teratomas, i.e., mesodermal mixed tumor (heterologous mixed müllerian tumors) of the uterus[62,71] (Fig. 3-112), Wilms' tumor,[604] malignant nerve sheath tumors,[647] medulloepithelioma,[653] medulloblastoma,[556] and malignant cytosarcoma phyllodes (Fig. 3-117). A primary rhabdomyosarcoma arising in the cerebrum was also recently reported.[648]

Smooth muscle tumors

The smooth muscle cell (leiomyocyte) is characterized by the following ultrastructural features:

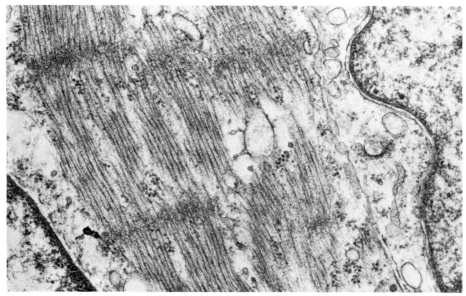

FIGURE 3-117
Malignant cystosarcoma phyllodes (breast, 16-year-old female). The tumor was growing mainly as a fibrosarcoma with foci of rhabdomyosarcoma. Portion of neoplastic rhabdomyoblast showing recognizable sarcomeres in the sarcoplasm. (×35,200.)

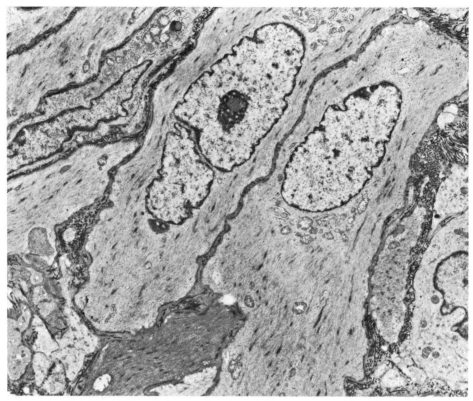

FIGURE 3-118
Normal smooth muscle (urinary bladder, 66-year-old male with superficially infiltrating epidermoid carcinoma). Smooth muscle cells in the muscular coat of the urinary bladder. Parallel arrays of intracytoplasmic 7-nm actin microfilaments (myofilaments) and scattered fusiform dense bodies dominate the cytoplasm of the leiomyocytes. (×5040.)

1. Parallel arrays of intracytoplasmic 6–7-nm actin microfilaments with interspersed fusiform dense bodies.
2. Plasmalemmal attachment plaques.
3. Surface pinocytotic vesicles.
4. Rare cell junctions.
5. An often discontinuous external lamina[399] (Figs. 3-118 to 3-120).

The above structures are expressed to varying degrees in neoplastic leiomyocytes[183,426] comprising leiomyomas (Fig. 3-119), leiomyosarcomas[249,443] (Fig. 3-120), leiomyoblastomas,[105,234,621] glomus tumors,[222,289] and uterine wall smooth muscle (also occasional stromal cell) tumors, e.g., plexiform tumors of the uterus.[447]

Not all the above-listed characteristics of leiomyocytes are evident in either leiomyoblastomas (low-grade epithelioid leiomyosarcoma)[124,234,514] or the more poorly differentiated leiomyosarcomas.[180] For example, along with Mackay and Osborne,[377] I have found that parallel arrays of actin myofilaments and associated fusiform structures are not always observed in leiomyosarcomas arising in the GI tract. A gradation from uncommitted mesenchymal cells to those with some leiomyocyte characteristics (Fig. 3-121), and finally to cells demonstrating unequivocal features of smooth muscle (Fig. 3-122), is found in most cases of leiomyosarcoma. Again, the irreducible minimum for ultrastructural diagnosis is the demonstration of bundles of myofilaments containing dense bodies.

Although both actin and muscle myosin have been demonstrated in vertebrate smooth muscle cells,[65,301] for some unknown reason the thicker 15-nm myosin fibrils are rarely preserved in the usual EM preparations. We recently found both types of myofilaments in smooth muscle cells located in the stroma of the prostate (Fig. 3-123) and in the neoplastic leiomyocytes comprising a rare leiomyosarcoma of bone[628] (note that sarcomeres

84

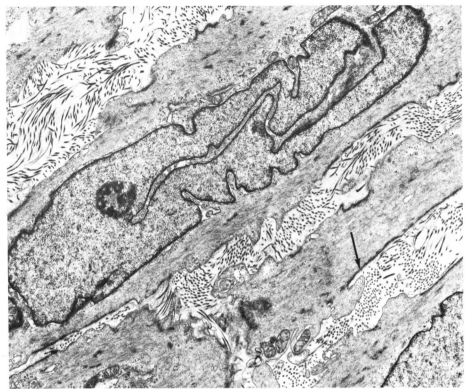

FIGURE 3-119
Leiomyoma (broad ligament, 46-year-old female). Plasmalemmal attachment plaques (*arrow*) and actin microfilaments with interspersed fusiform dense bodies are prominent in this specimen. Note that one of the benign neoplastic leiomyocytes has a markedly cleaved nucleus. Nuclear pleomorphism is not confined to malignant neoplastic cells. (×8400.)

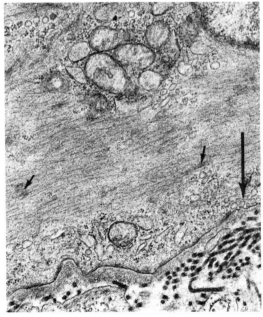

FIGURE 3-120
Leiomyosarcoma (right upper lobe lung, 36-year-old male). Portion of neoplastic leiomyocyte showing actin microfilaments, poorly developed fusiform dense bodies (*short arrows*), attachment plaques, pinocytotic vesicles (*long arrow*), and continuous external lamina. (×20,000.)

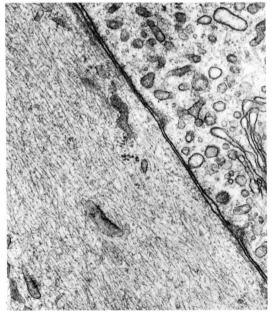

FIGURE 3-121
Leiomyosarcoma (colon, 75-year-old female). The actin microfilaments are more disorganized and lack fusiform densities. Although this is an obvious case of leiomyosarcoma by light microscopy, the EM findings are minimally diagnostic. (×28,800.)

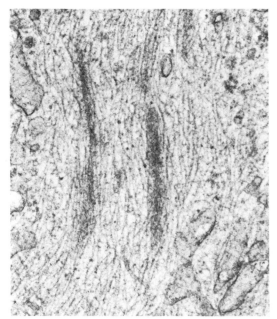

FIGURE 3-122
Leiomyosarcoma (duodenum, 52-year-old male). Portion of cytoplasm of neoplastic leiomyocyte illustrating 7-nm actin microfilaments and two fusiform dense bodies. (×60,000.)

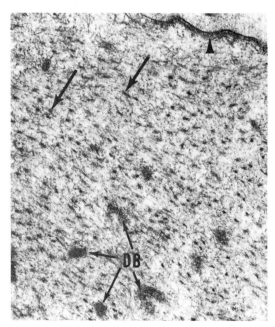

FIGURE 3-123
Normal prostate gland (55-year-old male). Portion of cytoplasm of smooth muscle cells. Tangential section showing actin microfilaments, 15-nm myosin fibrils (*arrows*), fusiform dense bodies (DB), and surface attachment plaques (*arrowhead*). (×40,000.)

are not found in smooth muscle tumors). To further complicate matters, 10-nm intermediate-size filaments (see below) are also found in leiomyocytes. Hubbard and Lazarides[264] showed that the chicken gizzard smooth muscle protein desmin or skeletin, the major protein subunit of intermediate filaments in smooth muscle cells, may form nonstoichiometric complexes with actin. Many human anti-smooth muscle antisera display activity not only toward actin-containing microfilaments, but toward intermediate filaments as well.[330]

Intermediate Filaments

The most diversified class of intracytoplasmic fibers found in both normal and neoplastic vertebrate cells is the heterogeneous group of morphologically similar intermediate filaments, with diameters of 8–12 nm (average diameter, 10 nm)[341] (Fig. 3-124). These chemically and immunologically dissimilar proteinaceous filaments are designated neurofilaments in neurons, glial filaments (Fig. 3-125) in astrocytes, and tonofilaments in keratinocytes[43,138,264] (Fig. 3-126) and thymic epithelial cells[37,498] (Fig. 3-127). Cell biologists have determined the protein subunits of many of these filaments by means of polyacrylamide gel electrophoresis and indirect immunofluorescence

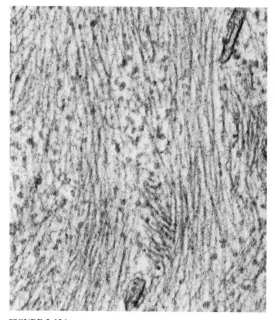

FIGURE 3-124
Meningothelial meningioma (dura, left frontal lobe, 62-year-old female). Portion of cytoplasm of neoplastic meningothelial cell. Note the disorganized bundles of intermediate filaments. The filaments range in diameter from 8.5 to 10 nm. (×74,000.)

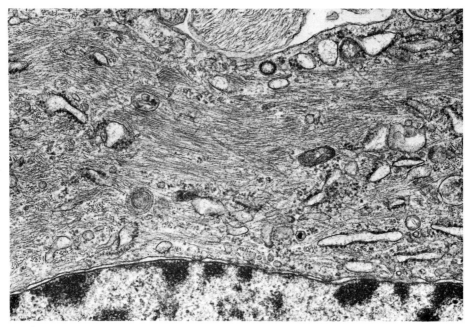

FIGURE 3-125
Malignant (grade 3) astrocytoma (cerebellum, 17-year-old female). Intermediate filaments composed of glial fibrillary acidic protein in the cytoplasm of the neoplastic astrocyte. (×27,000.)

microscopy (see Franke et al., ref. 191). For example, tonofilaments contain prekeratinlike proteins or cytokeratins; smooth muscle cell intermediate filaments contain a major protein called skeletin or desmin, whereas skeletal muscle cells contain desmin, vimentin, and synemin[226]; those found in most nonmuscle mesenchymal cells contain a protein termed vimentin; and glial filaments are composed largely of glial fibrillary acidic protein.[154,218,620] Rosenthal fibers most likely consist of tightly packed aggregates of these filaments.[250] The chemically distinct neurofilament proteins are still unnamed. Undoubtedly, many more distinct subtypes will be characterized.

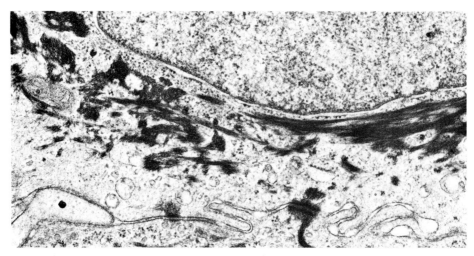

FIGURE 3-126
Arsenic-induced basal cell carcinoma (skin of anterior thigh, 79-year-old male). Portions of two neoplastic keratinocytes joined by desmosomes. Note the dense bundles of cytoplasmic tonofilaments. (×24,500.)

Epidermoid (squamous cell) carcinoma

Epidermoid carcinomas arise from keratinocytes
(epidermis of the skin), squamous epithelial cells
(mucous membranes), and from pluripotential
progenitor cells in nonsquamous epithelia, e.g.,
epidermoid carcinoma of the lung and areas of
squamous metaplasia in neoplasms (Fig. 3-128).
Neoplastic keratinocytes or squamous epithelial
cells are characteristically joined by well-formed
desmosomes and usually contain prominent bundles of tono- or cytokeratin filaments (Figs. 3-126
and 4-30). The latter term is more accurate, as the
filaments consist of prekeratinlike protein subunits.
In the more differentiated tumors, the cytokeratin
filaments are usually found in the perinuclear
cytoplasm and are a component of desmosomes
(Figs. 4-28 to 4-31). Anaplastic squamous cell
carcinomas contain few if any bundles of cytokeratins and are joined by rare primitive cell
junctions (see p. 111).

Cytokeratin filaments are easy to recognize, as
they are characteristically organized into electron-dense short curvilinear bundles of tightly
packed 10-nm filaments (Figs. 3-126 to 3-128).
When they are not in this configuration, they
should not be called cytokeratin filaments unless

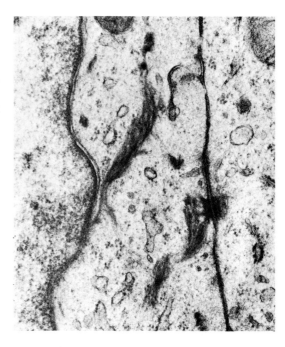

FIGURE 3-127
Thymoma (anterior mediastinum, 55-year-old male). Portions
of two neoplastic thymic epithelial cells joined by a desmosome.
Bundles of tonofilaments, one associated with the desmosome,
are evident in the cytoplasm. (×30,000.)

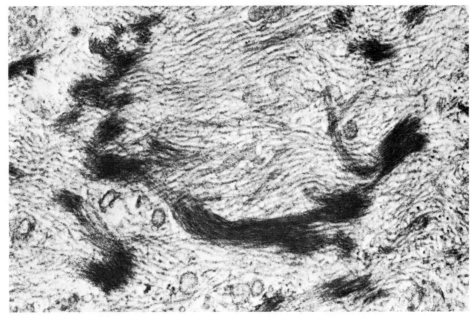

FIGURE 3-128
Malignant myoepithelioma of the breast (breast, 60-year-old female). Densely packed and loosely arranged
10-nm cytokeratin filaments (tonofilaments) in the cytoplasm of the neoplastic infiltrating myoepithelial cell.
This is an extremely rare spindle cell malignant tumor of the breast. (×42,000.)

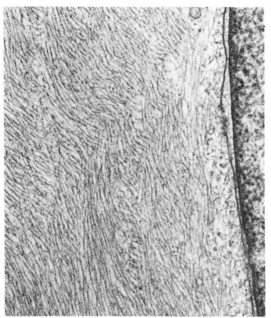

FIGURE 3-129
Chondrosarcoma (antrum, 14-year-old female). The cytoplasmic organelles in many of the neoplastic cells are displaced by dense bundles of 10-nm intermediate filaments. (×52,000.)

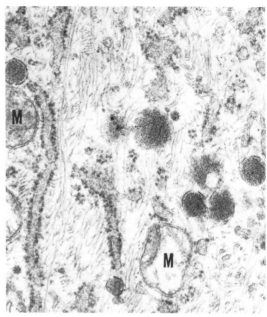

FIGURE 3-131
Hemangioendothelioma (femur, 45-year-old male). Loosely organized intermediate filaments, RER cisternae, mitochondria (M), and electron-dense lysosomes are illustrated. (×39,200.)

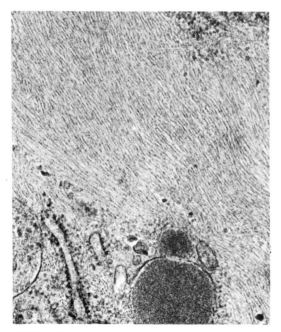

FIGURE 3-130
Angiosarcoma (ilium, 33-year-old male). Portion of cytoplasm of neoplastic endothelial cell largely occupied by masses of intermediate filaments most likely composed of the polypeptide vimentin. The membrane-limited dense bodies (*bottom*) probably are lysosomes. (×38,400.)

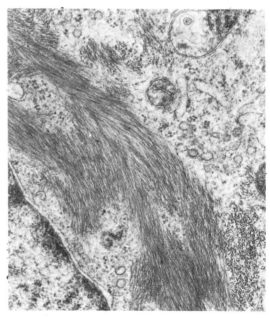

FIGURE 3-132
Infiltrating duct carcinoma (breast, 60-year-old female). Perinuclear bundles of 8-nm intracytoplasmic fibrils in the cytoplasm of a neoplastic ductular epithelial cell. Are these fibrils cytokeratin filaments (morphology) or microfilaments (size)? (×27,000.)

special studies are performed, e.g., indirect immunofluorescence using antiprekeratin antibodies.[37,191] It is noteworthy that most of the intermediate-size filaments found in human neoplastic cells have been erroneously labeled tonofilaments, microfilaments (I used to call nonspecific intermediate filaments microfilaments), or even myofilaments in the literature.

In mesenchymal tumors

The 10-nm intermediate filaments found in neoplastic mesenchymal tumors, e.g., chondrosarcomas (Fig. 3-129), malignant fibrous histiocytomas, and vascular tumors, e.g., angiosarcoma (Fig. 3-130) and hemangioendothelial sarcoma of bone (hemangioendothelioma) (Fig. 3-131), consist of large aggregates of filaments that do not resemble cytokeratins and frequently occupy most of the cytoplasm resulting in a hyalinelike appearance.[629] Using specific antibodies against various subtypes of intermediate filaments, Franke et al.[192] showed that intermediate-size filaments found in human endothelial cells are composed of the polypeptide vimentin, which is the predominant subunit of these filaments in cells of mesenchymal origin (excluding myocytes).

Because of their chemical diversity, widespread occurrence in different cell types, and the complex interactions between microfilaments and intermediate filaments, the electron microscopist should not attempt to subclassify the major classes of intracellular fibers unless well-known configurations are recognizable, e.g., in sarcomeres and cytokeratin filaments (tonofilaments). This is especially true if the sophisticated techniques of chemical analysis or indirect immunofluorescence are unavailable, which is usually the case. The nonspecific term "intracytoplasmic fibrils" should be used when the nature of the fibrils cannot be accurately determined (Fig. 3-132). Contrary to popular belief, it is not always easy to measure the diameter of the fibrils.

Hybrid Contractile Cells

Two interesting transitional or hybrid contractile cells, the myfibroblast and the myoepithelial cell, merit discussion because of their controversial role in tumor formation and behavior.

Myofibroblast

The myofibroblast, first described in contractile granulation tissue,[202,384] is a mesenchymal cell that shares fine structural features of both fibroblasts and smooth muscle cells, i.e., an elongated cell with bipolar cytoplasmic processes containing abundant

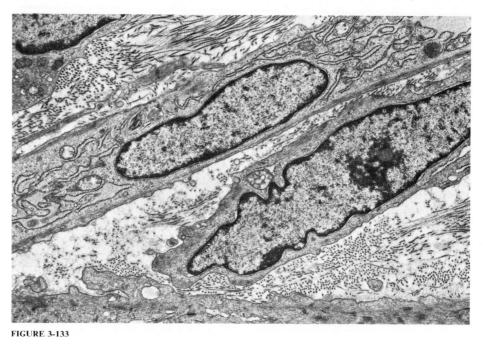

FIGURE 3-133
Myofibroblasts (cf. Fig. 3-128). Non-neoplastic myofibroblasts in stroma of malignant breast tumor of myoepithelial cell origin. Note the prominent branching RER and the peripherally located bundles of actin microfilaments with interspersed fusiform dense bodies. (×9200.)

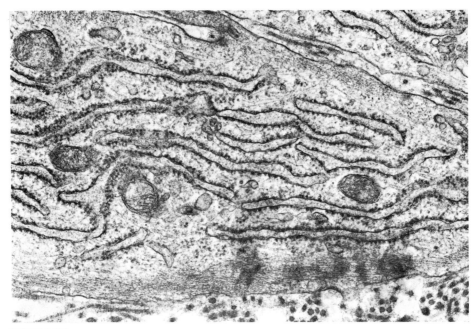

FIGURE 3-134
Portion of myofibroblast from same case (Fig. 3-133). Detail of cytoplasmic process showing well developed RER and subplasmalemmal actin microfilaments. The cell process is surrounded by stromal collagen fibrils. (×33,600.)

RER and a prominent Golgi apparatus (fibroblast), peripherally located bundles of actin myofilaments with fusiform densities arranged parallel to the long axis of the cell (Figs. 3-133 and 3-134) indented nuclei, and surface differentiations including rare scattered primitive cell junctions and irregular foci of basal lamina (leiomyocyte).[202,508] They represent a structural modulation of the fibroblast toward a contractile (smooth muscle) cell in response to a variety of stimuli.

Non-neoplastic myofibroblasts have been found in a variety of pathologic states, e.g., granulation tissue,[202,508] in the matrix of certain tumors, e.g., scirrhous carcinoma of the breast,[603] and in the stroma of invasive and metastatic carcinomas from diverse sites,[527] where they are probably responsible for overall tissue retraction.

Tumorlike lesions and benign fibroblastic neoplasms reported to be of myofibroblast origin include fibromatoses[201] nodular fasciitis,[643] and infantile digital fibroma.[50]

Neoplastic (?) myofibroblasts are more commonly found to be admixed with other mesenchymal cell types, e.g., primitive mesenchymal cells, fibroblasts, and histiocytes, in both benign and malignant neoplasms. Examples include desmoid tumors (low-grade fibrosarcoma),[217,564] desmoplastic fibroma of bone,[335] congenital mesoblastic nephroma,[535] malignant fibrous and fibrohistiocytic tumors,[113] cutaneous pseudosarcoma,[386] leiomyomatosis peritonealis disseminata,[466] parosteal osteogenic sarcoma,[485,625] and cardiac myxoma.[175] A low-grade spindle cell sarcoma of myofibroblasts has also been described.[619] (See Bhawan et al.[50] for additional references and discussion.) It is possible that the presence of numerous myofibroblasts in a particular neoplasm indicates a low level of malignancy and a better prognosis.

In my experience, myofibroblasts (both neoplastic or non-neoplastic) are rarely found in most of the above-mentioned tumors, and I have never seen a neoplasm composed solely of myofibroblasts or any cell junctions associated with these cells. According to Ghadially,[208] such tumors would be called myofibromas or myofibrosarcomas. Nevertheless, it is important that the electron microscopist recognize whether the myofibroblasts present in a particular tumor are reactive or neoplastic—no easy task in the case of mesenchymal tumors consisting of neoplastic spindle-shaped cells that resemble fibroblasts, e.g., parosteal osteogenic sarcoma.

Myoepithelial cell

Myoepithelial cells are stellate or spindle-shaped cells of ectodermal origin located at the periphery

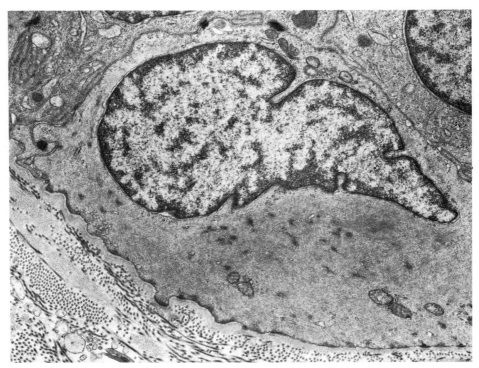

FIGURE 3-135
Florid sclerosing adenosis (breast, 42-year-old female). Hyperplastic myoepithelial cell joined to the overlying ductular epithelial cells by three desmosomes. Note the abundant cytoplasmic microfilaments, fusiform dense bodies, attachment plaques, pinocytotic vesicles (use hand lens), and well defined basal lamina. (×11,400.)

of secretory acini or smaller duct cells of salivary glands, mammary glands, sweat glands, lacrimal gland, and several other glands. They are not found, however, in the pancreas.[236] Ultrastructural characteristics of myoepithelial cells include (1) parallel bundles of 6-nm microfilaments with interspersed fusiform bodies that may terminate in hemidesmosomes or plaques on the basal cell membrane, (2) desmosomal junctions between each other and the overlying acinar or ductular cells, (3) basally located pinocytotic vesicles, and (4) a basal lamina separating the myoepithelial cells from the underlying stroma (Figs. 3-135 and 3-136).[236,574]

Myoepithelial cells participate in the formation of tumors in myoepithelium-containing organs. It is important to differentiate among compressed normal, hyperplastic, and neoplastic myoepithelial cells. An often interrupted single layer of compressed normal myoepithelial cells usually separates the proliferating mass of neoplastic ductular epithelial cells from the surrounding stroma in cases of lobular carcinoma *in situ* (LCIS) of the breast[6,598] (Fig. 3-136) and in other neoplasms arising in myoepithelial cell-containing structures

(see below). Myoepithelial cell hyperplasia is a frequent feature of fibrocystic disease of the female breast (cystic hyperplastic mastopathy) (Fig. 3-135) and intraductal papillomas.[6] According to Jao et al.,[275] focal multilayering of neoplastic (?) myoepithelial cells is a characteristic feature of fibroadenoma and adenosis of the mammary gland. Neoplastic, or more likely compressed normal or hyperplastic myoepithelial, cells quite possibly are also a component of some adenoid cystic carcinomas[236,263,265,517] adenomyoepitheliomas,[236] and apocrine cystadenomas.[241] In the above tumors, myoepithelial cells usually form an often interrupted single-layered cell sheath around neoplastic clusters of duct cells.

Several investigators have suggested that pluripotential neoplastic myoepithelial cells are responsible for the histologic complexity of mixed tumors (pleomorphic adenomas) of salivary gland origin.[145,236,265] Microscopically, these tumors consist of a diffuse proliferation of ductular epithelial cells, myoepithelial cells, and mesenchymal cells in a chondroid and myxoid–hyaline matrix or stroma. While reviewing more than 40 cases of mixed tumors of salivary gland origin, we noted

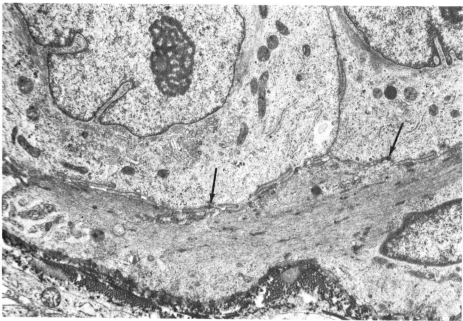

FIGURE 3-136
Lobular carcinoma in situ (breast, 43-year-old female). Two neoplastic ductular epithelial cells are separated from the collagenous stroma by a nonneoplastic myoepithelial cell. Note the small desmosomes (*arrows*) between the neoplastic cells and the myoepithelial cell and the perinuclear bundles of microfilaments in the neoplastic epithelial cells. (×8400.)

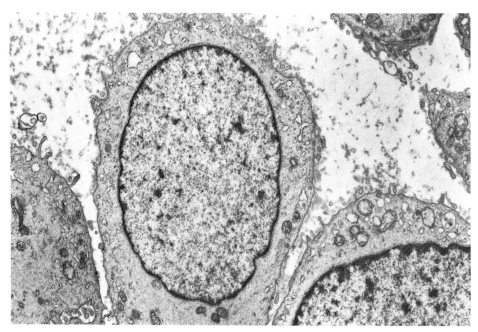

FIGURE 3-137
Benign pleomorphic adenoma (mixed tumor) (submandibular gland, 78-year-old female). Foci of transitional neoplastic myoepithelial cells in a myxoid stroma located between ducts and cartilagenous tissue. The cells contain numerous microfilaments in the organelle-free areas of the cytoplasm. (×7200.)

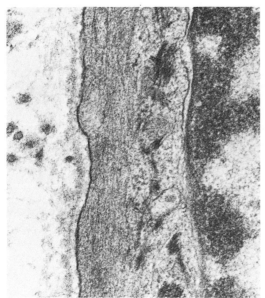

FIGURE 3-138
Benign pleomorphic adenoma (submandibular gland, 80-year-old female). Portion of neoplastic myoepithelial cell containing both short, dense perinuclear bundles of cytokeratin filaments (squamous metaplasia) and longitudinally oriented actin microfilaments in the ectoplasm. Note the basal lamina. (×52,000.)

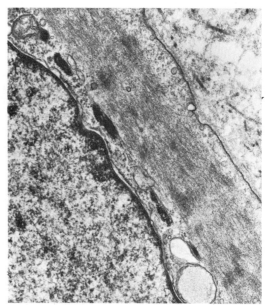

FIGURE 3-139
Malignant myoepithelioma of the breast (cf. Fig. 3-128). Features characteristic of myoepithelial cells (actin microfilaments, fusiform dense bodies, pinocytotic vesicles, and a basal lamina) are prominent. The presence of perinuclear bundles of cytokeratin filaments and the absence of a well-developed RER is helpful in distinguishing myoepithelial cells from myofibroblasts. (×21,000.)

that myoepithelial cells appear to transform into fibroblastic and chondrocytelike cells when separated from the ductal epithelial cells (Fig. 3-137). In our most convincing case, neoplastic myoepithelial cells, transitional cells, and chondrocytes all contained cytoplasmic glycogen, most prominently in the chondrocytes. A recent ultrastructural study of a chondroid syringoma, a mixed tumor of eccrine sweat gland origin, convincingly showed that the chondroid regions of the neoplasm consisted of modified myoepithelial cells rather than true chondrocytes.[618] The pseudocartilagenous areas contained cells similar to those found in the outer layers of the neoplastic ducts. Features that distinguished the metaplastic myoepithelial cells from true chondrocytes included a well-defined basal lamina, large numbers of intracytoplasmic fibrils, and no glycogen. This latter study lends further support to the contention that neoplastic mesenchymal cells are not a component of so-called mixed tumors.

A number of neoplasms termed myoepitheliomas were recently described as allegedly consisting entirely of a proliferation of neoplastic myoepithelial cells.[130,283,345,367,566,602] Essentially, these neoplasms consisted of loose masses of pleomorphic polygonal cells or spindle-shaped cells, or both, displaying most of the ultrastructural characteristics of myoepithelial cells, but lacking fusiform dense bodies. These bodies, however, were noted in the benign mammary myoepithelioma reported by Toth.[602] It must be emphasized that neoplastic cells frequently do not retain all the fine structural characteristics of the cell types from which they arise. A peculiarity of neoplastic myoepithelial cells is the loss of the fusiform dense bodies usually associated with their 6-nm actin micro(myo)filaments, the displacement of cytoplasmic organelles by large numbers of microfilaments (Fig. 3-137), or even the absence of these structures. Because many other neoplastic cells contain numerous nondescript intracytoplasmic fibrils as well, the myoepithelial origin of the mesenchymal elements in mixed tumor and so-called myoepitheliomas cannot be proved with certainty.

In addition to the 6-nm microfilaments minus the fusiform bodies, neoplastic myoepithelial cells in many benign mixed tumors of the parotid gland (Fig. 3-138) and also in a rare malignant myoepithelioma of the breast (Fig. 3-139) frequently contain short dense bundles of perinuclear cytokeratin filaments (tonofilaments). A myoepithelial cell with both cytokeratin filaments and longitudinally oriented microfilaments is illustrated in an apocrine cystoadenoma reported by Hassan and co-workers[241] (their Fig. 9). Franke et al.,[191] using electron and immunofluorescence microscopy, recently showed that all myoepithelial cells contain intermediate-size filaments heavily decorated with antibodies to prekeratin. These filaments are anchored to typical desmosomes and hemidesmosomes and are also intimately associated with microfilaments and their characteristic dense bodies. Vimentin and smooth muscle cell desmin fibrils are not present in myoepithelial cells. These observations show that the myoepithelial cell is derived from true epithelial cells and that cytokeratin filaments might function in contractile epithelial cells in a manner similar to that of desmin-containing filaments in myocytes.

Although myoepitheliomas of the breast are exceedingly rare in humans,[42] the presence of both linear arrays of microfilaments and cytokeratin filaments in the same cell as well as mature desmosomal intercellular junctions is helpful in distinguishing myoepithelial cells (Fig. 3-139) from myofibroblasts (Figs. 3-133 and 3-134) in breast neoplasms.[452] Apparently, myoepithelial cells can form a neoplasm in a monomorphic fashion or more commonly in conjunction with ductular epithelial cells.

CHAPTER IV

The Cell Surface

The presence of unusual cell surface configurations, modifications of the plasmalemma (cell membrane or unit membrane), cell surface specializations such a microvilli and cilia, and cell contacts or junctions frequently provides important clues to the cytogenesis of a particular neoplasm. This chapter explains the diagnostic significance of cell membrane specializations and intercellular junctions.

CELL MEMBRANE SPECIALIZATIONS

The following cell membrane specializations are covered in this section: (1) plasmalemmal configurations; (2) pinocytotic vesicles; (3) the asymmetric unit membrane of urinary bladder epithelium; (4) microvilli, the intracellular lumen, adenocarcinomas, and microvillar configurations; and (4) cilia.

Plasmalemmal Configurations

Irregular surface contours, pseudopods* (projections of membrane-enclosed ectoplasm), filopodia (Fig. 4-1) (finger-shaped protrusions considered by many investigators to be a type of microvillus), ruffled borders, and interdigitation of adjacent cell membranes may be evident in tumors of diverse origin and are of limited diagnostic significance. Neoplastic lymphocytes comprising non-Hodgkin's lymphomas frequently display irregular surface configurations (Fig. 4-2). Interdigitating cell membranes are not only a diagnostic feature of tumors derived from glandular epithelia, e.g., parathyroid adenoma[115] (Fig. 4-3), but are also found in epithelioid sarcomas (Fig. 4-4). Complexly tangled cytoplasmic processes from adjacent

cells are particularly prominent in meningothelial meningiomas (Fig. 4-5) and in the compact Antoni type A tissue of benign schwannomas (Fig. 4-6), consisting of neoplastic Schwann cells. Neoplastic chondrocytes frequently have a scalloped cell membrane[159,519,560] (Fig. 4-7).

Pinocytotic Vesicles

Pinocytotic vesicles are minute flask-shaped invaginations of the plasmalemma in which small extracellular particles and fluids are taken into or transported across the cell.[167] These surface vesicles are particularly prominent in perineurial cells (Fig. 4-8), endothelial cells (Fig. 4-9), pericytes (Fig. 4-9), and leiomyocytes (Fig. 3-120). The presence of pinocytotic vesicles in addition to other ultrastructural markers of one of these cell types is occasionally helpful in diagnosis. For example, neoplastic perineurial cells, the principal neoplastic cell comprising many neurofibromas[163,343,546,634] have long, straight, extremely thin cytoplasmic processes coated with a discontinuous external lamina. Clusters of pinocytotic vesicles are also often associated with their plasmalemmas (Fig. 4-8).

Asymmetric Unit Membrane (Urinary Bladder Urothelium)

The unique asymmetric unit membrane of the apical surface of superficial epithelial cells in the urinary bladder has a distinct scalloped appearance. As opposed to the usual cell membrane, the outer leaflet of the tripartite membrane is denser than the inner one[253,320,473] (as illustrated in Fig. 4-10). The asymmetric membrane is therefore thicker (12 nm) than the symmetric unit membrane (8–10 nm) or plasmalemma. The classic (symmetric) unit membrane of other cell types consists of two electron-dense layers about 2.5–3 nm thick, separated by a 3-nm clear space (Fig.

---

* Pseudopods, attentuated pleomorphic filopodia, and the broad ruffled extensions of the cell surface participate in cellular movements and the uptake of foreign materials.

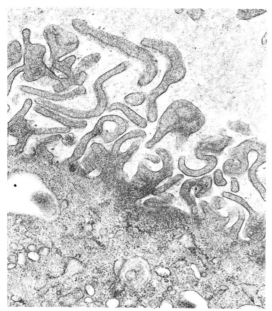

FIGURE 4-1
Malignant giant cell tumor (distal femur, 33-year-old female).
Ruffled border of multinucleated giant cell illustrating numerous pleomorphic projections of membrane-enclosed ectoplasm occasionally called filopodia. (×20,400.)

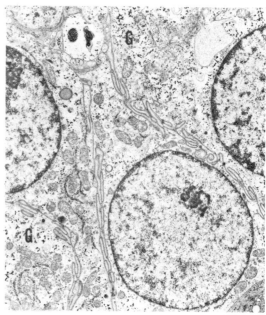

FIGURE 4-3
Parathyroid adenoma, chief cell type (parathyroid gland,
59-year-old male). The cell membranes of adjacent chief cells
are interdigitating. Glycogen (G). (×6000.)

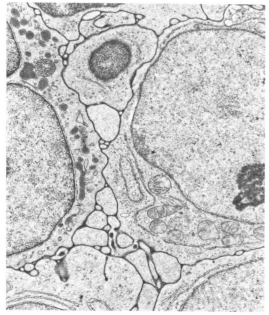

FIGURE 4-2
Malignant lymphoma, lymphoblastic T cell type (cf. Fig. 2-13).
Cluster of neoplastic lymphoblasts. Note the irregular surface
configurations and transversely sectioned pseudopods
(×7200,)

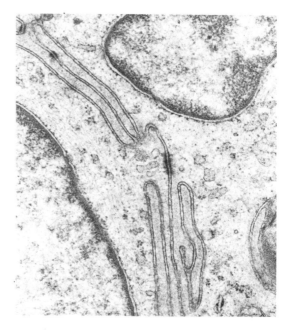

FIGURE 4-4
Epithelioid sarcoma (subcutaneous tissue, upper arm, 26-
year-old male). Portions of two neoplastic epithelioid cells with
interdigitating cell membranes joined by rudimentary cell
junctions (×24,000.)

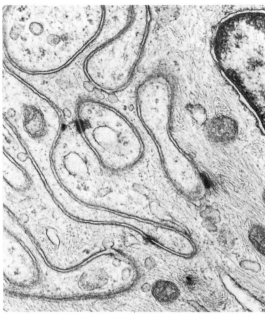

FIGURE 4-5
Meningothelial meningioma (dura, frontal lobe, 62-year-old female). Complexly tangled meningothelial cell processes joined by small desmosomes. Note the 10-nm glial filaments in the cytoplasm. (×24,000.)

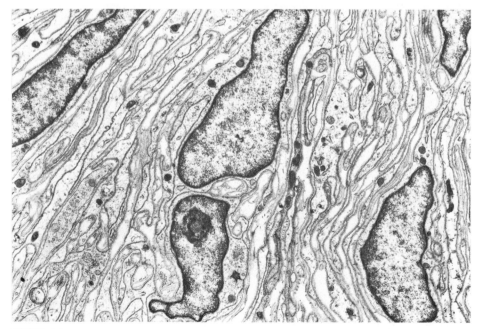

FIGURE 4-6
Benign schwannoma (groin, 72-year-old female). Neoplastic Schwann cells in Antoni type A tissue. Numerous complexly tangled attenuated cell processes are evident. (×7200.)

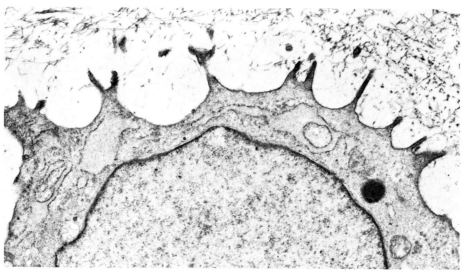

FIGURE 4-7
Low-grade chondrosarcoma (femur, 65-year-old male). Portion of neoplastic chondrocyte lying within a lacunae. Note the prominent scalloped cell membrane. (×13,200.)

4-14). Numerous fusiform or discoid vesicles derived from the Golgi apparatus[253,320] and also bounded by an inside-out asymmetric membrane (Fig. 4-10) usually reside within the apical cytoplasm. Koss[320] showed that these vesicles are incorporated within the asymmetric surface membrane. Properly prepared and oriented tissue specimens are required for resolving the fine structural details of the plasmalemma (Fig. 4-14).

In my experience, both discoid vesicles and an asymmetric unit membrane are lacking in papillary and poorly differentiated carcinomas of the urinary bladder in adult humans. These findings have been substantiated by other investigators.[197,321,404] The free surface facing the lumen is lined with a symmetric plasmalemma that forms stubby microvilli.

It is also interesting to note that the superficial urothelial cells of elderly persons (aged 61–82 years) lack the asymmetric unit membrane and precursor discoid vesicles found in younger persons[15,272] (Fig. 4-11). Because bladder carcinomas rarely occur in children and young adults, the diagnostic significance of this unique membrane is trivial.

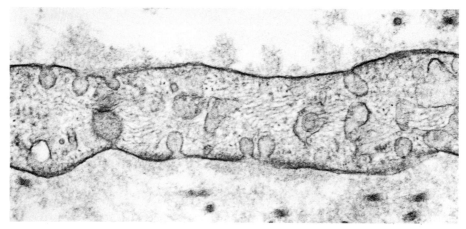

FIGURE 4-8
Neurofibroma (dermis, cheek, 55-year-old male). Perineurial cell process irregularly coated by external lamina substance. Note the prominent flaskshaped invaginations of the plasmalemma (pinocytotic vesicles) and cytoplasmic microfilaments. (×58,000.)

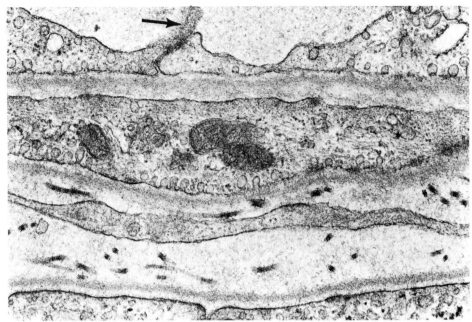

FIGURE 4-9
Parathyroid adenoma (parathyroid gland, 60-year-old female). *Top to bottom*, Capillary lumen, endothelial cell processes with basal lamina, pericyte surrounded by external lamina, thin fibroblast process surrounded by scattered collagen fibrils, and basal lamina of neoplastic chief cell. Pinocytotic vesicles are found on both surfaces of the endothelial cells and are particularly abundant on the basal surface of the pericyte process. Note the marginal fold (*arrow*) projecting into the capillary lumen, where the two endothelial cell processes meet. (×37,800.)

Microvilli

The free surface of many epithelial cells, particularly those of the small intestine and renal proximal tubule, form cylindrical processes called microvilli, approximately 90 nm in diameter and 1 μm in length. The rigid microvilli forming the striated or brush border of intestinal absorptive cells (Figs. 4-12 to 4-14) have numerous branching surface excrescences consisting of glycoproteins (the glycocalyx).[59,271] The microfilamentous core contains a number of proteins in addition to actin, e.g., villin and fimbrin,[81,82,393] and extends into the ectoplasm, contributing to the apical zone of the terminal web (Fig. 4-20) (see p. 108). Other microvilli, e.g., respiratory ciliated columnar epithelial cells, are more pleomorphic and may not exhibit a glycocalyx or obvious microfilamentous core in routine preparations (Figs. 4-22 and 4-23).

Intracellular lumen—adenocarcinoma

Neoplasms derived from glandular epithelial cells frequently possess ductular or acinar lumens lined with variable numbers of microvilli (Figs. 4-15 and 4-16). The ultrastructural demonstration of a so-called "intracellular lumen" with associated microvilli in a poorly differentiated tumor (Figs. 4-17 and 4-19) is generally diagnostic of adenocarcinoma.[13] Note the absence of a junctional complex (see p.108) always found adjacent to extracellular or true lumens (Figs. 4-28 and 4-29). Although intracellular lumens are a prominent feature of many adenocarcinomas of the breast[36] (Fig. 4-17),

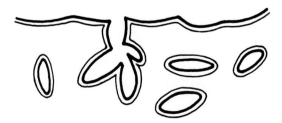

FIGURE 4-10
A highly schematic diagram showing the location and morphology of the asymmetric unit membrane and the fusiform vesicles that can be incorporated into the surface plasma membrane when the urinary bladder is distended with urine.

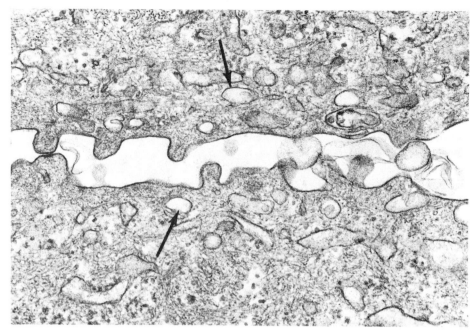

FIGURE 4-11
Normal urinary bladder epithelium (carcinoma of the prostate gland, 70-year-old male). Possible remnants of asymmetric unit membrane lining the apical surface and discoid vesicles (*arrows*). It is difficult to resolve the tripartite structure of the plasmalemma in most specimens. (×50,000.)

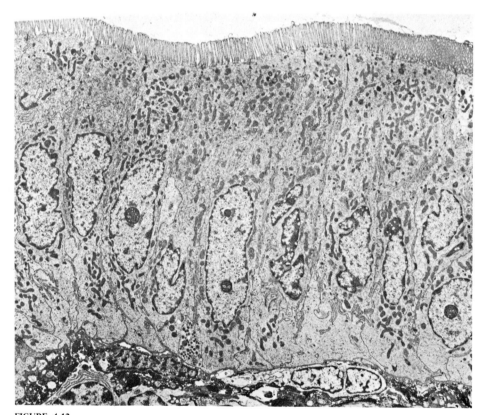

FIGURE 4-12
Normal jejunum (adjacent to jejunal adenocarcinoma, 53-year-old male). Columnar absorptive cells of the jejunum (longitudinal section of a portion of a villus). The free surface (*top*) or striated border consists of numerous closely packed microvilli. The core of the villus (*bottom*) consists of the connective tissue elements of the lamina propria. (×3040.)

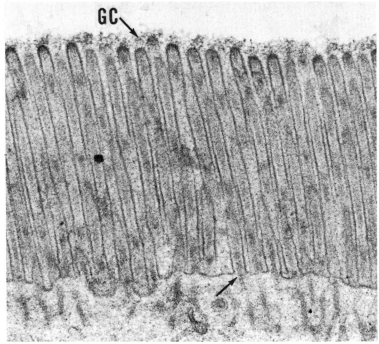

FIGURE 4-13
Higher-magnification electron micrograph of a portion of the striated border. Not all of the long microvilli are in the plane of the section. Note the microfilamentous core extending into the ectoplasm (*arrow*) and the glycocalyx (GC). (×29,600.)

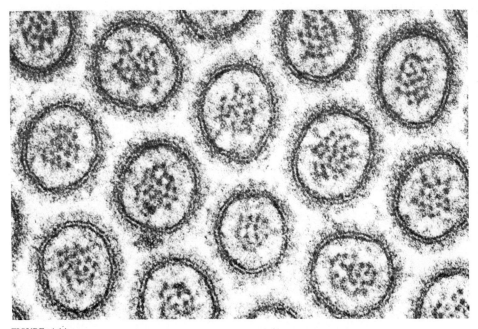

FIGURE 4-14
Transversely sectioned microvilli of intestinal absorptive epithelial cell (normal ileum, 58-year-old female). Note the surface excrescences or glycocalyx, tripartite structure of plasmalemma (unit membrane), and internal (core) bundles of microfilaments. (×198,000.)

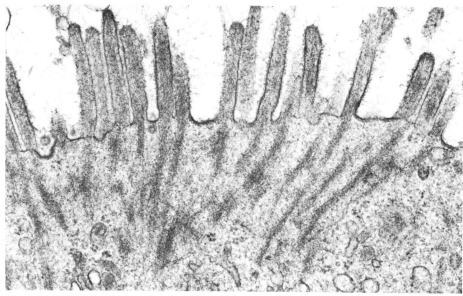

FIGURE 4-15
Well-differentiated adenocarcinoma (ampulla of Vater, 60-year-old male). Luminal surface of neoplastic ductular epithelial cell showing numerous microvilli. The core microfilaments extend well into the apical cytoplasm. (×36,000.)

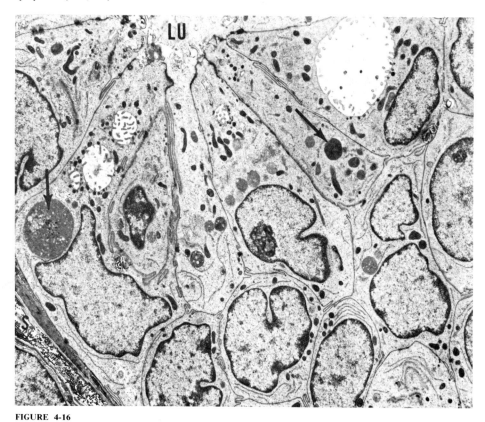

FIGURE 4-16
Infiltrating duct and *in situ* carcinoma (breast, 55-year-old female). Cluster of neoplastic ductular epithelial cells from an area of *in situ* carcinoma. Note the true extracellular lumen (LU) delineated by junctional complexes, the five microvillus-lined intracellular lumens, interdigitating lateral cell membranes, and increased numbers of basal cells. The large dense structures are secondary lysosomes (*arrows*). Stroma (S). (×4320.)

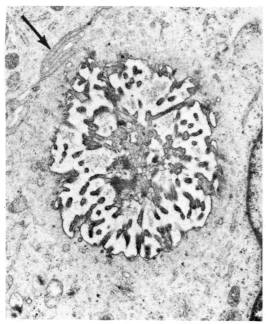

FIGURE 4-17
Metastatic poorly differentiated mammary carcinoma (anterior chest wall, 23-year-old female). Intracellular lumen. Note the presence of numerous filiform microvilli and the interdigitating cell membranes (*arrow*). (×10,500.)

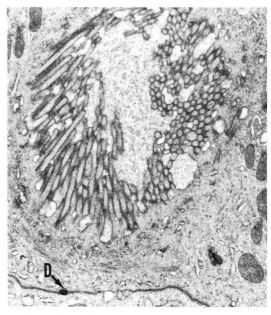

FIGURE 4-19
Anaplastic adenocarcinoma of lung origin (pleura, 64-year-old male). Portion of an intracellular lumen lined with numerous long slender microvilli in a large, pleomorphic tumor cell. The lumen contains a fine flocculent material. Desmosome (D). (×13,600.)

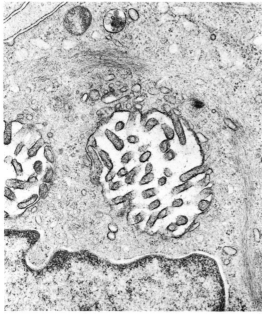

FIGURE 4-18
Infiltrating lobular carcinoma (breast, 44-year-old female). Two small intracellular lumens with associated microvilli. Note the fine bundles of intracytoplasmic microfilaments. (×24,000.)

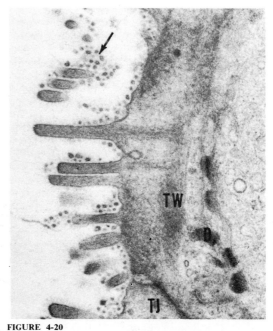

FIGURE 4-20
Adenocarcinoma, grade II (sigmoid colon, 66-year-old male. Cf. Fig. 1-1). Free surface of neoplastic colonic absorptive epithelial cell showing rigid microvilli with prominent core microfilaments continuous with the ectoplasmic terminal web (TW). Small glycocalyceal bodies (*arrow*) are associated with the external surface of the microvilli. Desmosomes (D) are seen in tangential section. Tight junction (TJ). (×21,600.)

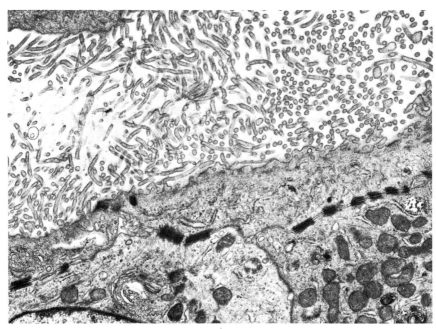

FIGURE 4-21
Epithelial mesothelioma (parietal pleura, 58-year-old male). Note the large numbers of tortuous microvilli in the extracellular space between tangentially sectioned neoplastic mesothelial cells. The cells are joined by numerous desmosomes. (×9200.)

e.g., secretory carcinoma[588] and infiltrating lobular carcinoma[6,36] (Fig. 4-18), and lung[160] (Fig. 4-19) origin, they are also seen occasionally in normal breast epithelial cells and in gynecomastia.[242] Intracellular lumens may or may not communicate with the cell surfaces.[13,36]

Other structures variously found in the cytoplasm or surface features of cells comprising adenocarcinomas, include mucigen granules, intracytoplasmic fibrils, interdigitating cell membranes, a prominent Golgi apparatus, glycogen, and mature intercellular junctions. In the more differentiated tumors, the cells are separated from the stroma by a well-defined basal lamina.

Microvillar configurations

The recognition of a particular morphologic microvillar configuration is often diagnostic for tumors of mesothelial cell origin and for pinpointing distinct types of adenocarcinomas.

Rigid microvilli with prominent core microfilaments extending into the ectoplasm (contributing to the terminal web), with or without either an external branching glycocalyx or glycocalyceal bodies (Figs. 4-15 and 4-20), are frequently found in cells comprising "intestinal-type carcinomas,"[389] e.g., most carcinomas derived from ep-

ithelial lining cells from the stomach, intestines, pancreatic ducts, gallbladder, endocervix, and mucinous bronchiolar and ovarian neoplasms. Recognition of this particular configuration is helpful for distinguishing between intestinal and nonintestinal metastatic adenocarcinomas. For example, prominent core microfilaments extending deep in the ectoplasm, glycocalyx bodies, and apical membrane-limited dense bodies (small mucigen granules?) are ultrastructural markers of colonic adenocarcinoma[252] (Figs. 3-47 and 4-20).

The diagnosis of diffuse, malignant, pleural epithelial mesotheliomas is frequently confirmed by the fine structural visualization of the long, tortuous or shaggy microvilli characteristic of the pluripotential mesothelial cell[67,312,626] (Fig. 4-21). The epithelioid and sarcomatous types, however, consist, respectively, of round and spindle-shaped cells without surface microvilli. Electron microscopy contributes little to the diagnosis of those latter variants unless foci of epithelial cells with long, tortuous microvilli are identified. We are of the opinion that there is a separate entity—a fibrosarcomatous mesothelioma—having clinical, histologic, and ultrastructural features similar to those of low-grade fibrosarcomas arising elsewhere in the body. These tumors most likely derive from submesothelial fibrocytes. Rare, benign, cystic peritoneal mesotheliomas resemble the pleural epithelial mesotheliomas.[423] Adenomatoid tumors, or genital tract neoplasms derived from serosal mesothelium, are also composed of cells having the long, bushy microvilli characteristic of neoplastic pleural mesothelial cells.[375,592] Similar microvilli line the apical surface of the distinct ependymal cells comprising choroid plexus papillomas.[101]

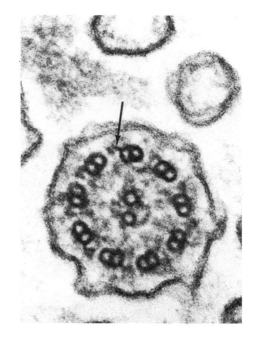

FIGURE 4-22

Ciliated columnar epithelium (normal nasopharynx, 58-year-old female). Cross-sectioned cilium. The axoneme consists of nine pairs of microtubules symmetrically arrayed around the two central microtubules. One or two short dynein arms (*arrow*) extends from one of each of the doublet microtubules. The transversely sectioned microvilli (*top*) lack a discernible microfilamentous core (×148,000).

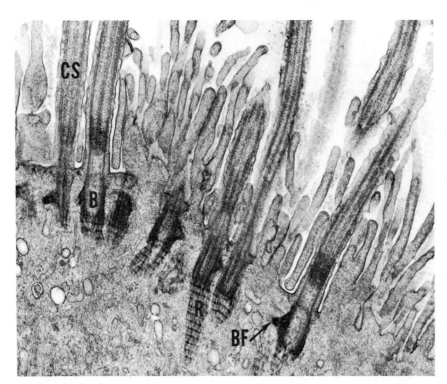

FIGURE 4-23

Ciliated columnar epithelium (normal nasopharynx, 31-year-old female). Apical surface of ciliated respiratory epithelial cell showing longitudinally sectioned cilia and microvilli. Ciliary shaft (CS), basal body (B), basal feet (BF), and rootlet (R). Note that the microvilli are more pleomorphic compared with those of intestinal-type epithelial cells. They also lack a discernible microfilamentous core. (×28,000.)

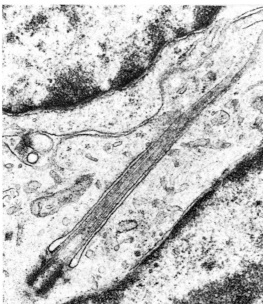

FIGURE 4-24
Anaplastic malignant spindle cell tumor (axilla, 70-year-old female). Cilium arising from a basal body deep in the cytoplasm. The tip of the shaft, which unfortunately is not in the plane of the section, most likely exits at the cell surface. (×23,000.)

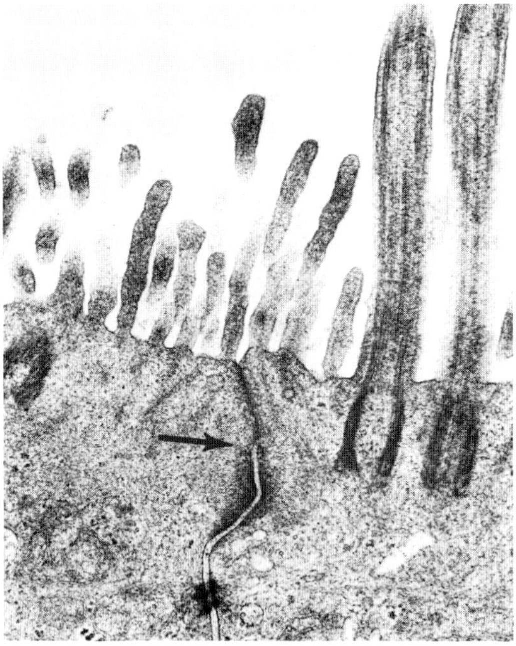

FIGURE 4-25
Low-grade papillary serous cystoadenocarcinoma (ovary, 65-year-old female). Two cilia, one basal body without a ciliary shaft, and numerous microvilli are evident. Ciliated cells were seen in only a few of the coelomic mesothelial cells comprising this tumor. Note the junctional complex (*arrow*). (×28,800.)

Cilia

Cilia are long, cylindrical motile processes having a complex internal component known as the axoneme. This latter structure consists of a highly characteristic circular arrangement of nine pairs of microtubules (doublets) composed of proteins called tubulins symmetrically arrayed around two central microtubules. Two short dynein arms extend from one of the microtubules (tubule A) of the doublets, each containing an axonemic protein called dynein whose ATPase activity is essential for ciliary motility (cilia without dynein are nonmotile).[4] Microtubule A is connected by radial spokes to a sheath surrounding the two central microtubules. These structures are easily identified in transverse sections of the ciliary shaft (Fig. 4-22). In longitudinal sections (Fig. 4-23), it is evident that the ciliary shaft terminates on a basal body (kinetosome) with a substructure nearly identical to that of the centriole (the centriole consists of nine triplet microtubules arranged in a circle). In favorable sections, electron-dense processes called basal feet project laterally from the basal body, and tapering striated rootlets extending into the ectoplasm are often visible[19,140,170] (Fig. 4-23).

Ciliated epithelial cells are particularly prominent in the Schneiderian membrane (nasal and paranasal mucosas),[490] including olfactory epithelium, the nasopharynx (Figs. 4-22 and 4-23), the upper respiratory tract (trachea and larger bronchi), and are also found in the endometrium, fallopian tubes, surface cells of the ovary,[57] ductuli efferentes (testis), and ependymal cells. Cells with a few surface cilia are occasionally found in various ductular epithelia, e.g., ductal and centroacinar cells of the human pancreas.[304,586] Microvilli are intermixed with the cilia in all the above-mentioned cells. So-called solitary "intracellular cilia,"[8] single cilia that grow out of interphase centrioles or abortive basal bodies in unciliated animal cells, are occasionally found in neoplasms of diverse origin. They are actually immature cilia that extend to the cell surface (Fig. 4-24).

Because ciliated cells are confined to only a few organs of the human body, the demonstration of these motile structures in poorly differentiated or metastatic tumors is theoretically significant. Unfortunately, however, they are rarely found in neoplasms derived from ciliated epithelial cells,

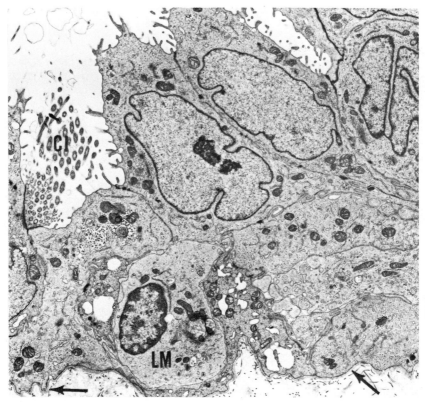

FIGURE 4-26
Cystoadenofibroma (ovary, 66-year-old female. cf. Fig. 2-4). Papillary formation of benign neoplastic coelomic mesothelial cells separated from the stroma by a well-defined basal lamina (*arrows*). Note the tangentially sectioned cilia (CI). Lymphocyte (LM). (×4560.)

e.g., bronchogenic or bronchiolar carcinomas,[41,306] Schneiderian papillomas,[490] endometrial carcinoma *in situ* or adenocarcinoma,[180,181] and fallopian tube carcinoma.[280] Occasional columnar epithelial cells with microvilli and cilia are seen in the benign glandular component of adenosarcoma of the uterus and ovary,[612] but are rarely found in ovarian serous cystadenocarcinoma[220,494] (Fig. 4-25). Nevertheless, ciliated cells are commonly noted in benign serous cystadenoma of the ovary and cases of borderline malignancy[177,178] and in ovarian cystadenofibromas[455] (Fig. 4-26). Ciliated cells are also present in Brenner tumors of the ovary. These distinctive tumors consist of scattered epithelial nests surrounded by a fibrous stroma. According to Klemi and Nevalainen,[310] Brenner tumors develop by direct metaplasia of ovarian surface epithelium.

Whereas cilia are rarely demonstrated in neoplastic cells comprising ependymomas and choroid plexus papillomas,[101,193] blepharoplasts (an archaic name for ciliary basal bodies) are almost always found in the apical cytoplasm[506] (Fig. 4-27) (see Chapter 6, case 2).

Cilia having an abnormal morphology are occasionally found in non-neoplastic and neoplastic epithelial cells.[190,400] For example, club-shaped giant cilia with a 9 + 0 axoneme, a feature of nonmotile cilia, were recently described in palisade and rosette-forming cells in a pineoblastoma[313] and projecting into the central lumen of the Flexner-Wintersteiner rosette in retinoblastomas.[471,608] These abnormal cilia are not diagnostic unless they are found in all or most cases of a particular tumor.

CELL JUNCTIONS

Cell junctions are defined as structurally specialized domains formed at regions of contact between two cells, and to which both cells contribute a part.[633] Different functional categories of intercellular junctions are present on the lateral surface

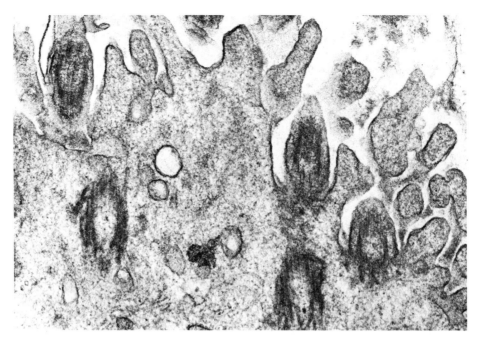

FIGURE 4-27
Metastatic myxopapillary ependymoma (right middle lobe lung, 37-year-old male). Ciliary basal bodies, also called blepharoplasts, in the apical cytoplasm of a metastatic ependymal cell. (×52,000.)

of simple epithelial cells: (1) impermeable, e.g., tight junction; (2) adhering, e.g., intermediate junction and desmosome; and (3) communicating, e.g., gap junction. These intercellular junctions and the hemidesmosome that anchors the cell to the underlying basal lamina are commonly found in neoplastic tissue.[633] The rarely encountered "septate junctions," recognized by periodic septa extending across the intercellular gap,[554] are currently nondiagnostic.

In this section, the fine structural morphology of intercellular junctions (including the hemidesmosome and excluding the septate junction) (Table 4-1) found in normal specialized epithelia are described before a commentary on the identification and interpretation of these surface specializations in neoplasms.

TABLE 4-1

Cell Junctions

Junctional complex
    Tight junction (zonula occludens)
    Intermediate junction (zonula adherens)
    Desmosome (macula adherens)
Gap junction (nexus)
Septate junction
Hemidesmosome (cell—basal lamina)

Junctional Complex

Ultrastructural examination of the apical "terminal web region" (the terminal web consists of a dense network of microfilaments located in the subluminal ectoplasm), of absorptive epithelial cells (Fig. 4-20), particularly in the small intestine, demonstrates the presence of a "junctional complex" (the light microscopist's terminal bar) consisting, from the lumen inward, of three distinct components: the tight junction, the intermediate junction, and the desmosome[166,267,554] (Figs. 4-28 and 4-29). In the tight junction (zonula occludens), the plasma membranes of two adjacent cells appear to be fused at a series of points. This juxtaluminal junction extends around the cell perimeter, sealing the intercellular space—an impermeable junction. The remaining two components of the junctional complex are adhering junctions called desmosomes. The intermediate junction (belt desmosome or zonula adherens) is recognized by the dense mats of actin-containing microfilaments adhering to the inner surfaces of adjacent membranes. Where "intestinal-type" surface microvilli are present, the core microfilaments connect with the belt desmosome (Fig. 4-28). Scattered cytokeratin filaments (tonofilaments) also contribute to the adherens zone. The

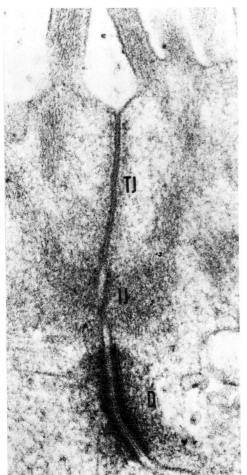

FIGURE 4-28
Junctional complex (cf. Fig. 1-1). The juxtaluminal junctional complex consists of a tight junction (TJ), intermediate junction (IJ), and desmosome (D). Note that the microfilaments of the intermediate junction are continuous with the core microfilaments of the microvilli. Cytokeratin filaments extend from the plaques of the desmosome a short distance into the cytoplasm. (×60,000.)

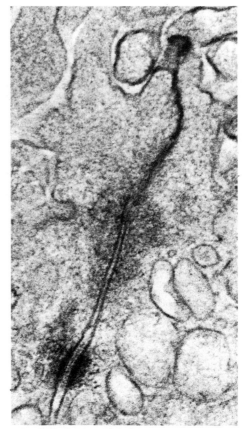

FIGURE 4-29
Junctional complex (cellular pleomorphic adenoma, parotid gland, 70-year-old female). Junctional complex adjacent to a microvillus-lined lumen, a portion of which can be seen at the *top*. It is very difficult to obtain a good longitudinal section through all three members of the junctional complex without using a gonimeter stage to tilt the plane of the section in the electron microscope. (×75,000.)

over the lateral cell surfaces. Intracellular desmosomes[352] (Fig. 4-32) are occasionally seen in both non-neoplastic and neoplastic epithelial cells.

Hemidesmosome and Gap Junction

Other types of cell junctions, although not as useful in diagnosis as the members of the junctional complex, merit brief mention. Hemidesmosomes join epithelial cells to the underlying basal lamina (Fig. 4-33). They also serve as anchoring sites for bundles of cytoplasmic cytokeratin filaments. In the gap junction or nexus (a communicating junction commonly found between smooth muscle cells), the intercellular space is narrowed from its normal width of about 25 nm to about 2–3 nm, and

last component of the junctional complex is the desmosome (macula adherens or spot desmosome) (Figs. 4-28–4-31). The classic desmosome consists of two disc-shaped plaques on the cytoplasmic surface of each plasma membrane flanking a dense line termed the central stratum that bisects the intercellular space (Fig. 4-31). Cytokeratin filaments characteristically extend from the plaques into the adjacent cytoplasm. Thinner filaments (transmembrane linkers) extend between the two cells, providing mechanical coupling between cytokeratin bundles of adjacent cells. Additional spot desmosomes are usually found scattered at random

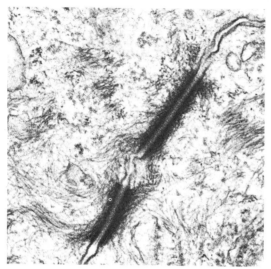

FIGURE 4-30
Metastatic anaplastic epidermoid carcinoma (peribronchial lymph node, 66-year-old female). Two mature desmosomes in a small focus of fairly well-differentiated tumor cells. Cytokeratin filaments (tonofilaments) extend from the plaques of the desmosome into the cytoplasm; small collections of these filaments are also seen scattered throughout the cytoplasm of the tumor cells. (×48,000.)

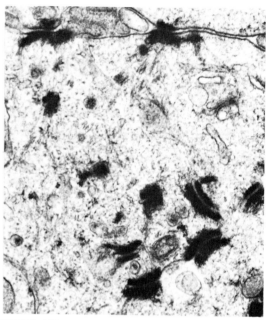

FIGURE 4-32
Thymoma (anterior mediastinum, 62-year-old male). Portions of two neoplastic thymic epithelial cells showing two typical desmosomes and a cluster of intracellular desmosomes. (×30,400.)

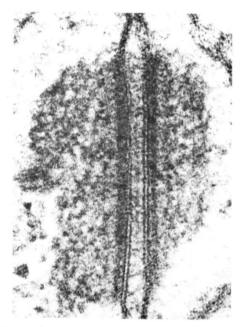

FIGURE 4-31
Desmosome (keratinocytes from skin of 48-year-old male with early case of mycosis fungoides). Note the intercellular central stratum, plaques, and dense bundles of cytokeratin filaments. (×186,000.)

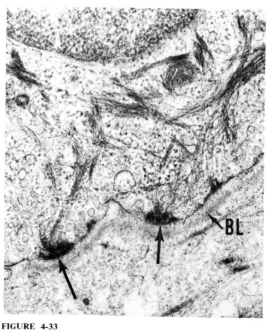

FIGURE 4-33
Actinic keratosis (skin of nose, 48-year-old female). Portion of basal keratinocyte and adjacent papillary dermis. Note the cytoplasmic cytokeratin filaments and the two mature hemidesmosomes (*arrows*). Basal lamina (BL) of keratinocyte. (×37,000.)

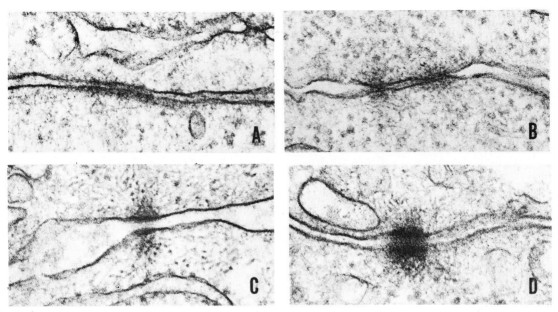

FIGURE 4-34
Primitive cell junctions. (*A*) Metastatic poorly differentiated epidermoid lung carcinoma (femur, 50-year-old female). Focal thickenings of opposing plasmalemmas. (*B*) Anaplastic mediastinal germ cell tumor (jugular lymph node, 34-year-old male). Two primitive cell junctions. Note the small filamentous mats associated with the junctions. (*C*) Poorly differentiated duct carcinoma (breast, 40-year-old female). Earliest recognizable desmosome. Note the plaques and the cross-sectioned 10-nm cytokeratin filaments. (*D*) *In situ* lobular carcinoma (breast, 66-year-old female). This intercellular junction is most likely a small desmosome. (*A–D*, ×80,000.)

in poorly resolved micrographs can be mistaken for a tight junction. Tangential sections, especially after staining with lanthanum (a heavy metal tracer), exhibit a highly ordered pattern of hexagonally packed cylindrical structures (connexons). These "intercellular channels" presumably permit the exchange of molecules between cells.[554,652] Because gap junctions are difficult to recognize without the help of special procedures (heavy metal tracers and freeze-fracturing), they are of limited diagnostic significance. McNutt and associates[403] reported that gap junctions occur rarely in dysplastic and neoplastic human cervical epithelial cells, but are fairly abundant in normal epithelial cells.

Primitive Cell Junctions

Whereas typical cell junctions are often found in various fairly well-differentiated epithelial neoplasms[633] incompletely developed cell contacts are more commonly found in anaplastic carcinomas, neoplasma simulating carcinomas, and certain sarcomas. We prefer to call these rudimentary intercellular junctions, which range from focal thickenings of adjacent cell membranes to what are probably poorly formed members of the junctional complex, "primitive cell junctions" (Fig. 4-34) These primordial poorly formed primitive cell junctions are commonly referred to as "tight junctions" or "desmosomes" in the literature on human tumors. When you are not sure what type of junction you are dealing with, do not give it a specific name. The same holds true for intracellular fibrils and other inclusions. In summary, less differentiated invasive carcinomas contain fewer cell junctions,[14] which are usually poorly developed (primitive).

In Neoplasms Other Than Typical Carcinomas and Sarcomas

Another common misconception is that intercellular junctions are only found in classic carcinomas, and their demonstration in a poorly differentiated or anaplastic tumor clearly establishes that the tumor is derived from squamous or glandular epithelia (including endocrine glands). On the basis of my own observations and on a critical review of the literature, either well developed, or

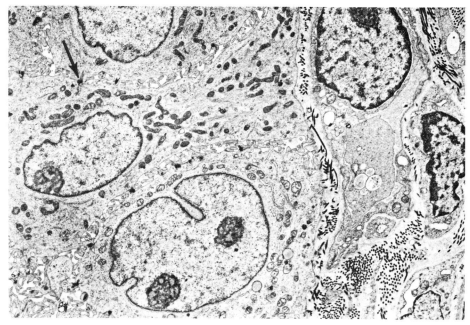

FIGURE 4-35
Brenner tumor (ovary, 54-year-old female). Portion of a nest of neoplastic epithelial cells separated from the stroma by a basal lamina. The cells have prominent surface microvilli and are joined by numerous small desmosomes (*arrow*). (×5300.)

more commonly, primitive cell junctions are found in a number of neoplasms that are neither classic carcinomas nor sarcomas.

Mesothelial cells are specialized cells of mesenchymal origin that line body cavities and viscera. Neoplasms derived from these cells may simulate metastatic carcinomas by light microscopy. Examples include (1) malignant pleural epithelial mesotheliomas[312,626] (Fig. 4-21); (2) adenomatoid tumors derived from genital tract serosal mesothelium[375,592]; and (3) ovarian neoplasms arising from the surface coelomic mesothelium, e.g., serous (Fig. 4-25) and mucinous cystadenocarcinoma[178,180,220]; cystadenomas[311]; and Brenner tumors (Fig. 4-35) (epithelial component).[77,310,526,504]

Thymomas are derived from neoplastic thymic epithelial cells that are often intermixed with varying numbers of non-neoplastic lymphocytes. The elongated cell processes contain bundles of cytokeratin filaments and are joined by numerous desmosomes[498] (Figs. 3-127 and 4-32). Thymic carcinoids (neurosecretory-type granules), lymphomas (no cell junctions or basal laminas), and seminomas (occasional intercellular junctions and conspicuous nucleolus), are also found in the anterior mediastinum (Table 1-2, p. 6).

Sex-cord stromal tumors derived from the specialized ovarian stromal cells often consist of cells

joined by primitive cell junctions. Examples include granulosa–theca cell tumors[205,219,374,505] (Fig. 4-36) and Sertoli–Leydig cell tumors[238,284,302,433,478] (Fig. 4-37). Intercellular junctions are also found in occasional ovarian and testicular germ cell tumors, e.g., seminoma, dysgerminoma, and gonadoblastoma.[54,282]

Many neoplasms arising in the central nervous system (CNS) are composed of cells joined by primitive or occasionally well-formed intercellular junctions. The differential diagnosis of CNS tumors often poses a challenge to the electron microscopist. Examples of some of these histologically complex neoplasms follow.

Meningiothelial meningiomas arise from neuroectodermally derived cells (meningocytes) lining the dura-arachnoid interface.[364,518] They characteristically form complex interdigitating cell processes joined by well-developed desmosomes (Fig. 4-5)[104,123,309,438,581] (see Chapter 6, case 1).

Ependymomas, which have a wide range of morphology, arise from ependymal cells lining the ventricular wall of the brain and the central canal of the spinal cord. The neoplastic cells in ependymoblastoma are often structurally similar to the cells that line the normal embryonic neural tube.[254] Both glial and ependymal cells originate from one primitive progenitor, the ependymoglia (tanocytic

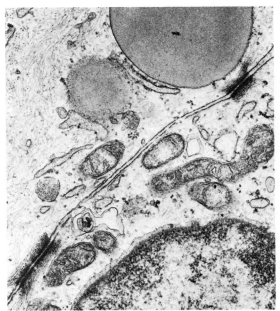

FIGURE 4-36
Granulosa cell tumor (ovary, 62-year-old female). Portions of two neoplastic cells joined by three desmosomes. Note the lipid droplets and randomly dispersed microfilaments. (×24,000.)

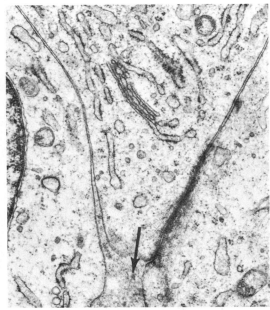

FIGURE 4-37
Sertoli–Leydig cell tumor (ovary, 21-year-old female). Neoplastic cells joined by a long cell junction that superficially resembles a tight junction or possibly an intermediate junction—note the intercellular space (*arrow*). (×19,200.)

ependyma).[193] The ependymal cells derive from ependymoblasts developing directly from this primordial precursor. The ventricular wall is lined by a continuous layer of ependymal cells directly overlying glial fibers and ependymal glial cells.[194] Because these neoplasms arise from a multipotential progenitor cell, i.e., the ependymoglia, glial cells (astrocytes) with prominent cytoplasmic intermediate (glial) filaments may be found in some ependymal tumors. The neoplastic ependymal cells, particularly those forming the distinctive rosettes, are joined by a variety of intercellular junctions (see Chapter 6, case 2). In the more differentiated areas (the luminal surface), juxtaluminal junctional complexes are evident.[193,254,644] Intercellular junctions are also found in papillomas of the choroid plexus,[101] a specialized type of ependyma.

Cerebellar medulloblastomas are highly cellular malignant tumors composed of closely packed spherical or oval cells with scanty cytoplasm that on occasion form Homer-Wright pseudorosettes indicative of neuroblastic differentiation. They are most likely neuroepithelial tumors of embryonic origin that may remain undifferentiated or may differentiate along astrocytic or neuronal lines. Primitive cell junctions and well-developed intermediate junctions are noted, especially in the more differentiated areas of the neoplasm.[90,507] Such findings are helpful in distinguishing these tumors from other small cell neoplasms arising in, or metastatic to, the brain, e.g., cerebellar sarcomas and non-Hodgkin's lymphomas.

Medulloepitheliomas are extremely rare, highly malignant tumors that probably originate from the pluripotential epithelium of the primordial neural tube differentiating along neuroectodermal cell lines. They consist of a tubular or papillary arrangement of columnar cells joined by numerous primitive cell junctions. The luminal surface of the cell lacks microvilli and cilia. Solid areas of tightly packed cells are also evident.[469]

Primitive neuroectodermal tumors of the CNS are composed of small undifferentiated cells with prominent nuclei and a generally scant cytoplasm containing few organelles. Careful ultrastructural examination often indicates that the cells are joined by rare primitive cell junctions.[63,392] These neoplasms have no specific ultrastructural features and are distinguished from the more well-established neuroectodermal neoplasms, e.g., medulloepitheliomas and cerebral neuroblastomas by their locations, clinical behavior, and histologic appearance.[63,239] I have examined a primitive neuroectodermal tumor arising in the cerebrum, in which the cells formed short neurites (axon or dendritic processes); however, no cell junctions

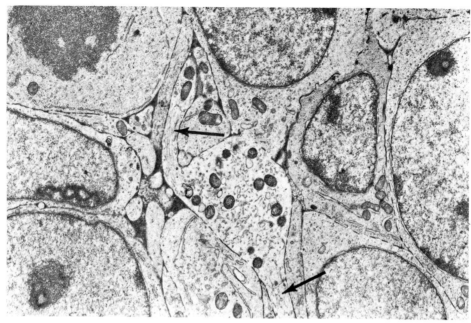

FIGURE 4-38
Primitive neuroectodermal tumor (cerebrum, 14-year-old female). Nest of primitive neuroectodermal cells showing early neuronal differentiation. Note the microtubules (neurotubules) in the neuritic processes (*arrows*) and the mitotic cell (*top left*). (×6400.)

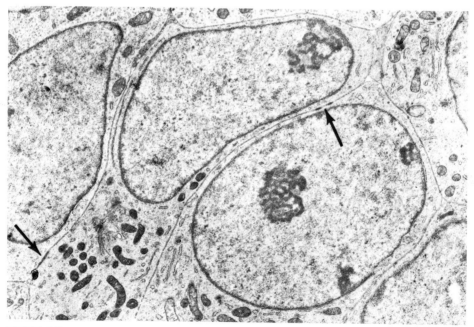

FIGURE 4-39
Metastatic primitive neuroectodermal tumor (lung, 8-year-old female). Nest of poorly differentiated small cells joined by widely scattered primitive cell junctions (*arrows*). Well-defined neuritic processes are not evident in this neoplasm. (×7600.)

were noted (Fig. 4-38). Seven cases arising outside the CNS consisted of poorly differentiated cells forming occasional neurites and joined by primitive cell junctions (Fig. 4-39)—no neurosecretory-type granules are evident in these neoplasms, thereby distinguishing them from neuroblastomas.

Retinoblastoma is a congenital malignant tumor of neuronal origin that arises from the nuclear layers of the retina.[471] The cells forming the characteristic Flexner–Wintersteiner rosettes are joined on their lateral surfaces by numerous intercellular junctions. They are most prominent in the juxtaluminal area.[471,608]

The large vacuolated physaliferous cells found in human chordoma, a neoplasm believed to arise from remnants of the embryonic notochord, are also joined by scattered small desmosomes.[162,298]

It should also be pointed out that neoplasms derived from neural crest cells that have migrated to various parts of the body, such as peripheral nerve sheath tumors (e.g., schwannomas and neurofibromas)[163] occasional malignant melanomas,[398] and apudomas or neuroendocrine tumors (see neurosecretory granule section), also exhibit varying numbers of intercellular junctions. It should be apparent that intercellular junctions are found in a wide variety of neoplasms derived from highly specialized cells originating from all three germ layers.

In Sarcomas

Although intercellular junctions, especially the primitive types, have been reported in fetal connective tissues,[196,502] in both normal and neoplastic (?) myofibroblasts,[485,603] and smooth muscle cells (nexus),[338] they are not commonly seen in neoplasms derived from mesenchymal cells—sarcomas—excluding those discussed in the previous section (see below).

Rare "intermediate junctions" have been described in a primary fibrosarcoma of the thyroid gland,[536] giant cell tumors of bone[562] and soft tissues,[9] and in occasional cases of other neoplasms composed of "fibroblastic" cells with a prominent RER, e.g., osteogenic sarcoma[524] and parosteal osteogenic sarcoma.[485] Nevertheless, except for rare focal thickening of opposing plasmalemmas,

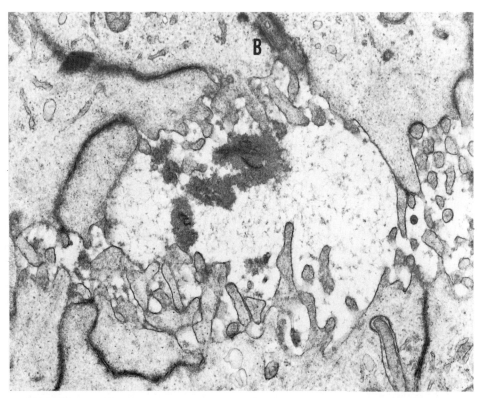

FIGURE 4-40
Synovial sarcoma (knee, 19-year-old female). Small lumen within a sheet of spindle-shaped neoplastic epithelioid cells. Note the surface microvilli, abortive junctional complexes, and the ciliary basal body (B). (×24,000.)

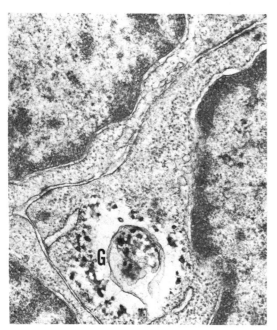

FIGURE 4-41
Ewing's sarcoma (midshaft of fibula, 16-year-old female).
Portions of three neoplastic cells joined by primitive cell junctions. Glycogen (G). (×24,000.)

I have not seen a single intercellular junction in 21 fibrosarcomas (all grades), 11 malignant fibrous histiocytomas, 20 osteogenic sarcomas, and 20 giant cell tumors (including two arising in soft tissues), or any other benign or malignant neoplasms derived from mesenchymal cells showing fibroblastic differentiation. For all practical purposes, it must be concluded that mature and well-defined rudimentary intercellular junctions are not found in such tumors. Primitive cell junctions, however, are evident in neoplasms derived from muscle cells, e.g., leiomyosarcoma[183,443,627] and rhabdomyosarcoma.[114,319]

Intercellular junctions of various types are more prevalent in a number of neoplasms arising from a variety of specialized mesenchymal cells, e.g., endothelial cells, and in tumors of uncertain histogenesis traditionally classified as "sarcomas", e.g., synovial sarcoma.

Endothelial cells are essentially mesenchymal cells adapted to lining the blood vessel lumen. Occasional primitive cell junctions and tight junctions are found in the following vascular tumors: (1) angiosarcoma[500] (Fig. 3-89), (2) hemangioendothelial sarcoma (hemangioendothelioma) of bone,[561] (3) lymphangiosarcoma,[408] (4) hemangiopericytoma,[35,150] and (5) Kaposi sarcoma.[78]

Synovial sarcomas are malignant neoplasms of obscure histogenesis characterized by a biphasic pattern of spindle-shaped cells and clefts lined by epithelioid cells. Monophasic synovial sarcomas consisting of sheets of spindle cells without the epithelioid component have also been described. Electron microscopic studies confirmed the epithelial nature of this tumor.[143,185,200,411,448,503] The closely packed spindle cells in the monophasic tumors and in the biphasic neoplasms are connected by intermediate and primitive cell junctions. Tight junctions delineate small abortive lumens (Fig. 4-40). The epithelioid cells lining the clefts, many of which are actually lumens, exhibit apical microvilli and lateral junctional complexes and often rest on a distinct basal lamina, features of true glandular epithelium.[411] Type A macrophagelike cells and type B fibroblastlike cells are found in normal human synovium.[32,209] As the human synovial membrane is obviously not a true "epithelium" (i.e., having no cell junctions and basal lamina), the origin of so-called synovial sarcomas remains a mystery.

Cell junctions are also seen occasionally in other neoplasms of unknown histogenesis bearing the connotation sarcoma essentially because they arise in mesenchymal tissues devoid of epithelial elements. For example, focal thickening of apposed cell membranes is found in most cases of Ewing's sarcoma of bone and soft tissues[360,380] (Fig. 4-41).

Epithelioid sarcoma is another soft tissue neoplasm with a peculiar histology that simulates either a squamous cell carcinoma or a granuloma.[155] The polygonal to spindle-shaped cells found at the periphery of the granulomatous-appearing tumor nodules often contain bundles of intermediate-size filaments and are joined by small desmosomes or primitive cell junctions (Fig. 4-4) in approximately one-third of cases. A number of investigators have suggested that they are derived from undifferentiated mesenchymal reserve cells or "synovioblastic mesenchyme" capable of differentiating along synovial or histiocytic lines.[60,458,515] The controversy regarding the histogenesis of these tumors is currently unresolvable because of the multipotential capabilities of the so-called undifferentiated mesenchymal reserve cells that remain in adult nonepithelial tissues. Nevertheless, because intercellular junctions are not commonly found in most neoplasms designated as sarcomas, and never in lymphomas, the absence of these structures in poorly differentiated or anaplastic tumors is often of diagnostic significance.

CHAPTER V

Extracellular Constituents

As previously stated, diagnostically significant structures are usually found within the cytoplasm of neoplastic cells (see Chapter 1, review and book list). Some extracellular constituents, especially the basal lamina, the subject of the first part of this chapter, are occasionally of diagnostic significance. The other formed extracellular components, e.g., collagen fibrils types I–V,[416] elastic fibers (elastin and microfibrils), amyloid,[213] psammoma bodies[184] (concentric laminae of calcium), and so forth, can be readily identified and characterized using special stains or histochemical methods, or both. For example, osteoid and reticulin fibrils (type III collagen) are physicochemical variants of collagen that cannot be confidently differentiated from ordinary collagen fibrils (Fig. 5-1) on the basis of fibril diameter and periodicity variations by routine TEM. These formed elements of the extracellular compartment are usually embedded in an amorphous or fibrillogranular ground substance. The diagnostic relevance of long-spacing collagen is discussed in the second part of this chapter.

BASAL LAMINA

The basement membrane the light microscopist sees (prominent in PAS-stained paraffin sections) encompasses the basal lamina and underlying collagen fibrils. Electron microscopically, the basal lamina is shown to be a granulofilamentous 50–80-nm-thick extracellular structure found whenever the plasmalemma of a parenchymal cell contacts collagen fibrils. A lighter zone, the lamina rara or lucida, separates the granulofilamentous lamina densa from the cell membrane (Fig. 5-2).[624] Some mesenchymal cells are often completely surrounded by a similar-appearing membrane more precisely called the external lamina.[208] The basal lamina consists essentially of equal amounts of collagenous glycoproteins, e.g., type IV procollagen, and noncollagenous glycoproteins, e.g., laminin and fibronectin, and glycosamino-glycans.[416,545,563,597]

In Neoplasms

Three important things to remember about the basal lamina with respect to neoplastic cells are:

1. Infiltrating or metastatic tumor cells often form a basal lamina (Fig. 5-3).
2. The basal or external lamina frequently has a patchy distribution (Fig. 5-4).
3. Neoplastic cells that are not epithelial in origin are often surrounded by an external lamina, e.g., muscle cells in leiomyosarcoma (Fig. 3-120) and embryonal rhabdomyosarcoma (Figs. 3-111 and 3-113).

The basal or external lamina may enclose clusters of tightly packed cells or encompass single cells lying free in the stroma. It is also important to be aware of so-called false basal laminas, resulting from stromal glyco- or mucoproteins adhering to the cell surface (Fig. 5-5).

The third item listed above is very important and requires further discussion. There are so many neoplasms derived from either the neural crest, e.g., schwannomas, or the mesenchyme, e.g., vascular tumors and liposarcoma, that consist of cells either partially or completely surrounded by an external lamina, that it would be more appropriate to list those neoplasms composed of cells that usually or definitely do not form this structure.

The following nosologic entities or broad categories of tumors consist of cells that are not surrounded (even partially) by a basal lamina or external lamina: (1) alveolar soft part sarcoma; (2) cartilaginous tumors; (3) chordoma (very rare); (4) eosinophilic granuloma; (5) epithelioid sarcoma; (6) Ewing's sarcoma; (7) all neoplasms composed of fibroblasts and fibroblastlike cells, excluding possibly myofibroblasts, and dermatofibrosarcoma protuberans (which consist of perineurial-like cells);[10] (8) endometrial stromal sar-

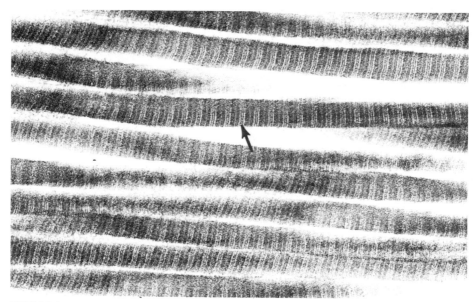

FIGURE 5-1
Collagen fibrils (skin of back, morphea, 32-year-old male). Interweaving bundles of collagen fibrils showing highly characteristic transverse bands (*arrow*) with a repeat distance of 64 nm. (×66,000.)

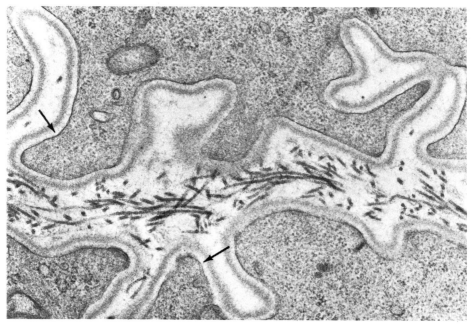

FIGURE 5-2
Papillary adenocarcinoma (kidney, 66-year-old male). Epithelial cell–stromal junction at the center of a papillae. A well-defined basal lamina separates the neoplastic epithelial cell basal plasmalemma from the stromal collagen fibrils. Lamina lucida (*arrows*). (×28,000.)

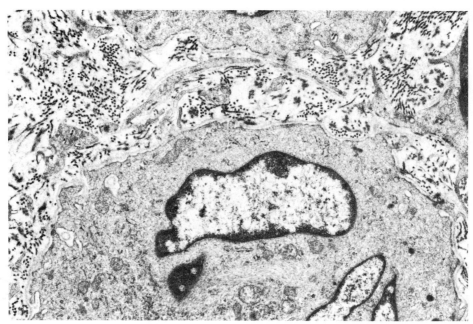

FIGURE 5-3
Hemangioendothelial sarcoma (hemangioendothelioma) (sternum, 30-year-old male). Portions of two isolated infiltrating neoplastic endothelial cells are illustrated. Note that these cells are surrounded by a basal lamina. (×11,600.)

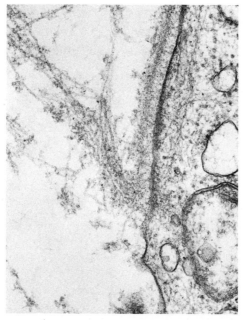

FIGURE 5-4
Benign pleomorphic adenoma (parotid gland, 45-year-old female). Portion of isolated myoepithelial cell in vicinity of neoplastic ducts showing detachment of the basal lamina from the plasmalemma. (×48,000.)

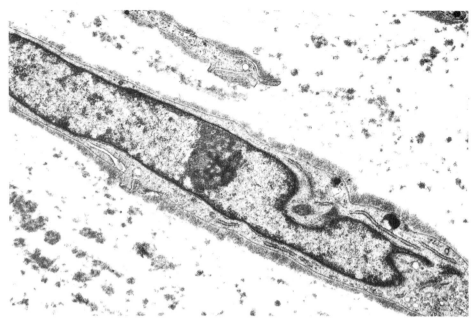

FIGURE 5-5
Low-grade myxoid fibrosarcoma (thigh, 78-year-old male). Granulofilamentous mucoprotein precipitate on the surface of a fibrocyte simulating a basal lamina. (×10,800.)

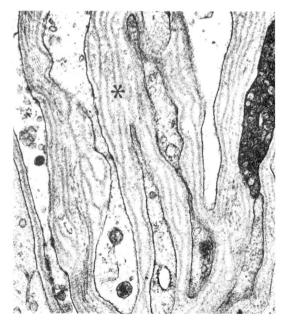

FIGURE 5-6
Benign schwannoma (posterior chest wall, 41-year-old male). Multiple (reduplicated) basal laminas (*asterisk*) are evident between the neoplastic Schwann cell processes. (×21,600.)

comas excluding endolymphatic stromal myosis[397]; (9) interstitial (Leydig) cell tumors and dysgerminomas (very rare); (10) all leukemias; (11) all lymphomas; (12) lymphangiosarcomas; (13) true histiocytic tumors, e.g., malignant histiocytosis; (14) neuroblastomas (excluding ganglioneuroblastoma) and primitive neuroectodermal tumors; (15) osteogenic sarcoma and benign osteoid-forming neoplasms (consist actually of fibroblastlike cells); (16) plasma cell tumors (multiple myeloma and plasmacytoma); (17) pure glial tumors, e.g., astrocytoma; (18) retinoblastoma; and possibly some other neoplasms not included in this listing.

Multilayering (reduplication) or thickening of the basal lamina may occur at the tumor–stromal interface of a variety of neoplastic epithelial cells, e.g., in benign schwannomas (Fig. 5-6); in fibroadenomas of the breast,[6,99,275] rare cases of infiltrating carcinoma of the breast (Fig. 5-7), and in clear cell carcinomas of the vagina.[142] Therefore, it is not diagnostic, with one exception. Highly replicated basal laminas are particularly prominent in the pseudocysts found in adenoid cystic carcinomas[322,572] (Fig. 5-8) and in dermal eccrine

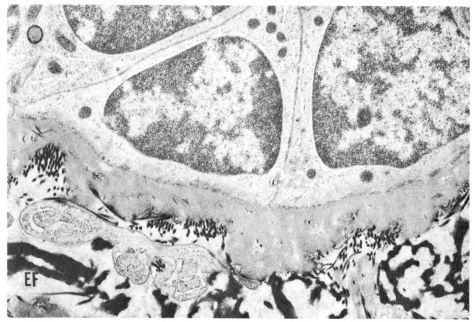

FIGURE 5-7
Infiltrating small cell duct carcinoma (breast, 53-year-old female). Portion of a cluster of small neoplastic ductular epithelial cells surrounded by a thickened basal lamina. Cell junctions and intracellular lumens were noted in the more centrally located cells. Elastic fibers (EF). (×11,600.)

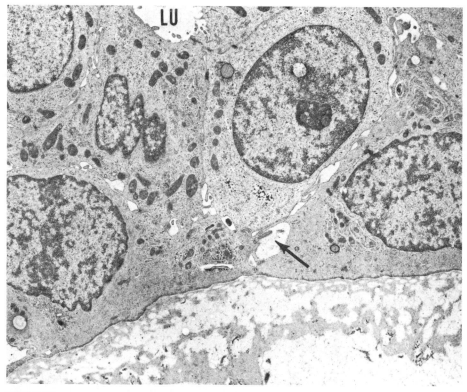

FIGURE 5-8
Adenoid cystic carcinoma (breast, 63-year-old female). Portion of tumor showing a pseudocyst with an irregular arrangement of replicated basal laminas. True lumen (LU), intercellular space (*arrow*). (×6480.)

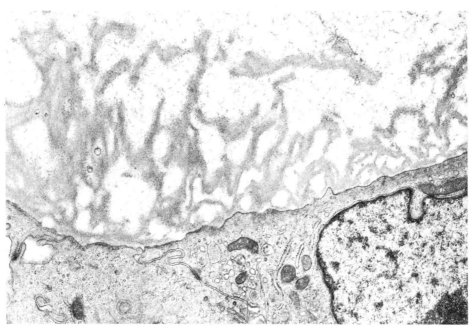

FIGURE 5-9
Dermal eccrine cylindroma (turban tumor of scalp: occipital scalp, 53-year-old male). Basal aspect of neoplastic duct. Abundant basal lamina substance is evident in the pseudocyst. By light microscopy these extracellular spaces may be mistaken for true lumens. (×12,000.)

cylindromas (Fig. 5-9); their identification is meaningful when the diagnosis of these entities is uncertain.

Reduplication or thickening of the capillary endothelial cell basal lamina is often noted in neoplastic conditions, e.g., in granular cell tumors,[121] and other pathologic conditions, e.g., in diabetes mellitus. It is of considerable importance in the diagnosis of many kidney diseases primarily involving glomeruli (the glomerular basement membrane), e.g., Alport's syndrome and membranous nephropathy. Excluding some of the glomerular diseases, accelerated cell death and replenishment may account for most of the accumulated layers of basal lamina.[624]

COLLAGEN

The formation of fusiform long-spacing collagen structures (Luse bodies)[368] with a highly characteristic periodicity of 120–150 nm is particularly prominent in benign schwannomas (Fig. 5-10) and occasional neurofibromas.[125,368,476] Although this type of collagen is supposedly not restricted to benign nerve sheath tumors,[476] I have found these banded collagen bodies mainly in the stroma of peripheral nerve sheath tumors. The presence of excess acid mucopolysaccharide-rich basal lamina substance may interfere with the production of normal collagen fibrils resulting in the formation of long-spacing collagen.[119,125,476] It is my opinion that the diagnostic efficacy of variations in fibril diameter and banding patterns is not yet firmly established.

Abnormal formation of banded collagen fibrils within cells, so-called intracellular collagen fibrils (Fig. 5-11), has been reported to occur in fibroblasts found in inflammatory tissue and in occasional mesenchymal neoplasms.[346,637] Intracellular collagen, usually found within membrane-bound vesicles that may fuse with lysosomes, has also been observed free in the cytoplasmic matrix. It has been suggested that these collagen fragments are the product of degradation of extracellular collagen fibrils by lysosomes within the tumor cell.[346] Intracellular collagen, although interesting, is not diagnostic.

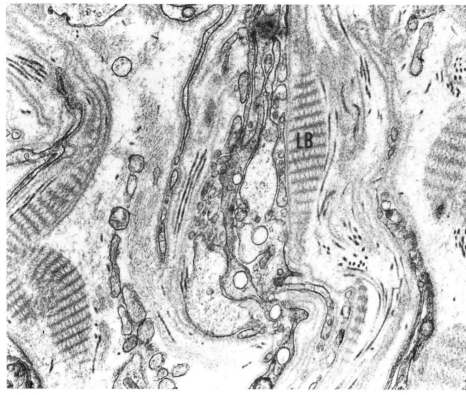

FIGURE 5-10
Benign schwannoma (groin, 72-year-old female). Numerous long-spacing collagen structures or Luse bodies (LB) are present in the interstitium of the Antoni type B tissue. (×18,400.)

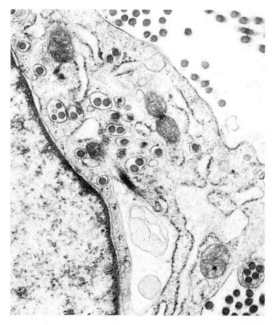

FIGURE 5-11
Epithelioid sarcoma (posterior neck, 49-year-old female). Cross-sectioned collagen fibrils are seen both in vacuoles within a fibroblastic cell and in the extracellular space. (×21,600.)

CHAPTER VI

Contribution of TEM to Tumor Diagnosis

This chapter presents 10 cases illustrating how TEM can contribute decisive, significant, or little information applicable to the accurate diagnosis of human tumors when the findings are correlated with available clinicopathologic data. A general summary of the monograph follows the case reports.

CASE REPORTS

The first two presentations are examples of tumors occurring in unusual locations. The third case is an example of a penile neoplasm that required ultrastructural evaluation in order to arrive at an accurate diagnosis. Cases 4 and 5 illustrate how electron microscopic findings confirm a diagnosis favored by the pathologist. Case 6 describes the problems encountered by the electron microscopist when studying small cell malignant tumors arising in the lung. Case 7 typifies the difficulty in interpreting the diagnostic significance of intracytoplasmic fibers. Cases 8–10 discuss tumors with fine structural characteristics that are not sufficiently distinctive to permit an accurate diagnosis despite a fairly certain diagnosis by light microscopy in case 8.

Case 1

A 41-year-old female first presented in 1972 with an 18-month history of vague chest discomfort and subsequent development of a right pleural effusion. Material obtained from thoracentesis was insufficient to make a diagnosis, so a right thoracotomy and total pleurectomy were performed. A large tumor mass measuring 12 cm in diameter and multiple smaller masses were found projecting into the pleural cavity. The tumors were incompletely excised. Histologic study indicated a malignant spindle cell tumor of unspecified type. A diagnosis of mesothelioma or a peculiar myosarcoma was

entertained. The patient was treated with radiation therapy. She remained free of symptoms due to tumor until 1979, when a computerized tomography (CT) scan for recurrent right-sided pain demonstrated the presence of a mass adjacent to the right crus of the diaphragm closely applied to the vertebral bodies of L1 and L2. In 1980, the patient underwent a laparotomy with partial resection of the paraspinal tumor. The remaining tumor was implanted with I-125 seeds. At this writing, the patient is back to normal activities with minimal symptoms.

Light microscopic examination

Specimens for histologic and electron microscopic studies were obtained from a lobulated mass of paraspinal tumor measuring 2.5 cm in maximum diameter. The cut surface was fleshy and pink with small foci of hemorrhage.

Light microscopically, the specimen consisted of a lobulated arrangement of round and fusiform cells with poorly defined boundaries surrounded by thick and thin fibrovascular septae (Fig. 6-1). Swirling patterns of cells were seen in some of the lobules. The nuclei were round or oval with stippled chromatin and inconspicuous nucleoli. Mitotic figures and psammoma bodies were not numerous. The tumor extended into the adjacent muscle and connective tissues. A tentative diagnosis of atypical cellular or low-grade malignant meningioma was made pending electron microscopic studies.

Toluidine blue stained 1-μm epoxy-embedded thick sections exhibited sheets of spindly cells with round or oval nuclei containing finely dispersed chromatin and one or two small round nucleoli (Fig. 6-2).

Electron microscopic examination

The electron microscopically examined specimen

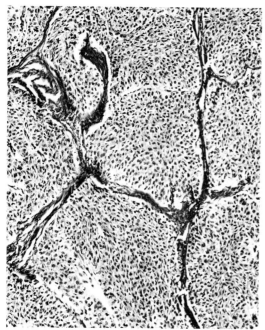

FIGURE 6-1
Case 1: Low-magnification photomicrograph showing clusters of oval and spindle-shaped tumor cells delineated by thin fibrovascular septae. (H&E, ×100.)

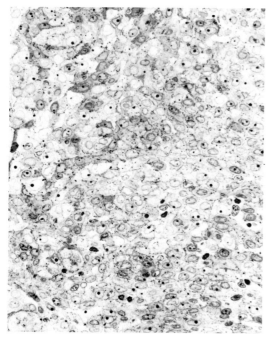

FIGURE 6-2
Case 1: Photomicrograph of epoxy-embedded tumor. Portion of a lobule of tumor cells showing finely dispersed chromatin and small, round, electron-dense nucleoli. (Toluidine blue, ×275.)

consisted of solid sheets of fusiform and spindle-shaped cells with relatively long, occasionally interdigitating cell processes, joined by numerous well-developed large desmosomes (Figs. 6-3 to 6-5). The nuclei were oval, irregular in contour, and slightly indented. The chromatin was generally finely dispersed, and one or two round, dense, centrally located or marginated nucleoli were evident. In addition to a normal complement of organelles, the cytoplasm contained small foci of glycogen particles and randomly oriented 6-nm microfilaments.

Discussion and conclusions

On the basis of the clinical and light microscopic findings, diagnoses of epithelial thymoma, mesothelioma, poorly differentiated squamous cell carcinoma, and meningioma were entertained. Epithelial thymomas composed of cells joined by numerous desmosomes usually contain numerous cytoplasmic cytokeratin filaments both as a component of the desmosomes and lying free in the cytoplasm. The absence of cytokeratin filaments ruled out a diagnosis of pure epithelial thymoma (a rare tumor), and the presence of large numbers of desmosomes is unusual in an anaplastic small cell epidermoid carcinoma. No long, shaggy microvilli characteristic of malignant epithelial mesotheliomas were found. Our findings were most consistent with a diagnosis of low-grade malignant meningothelial meningioma.

We are uncertain as to the origin of this tumor. The patient has a 8-year history of disease with no clinical evidence of intracranial tumor. The tumor most likely arose from a heterotopic arachnoid rest in the pleura, although origin in the thoracic or lumbar spinal canal with pleural extension cannot be ruled out. Extracranial and extraspinal meningiomas are rare lesions, usually occurring in the head and neck area (Wolff and Rankow, 1971). Ectopic meningiomas are known to arise in heterotopic brain and meningeal tissue that is occasionally found primarily in the midline of the head, neck, and trunk as a result of displacement of such tissue during fusion of the skull and spine in the embryo (So et al., 1978; Ho, 1980).

Final Diagnosis: Low-grade malignant meningothelial meningioma, most likely of pleural ectopic arachnoid cell rest origin.

Cited References

Ho, K-L.: Primary meningioma of the nasal cavity and paranasal sinuses.
   Cancer 46: 1442–1447, 1980.

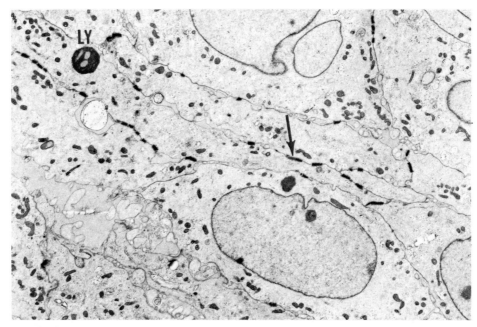

FIGURE 6-3
Case 1: Low-magnification electron micrograph showing sheets of neoplastic cells with long cytoplasmic processes. The cells are joined by numerous desmosomes (*arrow*). Note the finely dispersed chromatin, small nucleoli, and secondary lysosomes (LY). (×4320.)

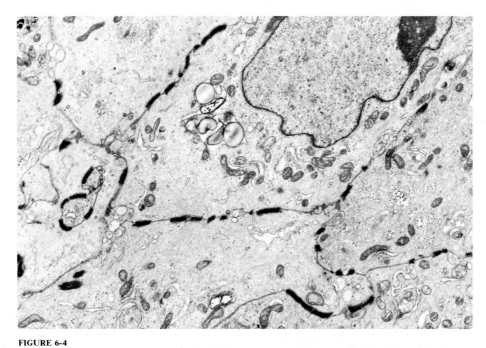

FIGURE 6-4
Case 1: Higher-magnification electron micrograph illustrating the interdigitating cell processes joined by numerous desmosomes. The organelle-free areas of the cytoplasm contain randomly oriented microfilaments. (×7200.)

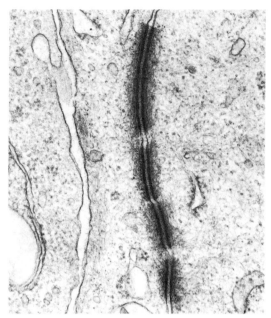

FIGURE 6-5
Case 1: Detail of four desmosomes. Note that the cytokeratin filaments extend only a short distance into the cytoplasm. (×38,000.)

So, S.C., Ngan, H., and Ong, G.B.: Ectopic meningiomas. Report of two cases and review of literature.
Surg Neurol 9: 231–237, 1978.
Wolff, M., and Rankow, R.M.: Meningioma of the parotid gland: an insight into the pathogenesis of extracranial meningiomas.
Hum Pathol 2: 453–458, 1971.

Case 2

A 37-year-old female was recently admitted to Memorial Hospital for Cancer and Allied Diseases (Memorial Hospital), New York City, with a complicated history of recurrent tumor since age 13, when a 9.5 × 6 × 6 cm right paraovarian cystic mass was excised. Histologic diagnosis was malignant papillary paraovarian cystoma. The lesion recurred when she was 23 years old as a large retroperitoneal mass measuring 18 cm in greatest diameter. A radical hysterectomy and pelvic cleanout, including bilateral salpingoophorectomy, was performed. The ovaries were uninvolved by tumor. Recently, exploratory laparotomy showed the presence of a large recurrent retroperitoneal mass that was deemed unresectable; the patient was admitted to Memorial Hospital, New York City. Further surgery demonstrated a 4 × 5 × 5-cm dumbbell-shaped retroperitoneal mass situated between the inferior vena cava and aorta. The surface of the mass was covered by a smooth, glistening membrane. A separate small implant in

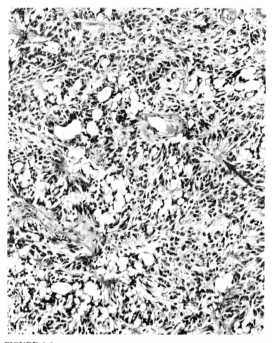

FIGURE 6-6
Case 2: Photomicrograph showing a complex histologic pattern. Perivascular pseudorosette (*arrow*). (H&E, ×110.)

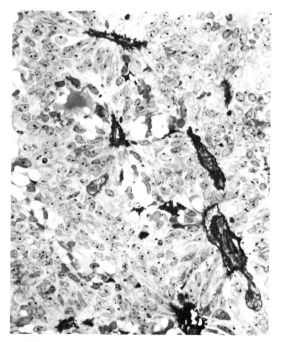

FIGURE 6-7
Case 2: Photomicrograph of epoxy-embedded tumor showing prominent perivascular pseudorosettes. (Toluidine blue, ×275.)

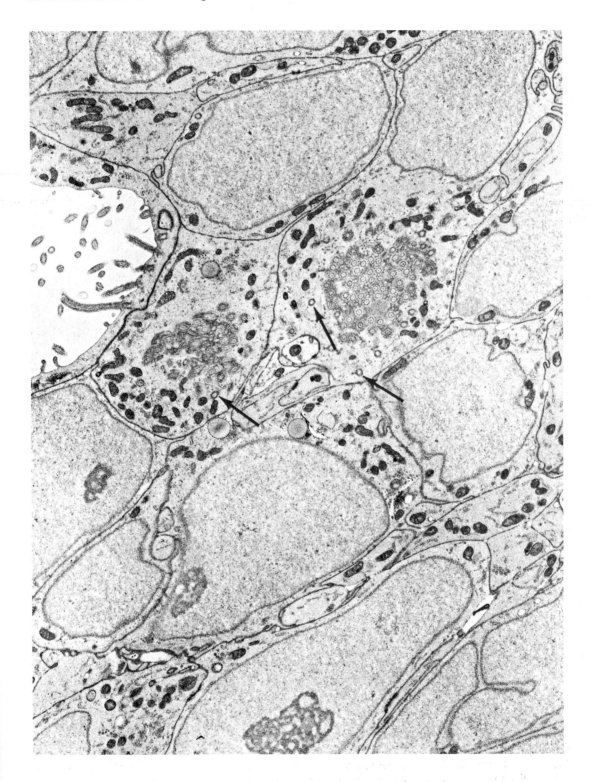

FIGURE 6-8
Case 2: Low-magnification electron micrograph of compactly arranged neoplastic ependymal cells. Note the finely dispersed nuclear chromatin, intracellular lumens (two of which are packed with cross-sectioned cilia), ciliary basal bodies (*arrows*), and the obliquely cut cytoplasmic processes sandwiched between adjacent cells. (×7200.)

the transverse mesocolon was also found. The patient was discharged in stable condition.

Light microscopic examination

The specimen submitted for pathologic examination consisted of a 5 × 8-cm soft, yellow-tan mass that was lobulated and partially cystic. The cysts contained an amber fluid, and the internal surface formed papillae.

Light microscopic examination exhibited a complex histologic picture of papillary structures lined by ciliated cuboidal or columnar cells with elongate nuclei and eosinophilic cytoplasm, solid foci of polygonal cells, scattered rosettes with small central lumens, and prominent perivascular pseudorosettes composed of capillaries with hyalinized walls surrounded by radiating, eosinophilic fibrillary tall columnar cell processes (Fig. 6-6). The elongate nuclei located at the distal pole contained small nucleoli and a moderate amount of fine chromatin particles. Mitotic figures were not numerous. Immunohistochemical staining for glial fibrillary acidic protein (Velasco et al., 1980) was focally positive. Positive staining by this process has been observed in astroglial and ependymal tumors. Review of all prior histologic material showed similar morphology. The light microscopic studies favored a diagnosis of an unusual cystic and papillary ependymoma of low-grade malignancy.

The histologic features of the tumor were shown in greater detail in the toluidine blue stained 1-μm epoxy-embedded specimens prepared for electron microscopic examination. Perivascular pseudorosettes were quite prominent (Fig. 6-7).

Electron microscopic examination

The electron microscopic features of the cells found in the solid areas and the pseudorosettes were sufficiently similar to allow a composite description. Unfortunately, papillary formations of tumor cells and true rosettes were not present in the submitted specimen. The compactly arranged elongated cells were joined by scattered primitive cell junctions. The moderately indented cigar-shaped nuclei contained finely dispersed chromatin and one or two relatively inconspicuous small round nucleoli (Fig. 6-8). Prominent intracellular lumens lined by variable numbers of rudimentary microvilli and cilia (Figs. 6-8 to 6-10) were a characteristic cytoplasmic feature. Subluminal ciliary basal bodies (blepharoplasts) (Fig. 6-8), small electron-dense mitochondria, randomly

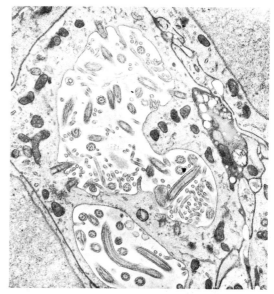

FIGURE 6-9
Case 2: Detail of two intracellular lumens showing longitudinally, tangentially, and cross-sectiond cilia and microvilli. (×8400.)

oriented microfilaments, and scattered bundles of intermediate-size glial filaments were also noted. Many transversely and obliquely cut peripheral cytoplasmic processes were sandwiched between adjacent cells. Long, straight cytoplasmic processes radiated from the central capillary wall in the pseudorosettes. The complexly folded bulbous basal surfaces were separated from the capillary endothelial cells by a tripartite structure that consisted of the thin basal lamina of the neoplastic cell, an amorphous substance containing randomly oriented collagen fibrils, and the thickened capillary basal lamina (Fig. 6-10). This structure corresponded to the hyalinized vascular wall seen in the histologic sections.

Discussion and conclusions

Both the histologic and ultramicroscopic findings strongly support a diagnosis of ependymoma of low-grade malignancy. These tumors are characterized by both perivascular pseudorosettes and true rosettes lined by columnar cells with occasional luminal cilia and blepharoplasts. A variant forming papillary structures has also been described. The absence of ovarian involvement by tumor rules out a low-grade papillary serous cystadenocarcinoma; these tumors almost always consist of nonciliated cells that do not form perivascular pseudorosettes (see p. 107).

Of interest is the site of origin of this tumor.

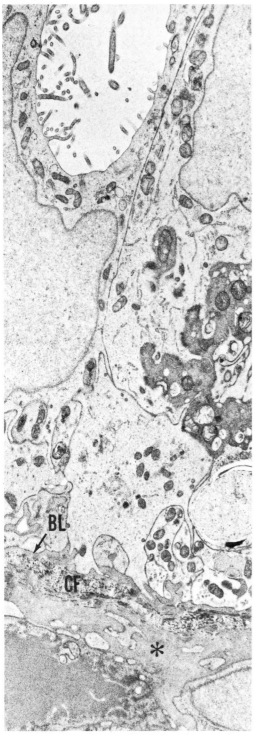

FIGURE 6-10
Case 2: Portion of a perivascular pseudorosette. Note (*top to bottom*): the intracellular lumen, nuclei containing finely dispersed chromatin, amorphous electron dense cellular debris (*right center*), complexly folded basal cell processes, thin basal lamina of ependymal cells (BL), collagen fibrils (CF), thickened (hyalinized) capillary basal lamina (*asterisk*), and capillary. (×7920.)

Careful clinical workup, including CT scans, demonstrated no intraventricular masses. In the spinal cord, a large percentage of the ependymomas originate in the lumbar and sacral regions, especially from the conus medullaris or the filum terminale. The latter is a unique structure that extends into the sacrum and consists of connective tissue derived from the pia mater, neural elements, neuroglial elements, and conspicuous ependymal cells. The most common type ependymoma arising in the filum terminale is the myxopapillary variant (Rubinstein, 1972; Wolff et al., 1972; Rawlinson et al., 1973). These tumors occasionally metastasize to the retroperitoneum. No involvement of the lower spinal regions was found, however. We suggest that this is a unique extraspinal low-grade malignant ependymoma arising in a paraovarian ependymal rest in the broad ligament with retroperitoneal metastases.

Final Diagnosis: Paraovarian ependymoma with retroperitoneal metastases.

Cited References

Rawlinson, D.G., Herman, M.M., and Rubinstein, L.J.: The fine structure of a myxopapillary ependymoma of the filum terminale.
Acta Neuropathol (Berl) 25: 1–13, 1973.

Rubinstein, L.J.: Tumors of the Central Nervous System. In: *Atlas of Tumor Pathology.* 2nd ser., fasc. 6. Armed Forces Institute of Pathology, Washington, D.C., 1972, pp. 104–126.

Wolff, M., Santiago, H., and Duby, M.D.: Delayed distant metastasis from a subcutaneous sacrococcygeal ependymoma. Case report with tissue culture, ultrastructural observations and review of the literature.
Cancer 30: 1046–1067, 1972.

Velasco, M.E., Dahl, D., Roessmann, U., and Gambetti, P.: Immunohistochemical localization of glial fibrillary acidic protein in human glial neoplasms.
Cancer 45: 484–494, 1980.

Case 3

A 59-year-old male was admitted to Memorial Hospital, New York City, in June 1979 with a 4–6-week history of splaying of urine and penile bleeding. He noticed a lesion developing on the dorsum of his meatus, which had grown rapidly during this period. The patient was otherwise completely asymptomatic. A Papanicolaou smear was positive for malignant cells, and subsequent biopsy demonstrated anaplastic malignant tumor consistent with either carcinoma or malignant melanoma. Partial penectomy and cystoscopy were performed. There was no lesion in the bladder or urethra other than the one at the meatus. Postoperatively, the patient did well and was discharged with a guarded prognosis.

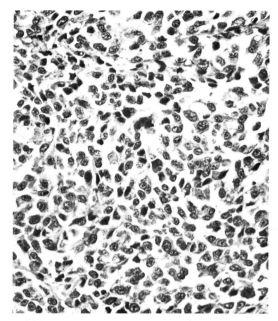

FIGURE 6-11
Case 3: Photomicrograph of randomly organized pleomorphic epithelioid cells infiltrating the corpora cavernosa. (H&E, ×250.)

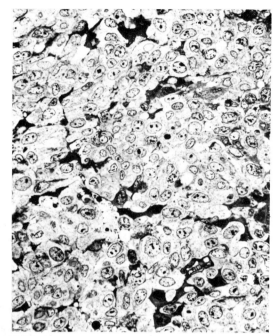

FIGURE 6-13
Case 3: Photomicrograph of epoxy-embedded tumor showing sheets of neoplastic cells and foci of electron-dense fibrous septae. Note the multiple nucleoli. (Toluidine blue, ×325.)

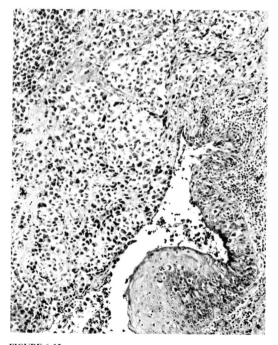

FIGURE 6-12
Case 3: Low-magnification photomicrograph showing ulcerated surface of glans penis infiltrated by tumor. Note the pagetoid changes in the intact squamous epithelium (*bottom right*). (H&E, ×90.)

Light microscopic examination

The surgical specimen consisted of the glans penis, surrounding soft tissues, and skin. An ill-defined, markedly indurated, glistening yellowish white tumor with focal areas of hemorrhage was found that involved the distal urethra (fossa navicularis) and infiltrated into the corpora cavernosa. The overlying skin of the glans penis was focally ulcerated. The tumor measured 2.3 × 1.5 × 0.5 cm.

Histologically, the tumor was composed of loosely organized pleomorphic epithelioid cells of varying size without any definitive cellular pattern (Fig. 6-11). The hyperchromatic nuclei varied in size and shape, and the cytoplasm was eosinophilic. Although pagetoid changes were evident in the stratified squamous epithelium adjacent to the ulcerated foci, no junctional changes were noted (Fig. 6-12). Mitotic figures were frequent. The Fontana-Masson silver stain and ferric ferricyanide reduction technique for melanin gave negative results. Light microscopic findings favored anaplastic squamous cell carcinoma over amelanotic malignant melanoma, pending ultrastructural studies.

The toluidine blue stained 1-µm-thick sections

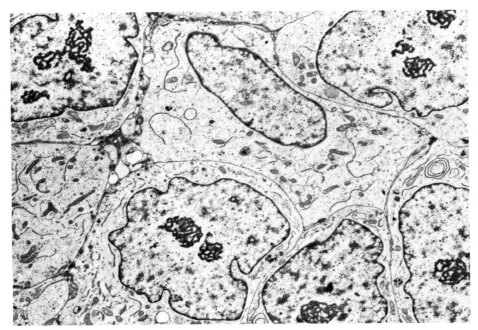

FIGURE 6-14
Case 3: Low-magnification electron micrograph showing sheets of neoplastic cells with pleomorphic nuclei containing multiple nucleoli. No cell junctions are evident. (×4320.)

showed solid clusters of tumor cells separated by delicate fibrous septae (Fig. 6-13). The round-to-oval nuclei were of variable size and contained finely clumped chromatin and multiple nucleoli; foci of spindle-shaped cells were also noted. The cytoplasm was abundant and focally granular.

Electron microscopic examination

The specimen consisted of aggregates of large polygonal and spindle-shaped cells with indented nuclei containing scattered small clumps of chromatin and multiple ropelike nucleoli (Fig. 6-14). The abundant cytoplasm contained scattered mitochondria, long cisternae of RER, ribosomes, small bundles of microfilaments, occasional lysosomes, and vacuoles (Fig. 6-14). High-magnification examination (20,000–40,000×) indicated widely dispersed foci of ellipsoidal lamellar (Fig. 6-15) and spiral premelanosomes (Fig. 3-104). No fully pigmented mature melanosomes or cell junctions were found.

Discussion and conclusions

The findings did not support a diagnosis of ana-

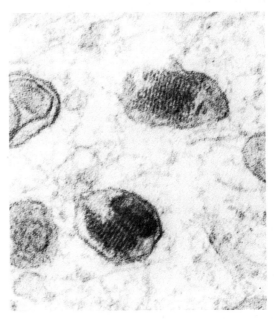

FIGURE 6-15
Case 3: High-magnification electron micrograph illustrating two ellipsoidal lamellar premelanosomes. Note the typical cross-banded (*striated*) pattern of the core. (×100,000.)

plastic carcinoma (Manglani et al., 1980), as no cytokeratin filaments or desmosomes were found. The demonstration of premelanosomes in the poorly differentiated epithelioid tumor cells clearly established the diagnosis of amelanotic malignant melanoma of the distal urethra. No junctional changes in the surface squamous epithelium were noted, and the bulk of the tumor involved the corpora cavernosa and the corpus spongiosum. This case represents a perfect example of a tumor that required electron microscopic evaluation to establish histogenesis. Malignant melanomas arising in the urethral mucosa are very rare (Guinn and Ayala, 1970; Bracken and Diokno, 1974).

The patient refused to undergo radical penectomy with perineal urethrostomy and bilateral prophylactic groin dissection. Metastasis subsequently developed and the patient was advised to have chemotherapy. The patient died of disease.

Final Diagnosis: Amelanotic malignant melanoma of the distal urethra.

Cited References

Bracken, R.B., and Diokno, A.C.: Melanoma of the penis and the urethra: 2 case reports and review of the literature. *J Urol 111: 198–200, 1974.*

Guinn, G.A., and Ayala, A.G.: Male urethral cancer: Report of 15 cases including a primary melanoma. *J Urol 103: 176–179, 1970.*

Manglani, K.S., Manaligod, J.R., and Biswamay, R.: Spindle cell carcinoma of the glans penis. A light and electron microscopic study. *Cancer 46: 2266–2272, 1980.*

Case 4

A 39-year-old-male sought medical attention in March 1973, when he noticed a sensation of tightness and pressure in his upper thorax just below the clavicles. Routine x-ray examination showed a large superior mediastinal mass. Bilateral simultaneous superior vena cavagrams showed displacement and obstruction of the superior vena cavae. Additional workup demonstrated no further disease. Mediastinoscopy suggested a primary superior mediastinal tumor. In April 1973 a sternotomy was performed; a large mass was removed that included the superior margins of the pericardium, a portion of the left lung, and tumor that extended in and around the large veins on both sides of the mediastinum. The lesion was removed in its entirety. The postoperative course was uneventful and the patient was discharged in early May 1973. The patient is free of clinical disease as of June 1980.

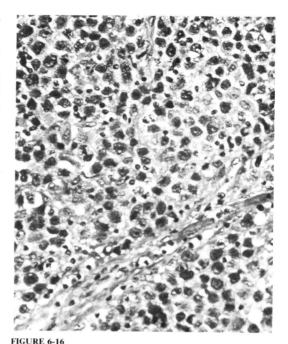

FIGURE 6-16
Case 4: Photomicrograph of viable areas of mediastinal tumor showing sheets of moderately large neoplastic cells with prominent round nuclei and scattered small lymphocytes located primarily in the region of the fibrous septae. (H&E, ×250.)

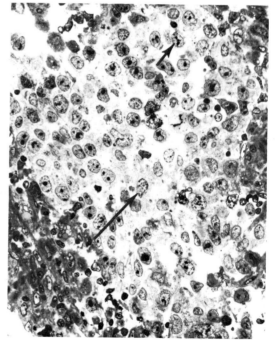

FIGURE 6-17
Case 4: Photomicrograph of epoxy-embedded tumor. Most of the neoplastic cells contain rounded nucleoli, although occasional elongated (*short arrows*) and fragmented (*long arrow*) nucleoli are also evident. (Toluidine blue, ×300.)

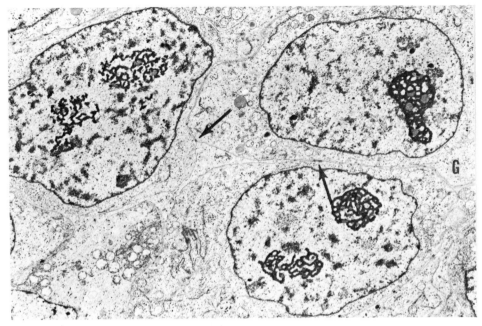

FIGURE 6-18
Case 4: Electron micrograph showing portions of four neoplastic cells. Three nucleoli consist of complexly twisted fibrous strands (nucleolonema). Note the primitive cell junctions (*arrows*) and widely scattered glycogen particles (G). (×6720.)

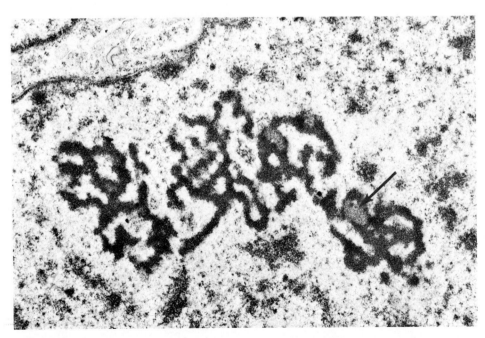

FIGURE 6-19
Case 4: Detail of nucleolar structure showing loosely organized fibrous strands and small granular component (*arrow*). (×16,800.)

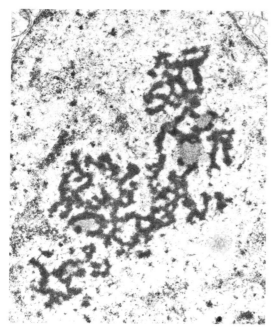

FIGURE 6-20
Case 4: Mediastinal seminoma (anterior mediastinum, 23-year-old man). Nucleolus from another patient with a typical mediastinal seminoma. Note the elongated and fragmented fibrous component. (×11,600.)

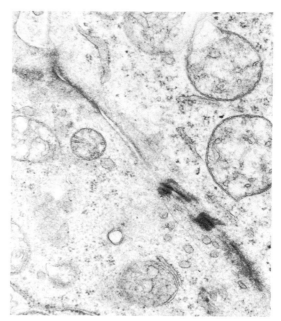

FIGURE 6-21
Case 4: Distorted junctional complex adjacent to a small lumen, a small part of which is evident (*top left*). (×25,200.)

Light microscopic examination

The specimen received for histologic study consisted of an irregular tumor mass measuring 14 × 11 × 8 cm and weighing 510 g. The external surface was covered with fibromuscular tissue and contained many irregular nodules measuring 0.1–3 cm in diameter. The cut surface was both firm and soft in consistency with finely granular and white-tan as well as yellowish-white fibrous areas. The tumor appeared to be completely covered by a very thin membranelike structure. The anterior chest wall and a biopsy of the left upper lobe of the lung showed no tumor.

Microscopically, the tumor consisted of sheets and cords of moderately large, round or polyhedral cells of uniform size separated by thin bands of collagen infiltrated with mature lymphocytes (Fig. 6-16). Extensive areas of necrosis were also noted. Mitotic cells were infrequent. The moderately large tumor cells contained a round, centrally located nucleus with coarsely stippled chromatin and a prominent slightly eosinophilic nucleolus. The relatively conspicuous cytoplasm was lightly stained with eosin. The cell borders were indistinct.

Cellular detail was more evident in the toluidine

blue stained 1-μm-thick sections of epoxy-embedded tissue. The relatively large round nuclei of the tumor cells variously contained either a large centrally located nucleolus or multiple, elongate, or fragmented nucleoli (Fig. 6-17). The surrounding collagenous trabeculae contained variable numbers of small lymphocytes. In other areas of the tumor, lymphocytes were scattered among the large neoplastic cells. A diagnosis of mediastinal seminoma was favored by most of the staff pathologists, although a histiocytic lymphoma or thymoma could not be ruled out.

Electron microscopic examination

The specimen submitted for electron microscopic examination was received fresh and consisted of sheets of large round or ovoid cells joined by an occasional cell junction (Fig. 6-18). The regularly shaped nuclei contained evenly scattered foci of heterochromatin and one or more prominent nucleoli. Although more typical rounded nucleoli with well-developed fibrous strands (nucleolonema) were found in approximately 60% of the cells, the remaining 40% had nucleoli with complex, elongated, fragmented fibrous strands that contained small foci of rounded granular masses (Figs. 6-18 and 6-19; see also Fig. 6-20). The abundant cytoplasm contained some small foci of glycogen particles in addition to a normal complement of organelles (Fig. 6-18). The cells were joined by widely scattered primitive cell junctions, although one section showed evidence of an abortive junctional complex (Fig. 6-21). Cytoplasmic fibrils were scant, and no basal lamina was noted. Scattered small collections of mature lymphocytes were seen both in the fibrous trabeculae and the sheets of tumor cells.

Discussion and conclusions

The ultrastructural characteristics of this tumor, i.e., fragmented nucleoli with a prominent fibrous component (nucleolonema), foci of cytoplasmic glycogen, and scattered rudimentary cell junctions, are similar to those found in testicular seminoma (Pierce, 1966; Schulze and Holstein, 1977; Janssen and Johnston, 1978; Damjanov et al., 1980), the closely related ovarian dysgerminoma (Ferenczy, 1976), and pineal germinoma (Markesberg et al., 1976). Our findings thus confirm the pathologists' tentative diagnosis of mediastinal seminoma (germinoma).

There is no question that electron microscopic examination can provide a definitive answer in cases for which the histologic evaluation of an anterior mediastinal tumor is equivocal (Levine, 1973; Rosai and Levine, 1976). The presence of well-developed fragmented nucleoli, and especially intercellular junctions, rules out a diagnosis of lymphoma. The absence of elongated cytoplasmic processes joined by well-formed desmosomes and curvilinear bundles of cytokeratin filaments (tonofilaments) eliminates the diagnosis of thymoma, whereas the rare thymic carcinoid tumors contain prominent dense-core endosecretory granules (Levine and Rosai, 1976). (See Table 1-2 and appropriate sections of the text for further explanation.)

Final Diagnosis: Mediastinal seminoma (germinoma).

Cited References

Damjanov, I., Niejadlik, D.C., Rabuffo, J.V., and Donadio, J.A.: Cribriform and sclerosing seminoma devoid of lymphoid infiltrates.
Arch Pathol Lab Med 104: 527–530, 1980.
Ferenczy, A.: The ultrastructural morphology of gynecologic neoplasms.
Cancer 38: 463–486, 1976.
Janssen, M., and Johnston, W.H.: Anaplastic seminoma of the testis. Ultrastructural analysis of three cases.
Cancer 41: 538–544, 1978.

Levine, G.D.: Primary thymic seminoma—A neoplasm ultrastructurally similar to testicular seminoma and distinct from epithelial thymoma.
Cancer 31: 729–741, 1973.
Levine G.D., and Rosai, J.: A spindle cell variant of thymic carcinoid tumor. A clinical, histologic, and fine structural study with emphasis on its distinction from spindle cell thymoma.
Arch Pathol Lab Med 100: 293–300, 1976.
Markesbery, W.R., Brooks, W.H., Milsow, L., and Mortara, R.H.: Ultrastructural study of the pineal germinoma in vivo and in vitro.
Cancer 37: 327–337, 1976.
Pierce, G.B.: Ultrastructure of human testicular tumors.
Cancer 19: 1963–1983, 1966.
Rosai, J., and Levine, G.D.: Tumors of the thymus. In *Atlas of Tumor Pathology*, 2nd ser., fasc. 13. Armed Forces Institute of Pathology, Washington, D.C., 1976.
Schulze, C., and Holstein, A.F.: On the histology of human seminoma. Development of the solid tumor from intratubular seminoma cells.
Cancer 39: 1090–1100, 1977.

Case 5

An obese 51-year-old female discovered a small nodule at the posterior aspect of the right elbow in July 1979. She was treated at another hospital for arthritis for 6 months, but the lesion continued to grow. In March 1980 she underwent a carpel tunnel release operation. Pathologic study exhibited a poorly differentiated small round cell tumor involving the mid-dermis and subcutaneous tissue. The patient underwent wide local excision and skin grafting in April 1980. Within 3 weeks the tumor recurred on the medial aspect of the right arm, and she was admitted to Memorial Hospital, New York City, for further evaluation and treatment in July 1980. She complained of burning progressive pain in the elbow down the forearm with numbness along the medial side of the forearm.

Physical examination found a large, diffuse tender swelling on the medial aspect of the right forearm and some fullness in the right axilla with tenderness. Radiologic studies indicated the presence of a tumor mass measuring approximately 5 cm in diameter just below the elbow on the medial and lateral aspects of the right upper extremity. The patient then received 1200 rads to the right elbow joint over a period of 5 days. She subsequently underwent a right arm forequarter amputation in late July 1980, as the tumor mass was unresectable. The patient's postoperative course was uncomplicated and she was discharged in satisfactory condition with a guarded prognosis. Follow-up examination in September 1980 showed no sign of recurrence or metastasis.

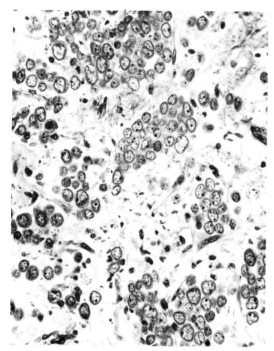

FIGURE 6-22
Case 5: Photomicrograph showing nests of moderately large round cells with a large nucleocytoplasmic ratio in edematous connective tissue. Note the rim of eosinophilic cytoplasm. (H&E, ×275.)

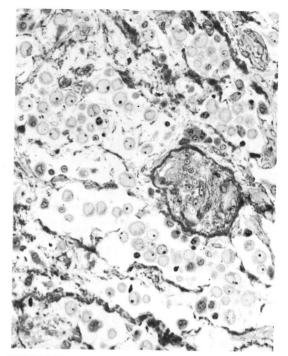

FIGURE 6-23
Case 5: Photomicrograph of epoxy-embedded tumor. Note the large nucleocytoplasmic ratio, finely dispersed chromatin, marginated nucleoli, and thin rim of cytoplasm. (Toluidine blue, ×275.)

Light microscopic examination

The specimen consisted of the right arm and scapula. Dissection of the amputated limb exhibited a large tumor mass measuring 10 × 5 × 5 cm located 5 cm from the anticubital fossa in the area of the biceps. Tumor was found adherent to nerves and fascia around the biceps, but did not grossly appear to involve the biceps, triceps, other muscle groups in the area, or the neurovascular bundle. Multiple lymph nodes ranging from 0.5 to 4.5 cm in diameter were identified in the axilla. Many of the larger nodes showed homogeneous white tissue when sectioned. Gross examination showed the bones of the arm and the scapula to be free of tumor.

Histologic study indicated that the tumor involved the dermis and subcutaneous tissue at the site of prior biopsy and the biceps muscle. Vascular involvement was also noted and multiple metastases were present in seven of 14 axillary lymph nodes. The margins of resection were free of tumor. Clusters of monomorphous round tumor cells were evident in the dermis, subcutaneous adipose tissue, and between bundles of skeletal muscle fibers. The

large round tumor cell nuclei contained finely dispersed chromatin and several small nucleoli. The nucleus was surrounded by a thin rim of eosinophilic cytoplasm (Fig. 6-22). Mitotic cells were fairly numerous. The cytologic features are seen in greater detail in the toluidine blue stained 1-μm thick sections of epoxy-embedded tissue. Note the distinct lack of nuclear heterochromatin, small marginated nucleoli, and scanty cytoplasm (Fig. 6-23). The Grimelius, Fontana-Masson, and mucicarmine stains were negative. A tentative diagnosis of Merkel cell carcinoma was made pending ultrastructural confirmation.

Electron microscopic examination

A small specimen of tumor in the dermis and subcutaneous tissue overlying the biceps muscle was submitted for ultrastructural evaluation. The specimen consisted of loosely organized clusters of uniformly round tumor cells embedded in a stroma composed of finely granular material and scattered collagen fibrils (Fig. 6-24). The nuclei were generally round or oval and had a smooth contour, except for one or two small cytoplasmic

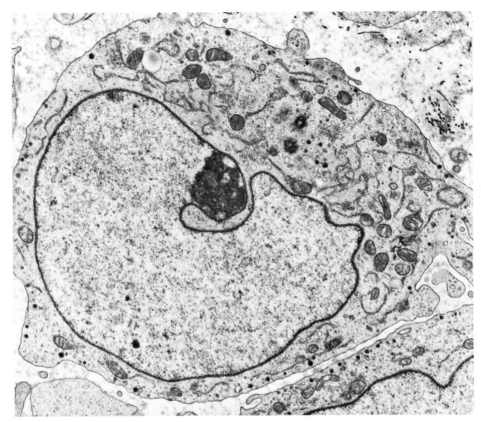

FIGURE 6-24
Case 5: Electron micrograph of one neoplastic cell and a portion of another. Dense-core neurosecretory-type granules are found in the Golgi cytoplasm (marked by two cross-sectioned centrioles) and just beneath the plasmalemma. Note the finely dispersed chromatin and the small nucleolus adjacent to the cytoplasmic indentation. (×9200.)

indentations. The chromatin was dispersed (euchromatin), and one or sometimes two small round marginated nucleoli were seen adjacent to the cytoplasmic herniations (Fig. 6-24). The nuclei were surrounded by a small amount of cytoplasm, except at the Golgi pole of the cell. The cytoplasm contained a moderately well-developed Golgi apparatus and scattered mitochondria and RER cisternae. In addition to the usual organelles, the cytoplasm also contained small (115–170-nm) round membrane-limited dense-core neurosecretory-type granules located both in the Golgi region and in the ectoplasm (Fig. 6-24). A distinct feature was the linear arrangement of the granules just beneath the plasmalemma (Figs. 6-24 and 6-25). No cytoplasmic fibrils, intercellular junctions, or basal laminas were identified.

Discussion and conclusions

The ultrastructural findings confirm the tentative diagnosis of so-called Merkel cell carcinoma (DeWolf-Peeters et al., 1980; Sibley et al., 1980; Sidhu et al., 1980). These primary cutaneous tumors are most likely derived from the Merkel cell (this has not been proved), a neuroendocrine or APUD cell presumably of neural crest origin and found as a component of the tactile hair disc of Pinkus, which forms complexes with slowly adapting mechanoreceptors (see Winkelmann, 1977; Sibley et al., 1980). Isolated Merkel cells are also occasionally found in the epidermis and dermis (Hashimoto, 1972). This recently described morphologically recognizable tumor was originally called "trabecular carcinoma of the skin" (Toker, 1972; Tang and Toker, 1978), and in a recent abstract was referred to as "small cell neuroepithelial tumor of the skin" (Silva and Mackay, 1980). Neoplastic Merkel cells frequently contain perinuclear bundles of 10-nm intermediate filaments in addition to the neurosecretory-type granules characteristically found both in the Golgi region

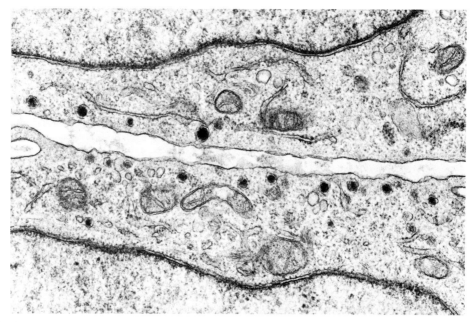

FIGURE 6-25
Case 5: Portions of two neoplastic cells showing 115–170-nm neurosecretory-type granules arranged in single file just beneath the plasmalemma. (×25,000.)

of the cytoplasm and in the ectoplasm. Although I have seen primitive cell junctions in other cases of Merkel cell carcinomas, none were found in this case.

The differential diagnosis of poorly differentiated cutaneous tumors composed of relatively small round cells includes anaplastic skin appendage tumors (cf. case 10), metastatic neuroendocrine tumors (apudomas), amelanotic melanomas, and non-Hodgkin's lymphoma. The presence of fairly numerous neurosecretory-type (endosecretory) granules and the absence of specific markers, e.g., premelanosomes, effectively eliminates all the above-mentioned entities, except metastatic apudoma. Careful workup ruled out the existence of a primary small cell neuroendocrine tumor, e.g., oat cell carcinoma, elsewhere in the body. The absence of neuritic processes makes an extremely rare cutaneous adult neuroblastoma unlikely (Mackay et al., 1976). The precise origin of this tumor, however, remains speculative, because it is possible that small cell carcinomas of skin adnexal origin can produce neurosecretory-type granules (Taxy et al., 1980).

Final Diagnosis: Merkel cell carcinoma.

Cited References

De Wolf-Peeters, C., Marien, K., Mebis, J., and Desmet, V.:

A cutaneous APUDoma or Merkel cell tumor? A morphologically recognizable tumor with a biological and histological malignant aspect in contrast with its clinical behavior.
Cancer 46: 1810–1816, 1980.
Hashimoto, K.: The ultrastructure of the skin of human embryos. X. Merkel tactile cells in the finger and nail.
J Anat 111: 99–120, 1972.
Mackay, B., Luna, M.A., and Butler, J.J.: Adult neuroblastoma. Electron microscopic observations in nine cases.
Cancer 37: 1334–1351, 1976.
Sibley, R.K., Rosai, J., Foucar, E., Dehner, L.P., and Bosl, G.: Neuroendocrine (Merkel cell) carcinoma of the skin. A histologic and ultrastructural study of two cases.
Am J Surg Pathol 4: 211–221, 1980.
Sidhu, G.S., Feiner, H., and Flotte, T.J.: Merkel cell neoplasms. Histology, electron microscopy, biology, and histogenesis.
Am J Dermatopathol 2: 101–119, 1980.
Silva, E.G., and Mackay, B.: Small cell neuroepithelial tumor of the skin.
Lab Invest 42: 151, 1980. (Abstr.)
Tang, C-K., and Toker, C.: Trabecular carcinoma of the skin. An ultrastructural study.
Cancer 42: 2311–2321, 1978.
Taxy, J.B., Ettinger, D.S., and Wharam, M.D.: Primary small cell carcinoma of the skin.
Cancer 46: 2308–2311, 1980.
Toker, C.: Trabecular carcinoma of the skin.
Arch Dermatol 105: 107–110, 1972.
Winkelmann, R.K.: The Merkel cell system and a comparison between it and the neurosecretory or APUD cell system.
J Invest Dermatol 69: 41–46, 1977.

Case 6

This 29-year-old male first noticed mild shortness

of breath and stridorous breathing in June of 1973. Respiratory symptoms progressed, and in October the patient began to cough up whitish sputum. Bronchoscopy at another hospital demonstrated the presence of a friable mass obstructing the left main stem bronchus. Biopsy disclosed oat cell carcinoma. The patient was admitted to Memorial Hospital, New York City, for further evaluation and treatment in early December 1973. X-ray examination showed left lower lobe atelectasis; pulmonary function studies showed moderate irreversible airway obstruction. No symptoms attributable to ectopic hormone production were evident. Bronchoscopy and left exploratory thoracotomy with pneumonectomy indicated a tumor 2 cm proximal from the carina obstructing the left main bronchus and involving hilar lymph nodes. Left hilar lymph nodes were submitted for histologic and electron microscopic study. The patient received radiation therapy and chemotherapy for known residual tumor. His disease progressed, and he died of respiratory failure within 1 year.

Light microscopic examination

The specimens received for histologic study consisted of fragments of grayish-tan tissues of varying size and a 2 × 1.5-cm left hilar lymph node that was tan, soft, and homogeneous. Histologic examination found two basic cell patterns: one consisting of elongated fusiform cells with hyperchromatic nuclei and scanty cytoplasm arranged in ribbons (Fig. 6-26), and another consisting of aggregates of varying size and shape of similar-appearing cells. No ductules or rosettes were evident. Only small disorganized aggregates of ovoid and spindle-shaped cells were present in the fragment of a left hilar lymph node submitted for electron microscopic evaluation (Fig. 6-27). The light microscopic diagnosis was metastatic malignant tumor with features of oat cell carcinoma and malignant carcinoid tumor in hilar lymph nodes.

Electron microscopic examination

The specimen submitted for electron microscopic examination consisted mainly of small aggregates of fusiform and spindle-shaped cells with a large nuclear–cytoplasmic ratio (Fig. 6-28). The nuclei were pleomorphic, filled with chromatin clumps of various sizes and small nucleoli. The scanty cytoplasm contained few organelles except for prominent polysomes. Isolated spherical neurosecretory-type granules of 90–110-nm diameter

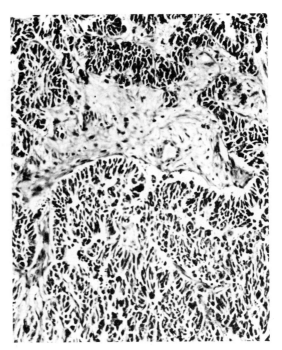

FIGURE 6-26
Case 6: Survey photomicrograph of more differentiated area of tumor showing ribbons of elongated cells as well as more disorganized clusters of neoplastic cells. (H&E, ×150.)

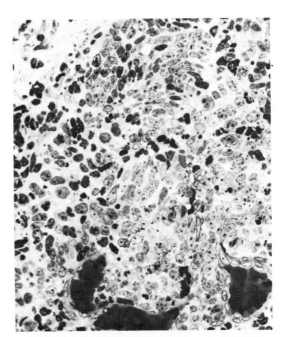

FIGURE 6-27
Case 6: Photomicrograph of epoxy-embedded tumor. The ovoid and spindle-shaped neoplastic cells are haphazardly arranged in the vicinity of congested blood vessels. (Toluidine blue, ×275.)

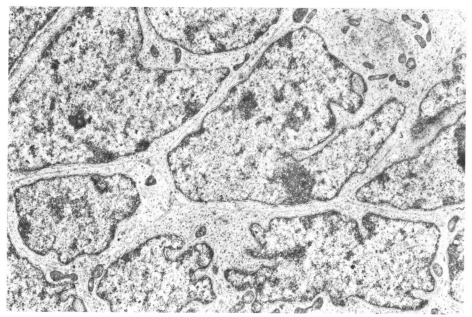

FIGURE 6-28
Case 6: Electron micrograph showing sheets of poorly differentiated neoplastic cells with pleomorphic nuclei.
(×7600.)

were found in the cytoplasm in a small focus of more differentiated cells (Figs. 6-29 to 6-31). The nuclear chromatin was more dispersed, and rudimentary cell junctions were found in only one section (Fig. 6-31). Mitotic cells were fairly prominent. No cytoplasmic fibers, e.g., cytokeratin filaments, or lumens with surface microvilli were identified.

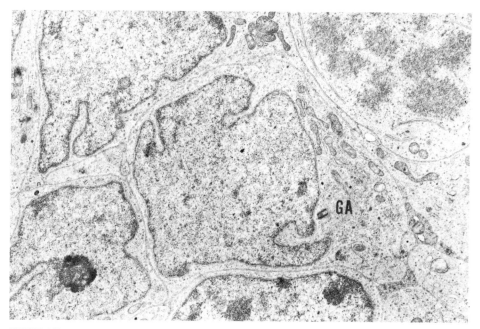

FIGURE 6-29
Case 6: Careful inspection will show the presence of scattered small neurosecretory-type granules, especially in the vicinity of the Golgi apparatus (GA), in this rare focus of more differentiated neoplastic cells. Note the mitotic cell (*top right*). (×11,200.)

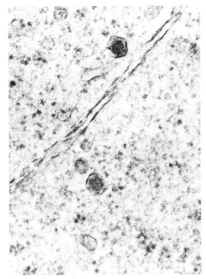

FIGURE 6-30
Case 6: High-magnification electron micrograph showing two neurosecretory-type granules measuring 100 nm in diameter. (×54,000.)

Discussion and conclusions

Whereas features of both malignant carcinoid tumor (ribbon pattern) and oat cell carcinoma (irregular aggregates of fusiform or lymphocyte-like cells) were evident in the histologically ex-

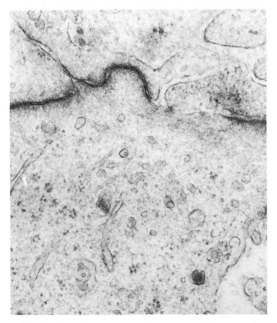

FIGURE 6-31
Case 6: Rare focus of primitive cell junctions. Note the lone neurosecretory-type granule (*bottom right*). (×35,200.)

amined sections, only the aggregates of the more poorly differentiated cells were present in the specimen submitted for ultrastructural evaluation.

This is a perfect example of the sampling problems encountered by the electron microscopist. Examination of the cells in the more differentiated trabecular areas might have revealed more neurosecretory-type granules or cell junctions. The demonstration of isolated neurosecretory-type granules and primitive cell junctions, however, in one small focus of tumor cells, was sufficient to support the tentative diagnosis of oat cell carcinoma.

As discussed in the text (p. 50), the term oat cell is descriptive. These tumors are not derived from Kultschitzky-type cells found in the lung unless scattered clusters of neurosecretory-type granules are identified by electron microscopic examination. The cells comprising the ribbonlike aggregates are large and spindled. A large spindle-cell variant of peripheral bronchial carcinoid tumor, although quite rare, has been described (Churg, 1977; Gillespie et al., 1979). The cells comprising these tumors are joined by desmosomes and contain abundant 80–160-nm spherical, dense-core neurosecretory granules.

It is generally recognized that oat cell carcinoma is a highly malignant variant of carcinoid tumor derived from Kultschitzky-type cells found in bronchial epithelium and glands, and that the neurosecretory granules are often larger and always more prominent in bronchial carcinoid tumors (Bensch et al., 1968; Hattori et al., 1972; McDowell et al., 1976; Fisher et al., 1978). It is important to recognize, however, that not all so-called oat cell lung carcinomas have neurosecretory-type granules (see Gould and Chejfec, 1978). Such tumors may be anaplastic bronchial basal cell tumors, poorly differentiated small cell variants of squamous cell carcinoma (Churg et al., 1980), or adenocarcinomas.

Final Diagnosis: Malignant tumor with features of malignant carcinoid tumor and oat cell carcinoma.

Cited References

Bensch, K.G., Corrin, B., Pariente, R., and Spencer, H.: Oat-cell carcinoma of the lung. Its origin and relationship to bronchial carcinoid.
Cancer 22: 1163–1172, 1968.
Churg, A.: Large spindle cell variant of peripheral bronchial carcinoid tumor.
Arch Pathol Lab Med 101: 216–218, 1977.

Churg, A., Johnston, W. H., and Stullbarg, M.: Small cell squamous and mixed small cell squamous-small cell anaplastic carcinomas of the lung.
  Am J Surg Pathol 4: 255–263, 1980.
Fisher, E.R., Palekar, A., and Paulson, J.D.: Comparative histopathologic, histochemical, electron microscopic and tissue culture studies of bronchial carcinoids and oat cell carcinomas of the lung.
  Am J Clin Pathol 69: 165–172, 1978.
Gillespie, J.J., Luger, A.M., and Callaway, L.A.: Peripheral spindled carcinoid tumor: a review of its ultrastructure, differential diagnosis, and biologic behavior.
  Hum Pathol 10: 601–606, 1979.
Gould, V.E., and Chejfec, G.: Ultrastructural and biochemical analysis of "undifferentiated" pulmonary carcinomas.
  Hum Pathol 9: 377–384, 1978.
Hattori, S., Matsuda, M., Tateishi, R., Nishihara, H., and Horai, T.: Oat-cell carcinoma of the lung. Clinical and morphologic studies in relation to its histogenesis.
  Cancer 30: 1014–1024, 1972.
McDowell, E.M., Barrett, L.A., and Trump, B.F.: Observations on small granule cells in adult human bronchial epithelium and in carcinoid and oat cell tumors.
  Lab Invest 34: 202–206, 1976.

Case 7

A healthy 16-year-old male presented to his physician with a 1-month history of three masses measuring up to 8 cm in greatest diameter on the left lower back over the ninth rib. The tumor was excised and reported as a small round cell sarcoma, possibly of neuroectodermal origin. The patient was admitted to Memorial Hospital, New York City, for further evaluation. On physical examination, two 3-cm nodules were found close to the ends of the surgical scar and a palpable lymph node was discovered in the lower left axilla. X-ray examination of the chest disclosed a left paravertebral mass below T10–T11, which probably represented the primary tumor. At surgery, the two nodules were reexcised and the enlarged axillary lymph nodes were removed. A thoracotomy performed at the same time found multiple pleural nodules in addition to a large unresectable paravertebral mass.

Light microscopic examination

Tissue from the subcutaneous tumor, an axillary lymph node, and a piece of pleura were submitted for pathologic examination. A portion of one of the tumor nodules was processed for electron microscopic evaluation.

Review of slides from the initial operation at another hospital showed a small cell malignant tumor that could not be precisely classified. A primitive neuroectodermal tumor was favored.

The specimens obtained from the back nodules

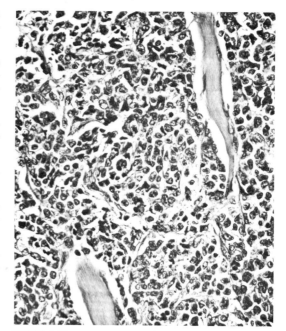

FIGURE 6-32
Case 7: Photomicrograph showing sheets of pleomorphic cells with no apparent organization infiltrating skeletal muscle. (H&E, ×300.)

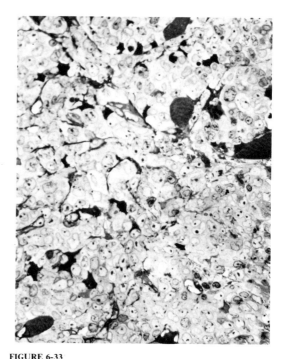

FIGURE 6-33
Case 7: Photomicrograph of epoxy-embedded tissue showing sheets of poorly differentiated neoplastic cells and fragments of striated muscle (larger, dense structures). (Toluidine blue, ×325.)

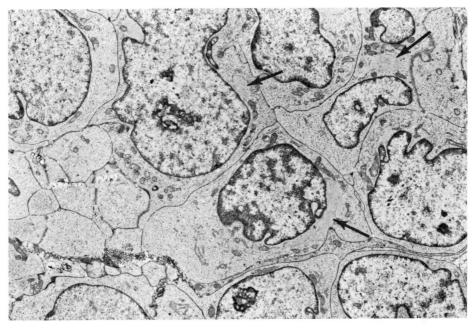

FIGURE 6-34
Case 7: Survey electron micrograph showing cohesive sheets of poorly differentiated cells containing numerous polysomes. Perinuclear bundles of intermediate filaments (*arrows*). (×4320.)

consisted of loosely organized sheets of small round, polygonal, and stellate cells with a high nucleocytoplasmic ratio infiltrating skeletal muscle (Fig. 6-32). The nuclei were pleomorphic and hyperchromatic and the scanty cytoplasm was eosinophilic and often indistinct. Mitotic figures were frequent. Similar-appearing tumor cells were also found in the enlarged axillary lymph node and in

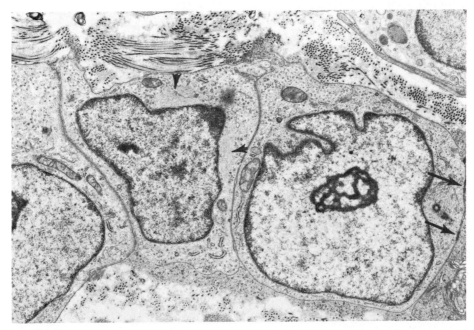

FIGURE 6-35
Case 7: Linear arrangement of four neoplastic cells surrounded by a collagenous stroma. Cell junctions (*arrows*), intermediate filaments (*arrowheads*). (×7600.)

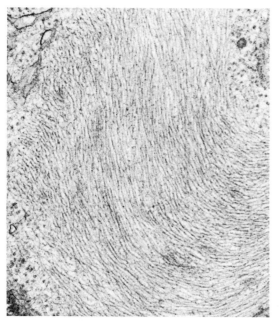

FIGURE 6-36
Case 7: Disorganized bundle of cytoplasmic intermediate filaments in nuclear depression. (×38,000.)

the pleural nodules. The light microscopic findings favored a diagnosis of embryonal rhabdomyosarcoma over primitive neuroectodermal tumor.

The toluidine blue stained 1-μm sections of epoxy-embedded tissue exhibited coherent sheets of moderate-size round and ovoid cells and fragments of normal skeletal muscle (Fig. 6-33). The tumor cell nuclei were round or slightly pleomorphic and contained a prominent centrally located nucleolus. The distinct cytoplasm of the cells appeared homogeneous and stained light blue.

Electron microscopic examination

The specimens submitted for electron microscopic evaluation consisted primarily of sheets of ovoid and fusiform cells joined by scattered primitive cell junctions (Fig. 6-34). Rare linear formations of similar-appearing cells surrounded by collagen on their free surfaces were also identified (Fig. 6-35). The tumor cell nuclei varied in size and shape and contained a moderate-size nucleolus that was usually centrally located. The chromatin pattern varied considerably from cell to cell.

The cytoplasm of the neoplastic cells contained prominent polysomes and bundles of nonspecific intermediate filaments measuring 8–10 nm in di-

ameter (Figs. 6-34 to 6-36). Actin microfilaments (6 nm), muscle myosin (15 nm), and Z discs were not identified.

Discussion and conclusions

This case is a classic example of the problems encountered in the differential diagnosis of small round cell tumors arising in adolescents. Cell shape and the presence of intercellular junctions rule out a diagnosis of non-Hodgkin's lymphoma. The absence of dendritic or axonic cell processes and conspicuous microtubules does not favor a primitive neuroectodermal tumor, although it is often difficult to make this diagnosis. It is generally agreed that the minimum ultrastructural criterion for the diagnosis of embryonal rhabdomyosarcoma is the demonstration of recognizable arrays of actin and myosin myofilaments usually associated with linearly arrayed ribosomes (see Figs. 3-111 to 3-115) (Morales et al., 1972; Gonzalez-Crussi and Black-Schaffer 1979). Identification of Z disc material is an added helpful feature.

These tumors are best classified as childhood sarcomas of undetermined histogenesis, even though it can be argued that these cells are destined to become rhabdomyoblasts, since animal studies show the presence of wavy bundles of intermediate filaments during the early stages of myogenesis (Granger and Lazarides, 1980). In a recent abstract, Newton and Soule (1976) stated that children with sarcomas of undetermined histogenesis tend to be older at diagnosis and that the tumors appear more frequently along the trunk. Survival of patients with these tumors treated with chemotherapy designed for embryonal rhabdomyosarcoma appears comparable to that observed in children or adolescents with that tumor. Although the prognosis is grave, the patient is responding to chemotherapy.

Final Diagnosis: Childhood sarcoma of undetermined histogenesis.

Cited References

Gonzalez-Crussi, F., and Black-Schaffer, S.: Rhabdomyosarcoma of infancy and childhood. Problems of morphologic classification. (Review.)
  Am J Surg Pathol 3: 157–171, 1979.
Granger, B.L., and Lazarides, E.: Synemin: A new high molecular weight protein associated with desmin and vimentin filaments in muscle.
  Cell 22: 727–738, 1980.
Morales, A.R., Fine, G., and Horn, R.C., Jr.: Rhabdomyosarcoma: an ultrastructural appraisal.
  Pathol Annu 7: 81–106, 1972.

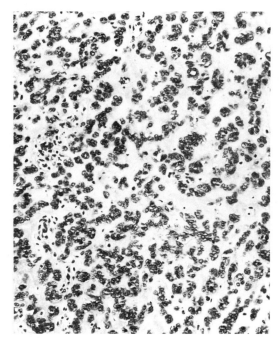

FIGURE 6-37
Case 8: Low-magnification photomicrograph showing variable-size clusters of neoplastic cells in a lightly stained chondromyxoid matrix. (H&E, ×130.)

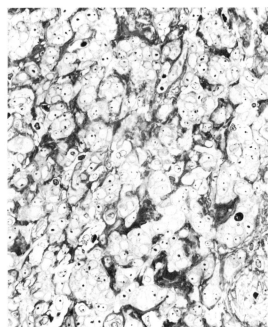

FIGURE 6-38
Case 8: Photomicrograph of epoxy-embedded tumor. The pale-staining cells lie within an amorphous densely stained matrix. Note the finely dispersed chromatin and the small round nucleoli. (Toluidine blue, ×325.)

Newton, W.A., and Soule, F.: Childhood sarcomas of undetermined histogenesis: Comparison with childhood rhabdomyosarcoma.
Am J Pathol 82: PPC-2, 1976. (Abst.)

Case 8

A 2.5-month-old male baby presented at another hospital in August 1975 with a lemon-size mass in the right outer thigh. Physical examination showed no other evidence of tumor. At surgery, a soft, tan, glistening, focally hemorrhagic tumor measuring approximately 4 × 6 cm was resected from the fascial planes of the vastus lateralis muscle about 20 cm (8 in.) below the femoral triangle. A diagnosis of embryonal rhabdomyosarcoma was suspected. Slides and formalin-fixed tissue were sent to Memorial Hospital, New York City, for consultation. The tumor recurred in the thigh and was reexcised in September 1975. The neoplasm was treated with actinomycin D, methotrexate, vincristine, cytoxan, and adriamycin (different combinations of drugs at different times). In April 1976 inguinal nodes were dissected for clinically metastatic disease. Pulmonary metastases were noted in August 1976, and the patient subsequently died from heart failure in May 1977.

Light microscopic examination

The predominant histologic pattern was that of collections of 2–10 rounded cells with relatively large vesiculated nuclei and scanty cytoplasm surrounded by a pale-staining lightly eosinophilic chondromyxoid matrix (Fig. 6-37). Sheets of closely packed cells of a similar histology infiltrating hemorrhagic muscle tissue were also evident. The ground substance stained positively with PAS with and without diastase pretreatment. The Alcian blue stain was more positive at pH 2.5 than at pH 1.0. The intensity of staining at both pH values was slightly reduced by hyaluronidase pretreatment.

On the basis of the histologic and histochemical findings, a diagnosis of malignant tumor with some chondroid features, most likely a mesenchymal chondrosarcoma, was made.

The toluidine blue stained 1-μm-thick sections of epoxy-embedded tumor exhibited irregular clusters of pale-staining uniform round and oval cells separated by an amorphous blue-violet matrix (Fig. 6-38). The smooth-contoured nuclei contained finely dispersed chromatin and one or two small nucleoli. Mitotic cells were not prominent.

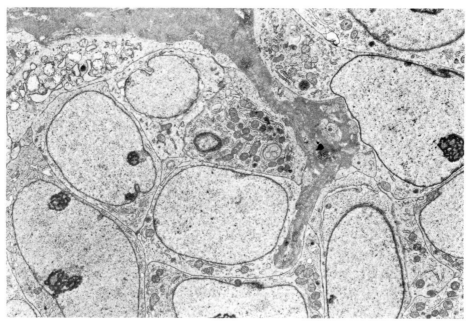

FIGURE 6-39
Case 8: Low-magnification electron micrograph of an irregular cluster of round-to-oval tumor cells delineated by a densely granular matrix. (×4320.)

Electron microscopic examination

Tissue for electron microscopic study was initially fixed in buffered formalin. Closely packed clusters of round-to-oval cells with large euchromatic nuclei and scanty cytoplasm embedded in a dense fibrillogranular matrix formed the bulk of the tumor (Figs. 6-39 and 6-40). The nuclei were smooth-surfaced or slightly notched and contained one or two relatively small nucleoli. The cytoplasm contained moderate numbers of mitochondria; a distinct Golgi apparatus; scattered, somewhat dilated, RER cisternae; ribosomes; rare small foci of glycogen particles; and lysosomes (Fig. 6-40). Lipid droplets and intercellular junctions were not identified. The intercellular matrix was homogeneous and densely granular and contained foci of fine collagen fibrils (Fig. 6-39).

Discussion and conclusions

Extraskeletal mesenchymal chondrosarcoma is a rare malignant tumor composed of small round-to-oval poorly differentiated cells arranged singly or in clumps with focal areas of cartilagenous or chondroid matrix. Only a few ultrastructural studies of this entity, and myxoid and chordoid variants of chondrosarcoma, have been reported

in the literature (Enzinger and Shiraki, 1972; Angerwall and Enerback, 1973; Steiner et al., 1973; Fu and Kay, 1974; Smith et al., 1976; Whelan Weiss, 1976; Mehio and Ferenczy, 1978). These studies support the finding of chondroblastic differentiation by findings of dilated RER, well-developed Golgi apparatus, lipid droplets, glycogen particles, rare cells with a scalloped surface, and areas of extracellular matrix characteristic of hyaline cartilage. It must be emphasized that most of the tumors are composed primarily of more poorly differentiated mesenchymal cells, whereas well-defined areas of mature cartilage are often absent.

The present case is a probable example of a poorly differentiated extraskeletal mesenchymal chondrosarcoma. Features compatible with chondroblastic differentiation include a well-developed often dilated RER and Golgi apparatus, foci of glycogen particles, and histochemical findings favoring a sulfated mucopolysaccharide matrix. Lipid droplets, a scalloped cell surface, and a matrix consisting of loosely dispersed randomly oriented fine fibrils lacking periodicity and proteoglycan granules—all characteristic of differentiated neoplastic chondrocytes—are not evident. The above-described cytoplasmic features for this tumor are nondiagnostic, all being manifested to varying degrees in other neoplasms.

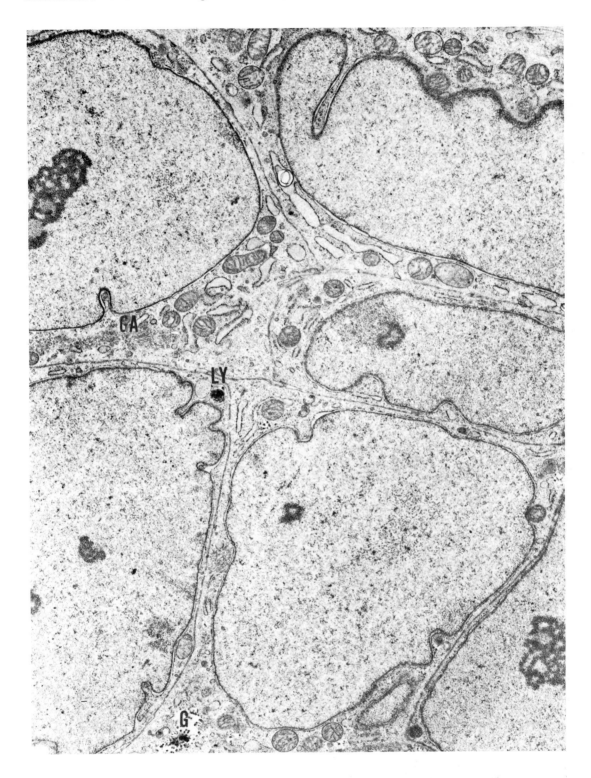

FIGURE 6-40
Case 8: Portion of a typical cluster of tumor cells with a large nucleocytoplasmic ratio. Mitochondria, partially dilated RER cisternae, a Golgi apparatus (GA), a secondary lysosome (LY), and a focus of glycogen particles (G) are evident in the cytoplasm. (×11,200.)

Highly cellular variants, as in this case, generally have a poor prognosis.

Three neoplasms that fulfill the morphologic criteria of mesenchymal chondrosarcoma have been examined in our laboratory. One, from the thigh of a 41-year-old female closely resembled the present case, although the cells were smaller. The second case, from the femur of a 37-year-old male, was also morphologically similar, but the matrix consisted of randomly oriented collagen fibrils. The third case, from the arm of a 65-year-old female, was unusual in that it consisted predominantly of well-differentiated chondrocytes with prominent cytoplasmic lipid and glycogen. The cells also had a scalloped plasmalemma.

Final Diagnosis: Malignant tumor with some chondroid features most consistent with a diagnosis of extraskeletal mesenchymal chondrosarcoma.

Cited References

Angerwall, L. Enerback, L., and Knutson, H.: Chondrosarcoma of soft tissue origin.
  Cancer 32: 507–513, 1973.
Enzinger, F.M., and Shiraki, M.: Extraskeletal myxoid chondrosarcoma. An analysis of 34 cases.
  Hum Pathol 3: 421–435, 1972.
Mehio, A.R., and Ferenczy, A.: Extraskeletal myxoid chondrosarcoma with "chordoid" features (chordoid sarcoma).
  Am J Clin Pathol 70: 700–705, 1978.
Smith, M.T., Farinacci, C.J., Carpenter, H.A., and Bannayan, G.A.: Extraskeletal myxoid chondrosarcoma. A clinicopathological study.
  Cancer 37: 821–827, 1976.
Steiner, G.C., Mirra, J.M., and Bullough, P.G.: Mesenchymal chondrosarcoma. A study of the ultrastructure.
  Cancer 32: 926–939, 1973.
Whelan Weiss, S.: Ultrastructure of the so-called "chordoid sarcoma." Evidence supporting cartilagenous differentiation.
  Cancer 37: 300–306, 1976.
Fu, Y-S., and Kay, S.: A comparative ultrastructural study of mesenchymal chondrosarcoma and myxoid chondrosarcoma.
  Cancer 33: 1531–1542, 1974.

Case 9

A 41-year-old male first presented in October 1973 with pain in the right calf followed by a painful swollen left arm, suggesting left subclavian thrombosis. In January 1974, extensive bilateral cervical lymphadenopathy developed and the patient was admitted to Memorial Hospital, New York City, for further evaluation. Incisional biopsy of an enlarged left cervical lymph node demonstrated metastatic poorly differentiated carcinoma

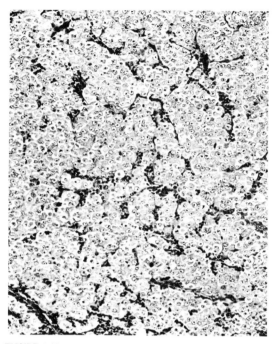

FIGURE 6-41
Case 9: Low-magnification photomicrograph showing sheets of uniformly large round cells effacing the lymph node. (H&E, ×180.)

which showed some epidermoid features. The nasopharynx and lung were considered possible primary sites. Examination and biopsy of the nasopharynx showed no tumor. Chest x-rays were inconclusive. The patient subsequently received 6000 rads to the neck. In June 1974 headache and drowsiness developed and neurologic workup demonstrated a mass in the right anterior cranial fossa. Biopsy of the right frontal lobe found metastatic poorly differentiated carcinoma. Physical workup showed firmness in the right upper quadrant. The patient subsequently received bleomycin therapy pushed to toxicity followed by 5-fluorouracil. Seizure activity and increasing dyspnea developed. The patient's condition progressively deteriorated, and he died in respiratory failure in November 1975. No autopsy was performed.

Light microscopic examination

Two cervical lymph nodes, one measuring 1.8 cm and the other 2.5 cm in greatest dimension, were submitted for histologic and electron microscopic evaluation. The lymph nodes were firm with a whitish homogeneous cut surface.

Histologically, the specimen consisted of ir-

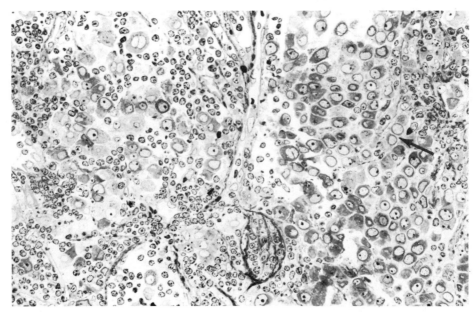

FIGURE 6-42
Case 9: Photomicrograph of epoxy-embedded tumor. The large round cells are arranged singly or in clumps. Note the more densely stained substance encircling the nucleus in some of the cells (*arrow*). (Toluidine blue, ×325.)

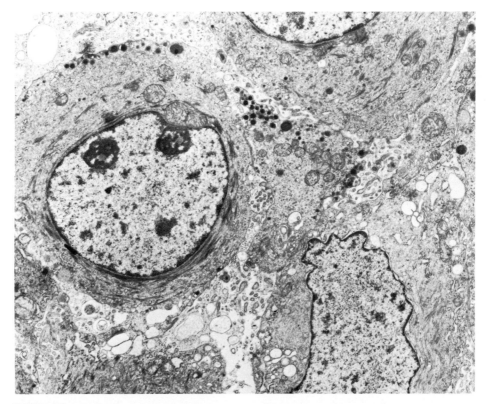

FIGURE 6-43
Case 9: Electron micrograph of typical tumor cells showing the prominent perinuclear profiles of cytokeratin filaments, peripherally located secretory granules, and foci of surface microvilli. (×6000.)

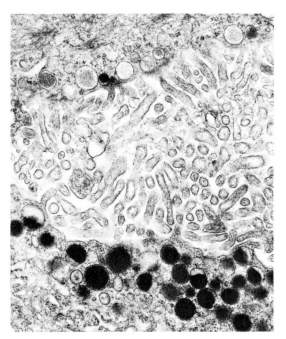

FIGURE 6-44
Case 9: Higher-magnification electron micrograph of a portion of the surface of two cells. Note the variously sectioned profiles of microvilli, the cytokeratin filaments, the more electron-lucent membrane-limited secretory granules (*top*), and the electron-dense membrane bound secretory granules (*bottom*). (×17,000.)

regular nests of uniform large round cells with centrally located nuclei and distinctly eosinophilic cytoplasm delineated by remnants of lymphoid tissue (Fig. 6-41). The large round nuclei had a fine chromatin pattern and contained a centrally located nucleolus. Melanin, Grimelius, and mucicarmine stains were negative. The neoplasm was diagnosed as a poorly differentiated carcinoma with some epidermoid features. Possible sites of origin include the paranasal sinus, nasopharynx, and lungs.

The light microscopic features were shown in greater detail in the toluidine blue stained 1-μm-thick sections. The nuclei of the neoplastic cells were encircled by a rim of dense blue-staining homogeneous material (Fig. 6-42).

Electron microscopic examination

The electron microscopic evaluated specimens consisted of uniform epithelial tumor cells exhibiting foci of surface microvilli (Fig. 6-43). The round nuclei contained irregularly dispersed clumps of chromatin of varying size and multiple small nucleoli. The intense perinuclear staining

noted in the thick sections was caused by curvilinear profiles of cytokeratin filaments (tonofilaments). Some cells contained large bundles of these filaments, occupying most of the cytoplasm. Another prominent feature of the tumor cells was the peripherally located secretory granules (Figs. 6-43 and 6-44). Most of the granules contained an electron-dense core and were limited by a membrane. They ranged in size from 140 to 400 nm, with an average diameter of 290 nm. Rare primitive cell junctions were noted in areas of cell contact.

Discussion and conclusions

The ultrastructural findings suggest that this tumor is most likely a metastatic adenocarcinoma derived from a serous or possibly a seromucous gland with extensive areas of squamous metaplasia. These glands are located in the lamina propria of the nasopharynx, paranasal sinuses, and in the primary and secondary bronchi up to the point at which the cartilage ends (Breeze and Wheeldon, 1977). Unfortunately, the site of origin of this tumor remains speculative, since permission for autopsy was not obtained.

This case is also a good example of the problems encountered by the electron microscopist when interpreting the nature of secretory granules. The granules have an average diameter of 290 nm, although some range up to 400 nm in size, well within the size range for neuro- or endosecretory-type granules. Small subsurface electron-dense mucigen (Fig. 3-47) and serous granules (Fig. 3-48) are seen, however, in mucin-producing and some serous adenocarcinomas, respectively. As special stains for mucin and neurosecretory granules are negative, and the histologic and ultrastructural findings of numerous cytokeratin filaments and prominent surface microvilli are not consistent with a neuroendocrine tumor (apudoma), we favor origin in a serous gland. Nevertheless, we cannot rule out a variant of small cell lung carcinoma derived from either the Kultschitzky cell or another cell type that has undergone squamous metaplasia (Churg et al., 1980) or multidirectional differentiation (Gould et al., 1981). It is also unlikely that the granules are primary lysosomes because of the subsurface distribution.

I have not seen a tumor with a similar morphology, and as far as I am aware none has been reported in the literature. An acinic cell tumor originating from a serous cell in a bronchial submucosal gland was studied by Fechner and associates (1972). The neoplastic cells comprising the latter tumor, however, contained numerous large serous granules distributed throughout the cytoplasm and no cytokeratin filaments.

Final Diagnosis: Poorly differentiated adenocarcinoma with extensive areas of squamous metaplasia, most likely originating in a bronchial submucosal serous gland.

Cited References

Breeze, R.G., and Wheeldon, E.B.: The cells of the pulmonary airways. (Review.)
Am Rev Resp Dis 116: 705-777, 1977.
Churg, A., Johnston, W.H., and Stulbarg, M.: Small cell squamous and mixed small cell squamous-small cell anaplastic carcinomas of the lung.
Am J Surg Pathol 4: 255-263, 1980.
Fechner, R.E., Bentinck, B.R., and Askew, J.B., Jr.: Acinic cell tumor of the lung. A histologic and ultrastructural study.
Cancer 29: 501-508, 1972.
Gould, V.E., Memoli, V.A., and Dardi, L.E.: Multidirectional differentiation in human epithelial cancers.
J Submicrosc Cytol 13: 97-115, 1981.

Case 10

A 74-year-old male was first seen by his physician in March 1976 with a chief complaint of suprapubic and left inguinal swelling. One month earlier he claimed he had injured his pubic region while lifting a table. The patient was advised to treat the area of swelling with hot sponges. In June 1976 the swelling increased again and he was admitted to Memorial Hospital, New York City. Workup showed a suprapubic mass and slightly enlarged left inguinal lymph nodes. He was in little pain, had no difficulty urinating and had no hematuria. Physical examination was otherwise unremarkable. The suprapubic mass and one left inguinal lymph node were surgically excised and submitted for histologic and ultrastructural evaluation. As of January 1978 the patient was free of clinical disease.

Light microscopic examination

The specimen from the suprapubic area consisted of an 11 × 8 × 7-cm encapsulated mass covered by an ellipse of skin and subcutaneous tissue. Sectioning of the tumor showed a moderately soft tan tissue with scattered foci with a more rubbery consistency and a few cysts filled with a thin mucoid fluid. The inguinal lymph node was uninvolved by tumor.

On histologic examination, the specimen was shown to consist of solid sheets of moderate-size

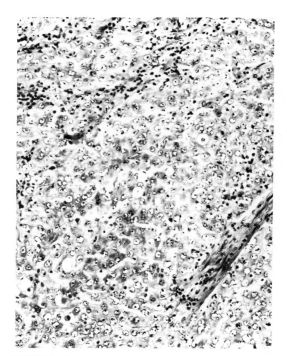

FIGURE 6-45
Case 10: Low-magnification photomicrograph showing sheets of polygonal tumor cells infiltrating loose connective tissue. (H&E, ×120.)

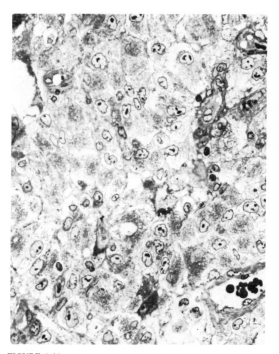

FIGURE 6-46
Case 10: Photomicrograph of epoxy-embedded tissue showing cellular structure in more detail. Note the relatively large areas of granular cytoplasm. Blood vessel (*bottom right*). (Toluidine blue, ×325.)

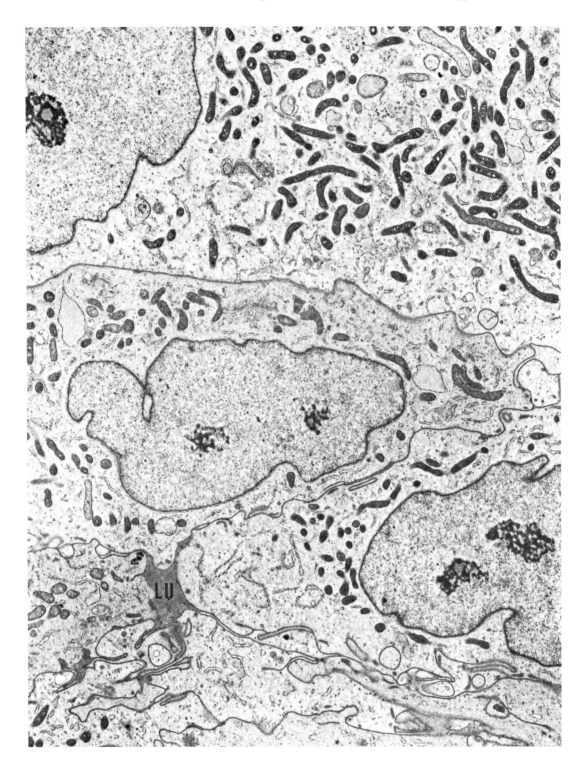

FIGURE 6-47
Case 10: Electron micrograph showing portions of large, pleomorphic, contiguous neoplastic cells. The abundant cytoplasm contains numerous elongated mitochondria. Note the lumenlike intercellular space (LU). (×6720.)

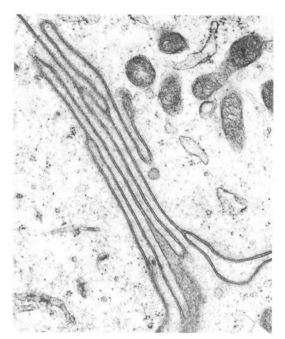

FIGURE 6-48
Case 10: Detail of interdigitating cell membranes.
(×24,000.)

uniform, round and polygonal cells containing one or sometimes two nuclei, and infiltrating loose connective tissue (Fig. 6-45). The abundant cytoplasm was focally granular and eosinophilic. The granular nature of the cytoplasm was more pronounced in the toluidine blue stained 1-μm-thick epoxy-embedded sections (Fig. 6-46). The nuclei contained two to three nucleoli and finely dispersed chromatin. Mucicarmine and melanin stains were negative. The histologic diagnosis was anaplastic malignant tumor, favoring carcinoma over sarcoma pending ultrastructural findings. The overlying skin was uninvolved by tumor.

Electron microscopic examination

The specimen submitted for electron microscopic examination consisted of sheets of large pleomorphic cells with irregularly shaped nuclei containing multiple small nucleoli and finely dispersed chromatin (euchromatin) (Fig. 6-47). In addition to a normal complement of organelles, the cytoplasm contained prominent foci of electron-dense mitochondria, accounting for the cytoplasmic granularity seen in the histologic sections. Lumenlike intercellular spaces containing an electron-dense granular substance (Fig. 6-47) and prominent interdigitating apposing cell membranes (Fig. 6-48)

were also evident. No cell junctions, secretory granules, or intracytoplasmic fibers were found, however. Mitotic cells were infrequent, and an occasional small capillary was noted. Small, rare intercellular spaces contained scattered collagen fibrils embedded in a granulofilamentous material.

Discussion and conclusions

Clearly, the light microscopic and ultrastructural findings are not sufficiently distinctive to establish an unequivocal diagnosis, although the histologic pattern and fine structural prominence of interdigitating cell membranes favor an anaplastic carcinoma over a sarcoma. As illustrated in the text discussion (Fig. 4-4), interdigitating cell membranes are also found in epithelioid sarcomas. The clinicopathologic setting and histologic findings rule out this entity, as these tumors of uncertain histogenesis always arise in the subcutaneous tissue or in the tendons and fascia of the extremities. They consist of distinctive irregular nodular masses of large eosinophilic polyhedral cells, often with necrotizing foci (resembling granulomas) surrounded by hyalinized collagen (Enzinger, 1970; Bloustein et al., 1976). Although ultrastructural features distinctive for squamous cell carcinoma (bundles of cytokeratin filaments and cytokeratin–desmosome complexes) or adenocarcinoma (secretory granules and abortive glandular lumens with projecting microvilli) are absent, we suspect that the neoplasms is a poorly differentiated skin appendage lesion (Hashimoto and Lever, 1969), since metastatic carcinoma was ruled out and the patient is currently free of clinical disease (the mass was excised with the margins free of tumor).

This is a classic example of a poorly differentiated tumor devoid of sufficiently distinctive histologic and fine structural features that could be used to determine cytogenesis and site of origin.

Final Diagnosis: Poorly differentiated carcinoma of skin appendage origin.

Cited References

Bloustein, P.A., Silverberg, S.G., and Waddell, W.R.: Epithelioid sarcoma. Case report with ultrastructural review, histogenetic discussion, and chemotherapeutic data. *Cancer 38: 2390–2400, 1976.*

Enzinger, F.M.: Epithelioid sarcoma: A sarcoma simulating a granuloma or a carcinoma. *Cancer 26: 1029–1041, 1970.*

Hashimoto, K., and Lever, W.F.: Histogenesis of skin appendage tumors. (Review.)
   Arch Dermatol 100: 356–369, 1969.

SUMMARY

This monograph has attempted to show how TEM contributes to the diagnosis of human tumors by the analysis of fine structural details. It is my contention that TEM is complementary to light microscopy and should be correlated with relevant clinicopathologic data whenever possible.

I would like to briefly summarize the contributions and limitations I have found using TEM.

Contributions

1. Transmission electron microscopy often helps the surgical pathologist resolve a difficult differential diagnosis.
2. Depending on the experience of the pathologist, a small but significant number of tumors are unequivocally diagnosable on the basis of ultrastructural findings.
3. Transmission electron microscopy can help the pathologist decide that an exact diagnosis is not possible and that the neoplasm may thus reasonably be classified in relatively general terms, such as "anaplastic sarcoma with spindle cell features," and so forth.

Limitations

The following technical problems encountered by the electron microscopist and difficulties in interpreting ultrastructural data serve to point out some serious limitations of this adjunct technique.

1. Lack of adequate sampling either quantitatively or by the submission of inappropriate material, i.e., normal tissue adjacent to a tumor.
2. Well-preserved representative areas of tumor is an essential prerequisite for effective ultrastructural interpretation. Many tumors cannot be adequately examined because of extensive anoxic changes (even within promptly prepared specimens), either because of therapy or because of an inadequate blood supply, or both.
3. A limited amount of time is available for examining specimens, e.g., looking for premelanosomes in a suspected case of malignant melanoma.
4. It may be difficult to differentiate among primary lysosomes, neurosecretory-type granules, and small mucigen or zymogen granules when only small numbers of the latter structures are present in a particular neoplasm. The use of histochemical or immunohistologic techniques occasionally helps. Unfortunately, many of the latter procedures require frozen sections of unfixed tissue, which may not be available.
5. Although I can usually determine that a primary or metastatic neoplasm is an apudoma or neuroendocrine tumor, I am often unable to establish the site of origin or the nature of the secretory product found in the dense-core granules.
6. The diagnostic significance of cell junctions and basal lamina is often diminished because these structures are found in many neoplasms that are not typical carcinomas, e.g., benign schwannomas, ovarian sex-cord tumors, angiosarcomas, and synovial sarcomas.
7. Some ultrastructural patterns are not yet completely understood in terms of their diagnostic significance (e.g., case 7).
8. Morphologic diversity sometimes limits the usefulness of TEM in evaluating tumors. For example, metaplastic changes may be confusing, hybrid cells such as myofibroblasts and myoepithelial cells express features of two differentiated cell types, and ultrastructural features of multidirectional differentiation are evident in many sarcomas.
9. It is not possible to determine the histogenesis of some sarcomas by TEM, even though they have fairly consistent, distinct ultrastructural features, e.g., alveolar soft part sarcoma, Ewing's sarcoma, epithelioid sarcoma, and synovial sarcoma.

CONCLUSION

Even though most neoplasms can be accurately and efficiently diagnosed by light microscopy, TEM examination always contributes detailed information regarding the ultrastructural features of a tumor and is confirmatory and even diagnostic in a large percentage of cases. Whereas application of TEM to the diagnosis of tumors has developed rather slowly, ultrastructural pathology is now widely accepted as a valid subspecialty of surgical pathology. Future achievements in this area are dependent on the development of more refined cytochemical, immunocytochemical, autoradiologic, x-ray analysis, and other techniques for determining the nature and chemical composition of subcellular structures.

Appendix A. Materials and Methods

The procedures described in this appendix are those used successfully in our laboratory for many years. Other techniques for fixing, embedding, and staining tissues may be used as well. For example, neoplasms may be fixed in phosphate-buffered glutaraldehyde solutions, postfixed with osmium in various buffers, embedded in one of the currently available epoxy resins, and stained with lead hydroxide (see general references).

Biopsy specimens of solid neoplasms were processed as soon as possible after surgery in order to minimize artifacts (Appendix B). Most specimens were cut into 1-mm cubes with a new scalpel blade and fixed for periods ranging from 2 to 72 hours in s-collidine-buffered (pH = 7.4) (Bennett and Luft, 1959) Karnovsky's fixative (Karnovsky, 1965) at 4°C (the active ingredients are formaldehyde and glutaraldehyde). Diagnostically difficult tissues that required quick processing were fixed for 45 min in a mixture of glutaraldehyde (5%) and acrolein (4 drops to 10 ml fixative) (Sanborn et al., 1964) prepared in phosphate buffer. Buffy coat specimens from leukemia patients were fixed *in situ* in the centrifuge tube for 30 min after the plasma was gently removed with a fine pipette. The fixed, hardened buffy coat was then gently separated from the packed red cells and handled like solid tissue. After rinsing in buffer, the aldehyde-fixed specimens were postfixed for 1 h in s-collidine-buffered 1% osmium tetroxide. In order to enhance contrast, small pieces of tissue from most of the tumors were rinsed in distilled water and left overnight in 0.25% aqueous uranyl acetate (Farquhar and Palade, 1965). This treatment may result in blocks with annoying soft centers, especially those of lymphoid tissues.

Following dehydration in ethyl alcohols of ascending concentration and passage through propylene oxide, the specimens were immersed in a mixture of a Maraglas-D.E.R. 732 epoxy resin (for at least 3 h), placed in Beem capsules, and polymerized overnight in a 57°C oven (Erlandson,

1964). For orientation, thick (also called semithin) 1-µm sections cut with glass knives were stained with a sodium borate buffered 1% toluidine blue solution for approximately 1 min on a hot plate (Björkman, 1962). Light gold, thin (60–90 nm) sections were cut with diamond knives on a Sorvall MT2-B Porter-Blum ultramicrotome and picked up on formvar:carbon-coated 200-mesh copper grids. They were then stained with methanolic uranyl acetate (Stempak and Ward, 1964) followed by lead citrate (Reynolds, 1963), and examined in a Siemens Elmiskop 101 TEM using an 80 KV accelerating voltage and a 50-µm objective aperture.

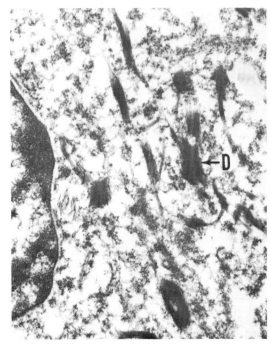

FIGURE A-1
Poorly differentiated epidermoid carcinoma (lung, 62-year-old male). The tissue was reprocessed from a paraffin block. The only recognizable cytoplasmic structures are dense bundles of cytokeratin filaments and desmosomes (D). (×22,800.)

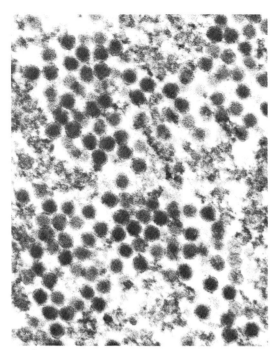

FIGURE A-2

Adenovirus (lung tissue from 21-year-old female who died after a bone marrow transplant for aplastic anemia). A piece of paraffin was cut out from a block showing numerous nuclear inclusions in necrotic lung tissue and reprocessed for electron microscopy. Note the excellent preservation of the 65-nm (average diameter) adenovirus virions. (×62,000.)

Electron microscopy fixatives (glutaraldehyde followed by osmium tetroxide) gave the best preservation of cell structures. The results obtained with buffered formalin fixation were variable, and usually less than ideal. It was often necessary, however, to retrieve formalin-fixed tissues for electron microscopic study. Pieces of tissue removed near the surface of the tumor usually were adequately fixed. Tissue obtained from formalin should be soaked in buffer for at least 1 day before osmium postfixation.

Reprocessing tissue recovered from paraffin blocks (by soaking in changes of xylene for up to 1 week) should be done as a last resort. Only the most hardy cell structures such as desmosomes (Fig. A-1), some secretory granules and inclusions, proteinaceous intracytoplasmic fibers (Fig. A-1), and virus particles (Fig. A-2) are adequately preserved.

Cited References

Bennett, H.S., and Luft, J.H.: s-Collidine as a basis for buffering fixatives.
J Biophys Cytol 6: 113–114, 1959.

Björkman, N.: Low magnification electron microscopy in histological work.
Acta Morphol Neerl Scand 4: 344–348, 1962.

Erlandson, R.A.: A new Maraglas, D.E.R. 732, embedment for electron microscopy.
J Cell Biol 22: 704–709, 1964.

Farquhar, M.G., and Palade, G.E.: Cell junctions in amphibian skin.
J Cell Biol 26: 263–291, 1965.

Karnovsky, M.J.: A formaldehyde-glutaraldehyde fixative of high osmolarity for use in electron microscopy.
J Cell Biol 27: 137A–138A, 1965.

Reynolds, E.: The use of lead citrate at high pH as an electron-opaque stain in electron microscopy.
J Cell Biol 17: 208–212, 1963.

Sandborn, E., Koen, P.F., McNabb, J.D., and Moore, G.: Cytoplasmic microtubules in mammalian cells.
J Ultrastruct Res 11: 123–138, 1964.

Stempak, J.G., and Ward, R.T.: An improved staining method for electron microscopy.
J Cell Biol 22: 697–701, 1964.

General References

Bloom, W., and Fawcett, D.W.: *A Textbook of Histology*, 10th ed. W.B. Saunders, Philadelphia, 1975.

DeRobertis, E.D.P., and DeRobertis, E.M.F., Jr.: *Cell and Molecular Biology*, 7th ed. Saunders College, Philadelphia, 1980.

Ebe, T., and Kobayashi, S.: *Fine Structure of Human Cells and Tissues.* John Wiley & Sons, New York, 1972.

Fawcett, D.W.: *The Cell*, 2nd ed. W.B. Saunders, Philadelphia, 1981.

Glauert, A.M. ed.: *Practical Methods in Electron Microscopy*. Elsevier North-Holland, New York, 1974–1980, vols. 2–8.

Ham, A.W., and Cormack, D.H.: *Histology*, 8th ed. J.B. Lippincott, Philadelphia, 1979.

Hayat, M.A.: *Principles and Techniques of Electron Microscopy: Biological Applications*, Vol. 1, 2nd ed. University Park Press, Baltimore, 1981.

Johannessen, J.V.: Use of paraffin material for electron microscopy. In: *Pathology Annual*, Vol. 12, part 2. S.C. Sommers and P.P. Rosen (eds.). Appleton-Century-Crofts, New York, 1977, pp. 189–224.

Krstić, R.V.: *Ultrastructure of the Mammalian Cell. An Atlas.* Springer-Verlag, New York, 1979. (Drawings.)

McDowell, E.M.: Fixation and processing. In: *Diagnostic Electron Microscopy*, Vol. 1. B.F. Trump and R.T. Jones (eds.). John Wiley & Sons, New York, 1978, pp. 113–139.

Porter, K.R. and Bonneville, M.A.: *Fine Structure of Cells and Tissues*, 4th ed. Lea & Febiger, Philadelphia, 1973.

Rhodin, J.A.G.: *Histology. A Text and Atlas.* Oxford University Press, New York, 1974.

Wischnitzer, S.: *Introduction to Electron Microscopy*, 3rd ed. Pergamon Press, New York, 1981.

Yang, G.C.H., and Morrison, A.B.: Wide-field electron microscopy. A rapid method for the study of histologic material that provides a bridge between light and electron microscopy.
Am J Clin Pathol 64: 648–654, 1975.

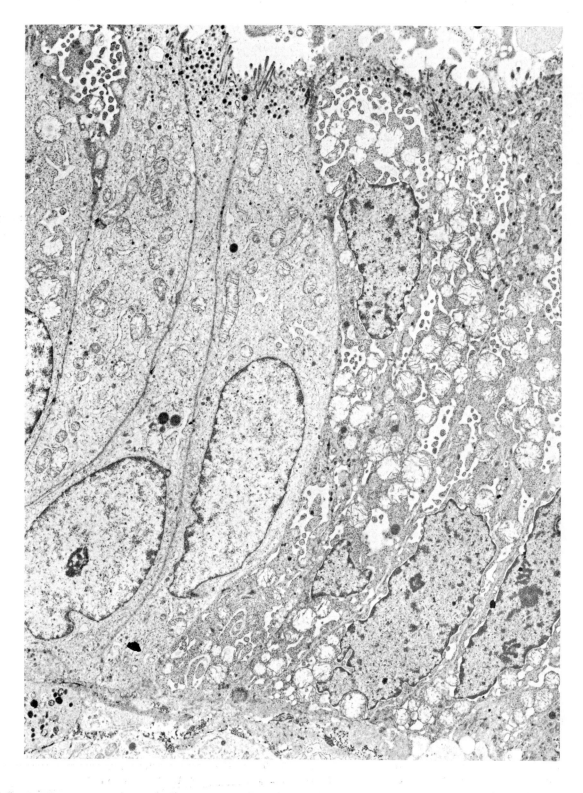

FIGURE A-3
Survey electron micrograph of neoplastic colonic epithelial cells (cf. Fig. 1-1). Necrotic neoplastic cells are at the right. See text description. (×5600.)

Appendix B. Artifacts

The first step in evaluating a biopsy specimen prepared for electron microscopy is to make sure that well-preserved representative tumor is present in the thin (60–90-nm) sections of epoxy-embedded tissue. Tissue that looks well preserved in hematoxylin and eosin- (H&E)-stained paraffin-embedded tumors is sometimes found to be necrotic when examined under the electron microscope. The poor preservation of promptly fixed neoplastic tissue results from autolysis and necrosis that occurs within the tumor mass, and not from inadequate fixation. Single cells (apoptosis) or groups of cells may be affected (Searle et al., 1975). Apoptosis is characterized by margination of chromatin and cytoplasmic condensation in its early stage. Such cells are often erroneously referred to as "dark cells" in the literature. True dark cells usually contain large numbers of tightly packed organelles, such as ribosomes, lysosomes, electron-dense mitochondria, and/or numerous dense aggregates of cytoplasmic fibrils.

Viable tumor cells adjacent to necrotic neoplastic cells from an adenocarcinoma of the sigmoid colon are illustrated in Figure A-3. The nuclei of the necrotic cells have an irregular outline and contain prominent foci of condensed chromatin. Dilated cisternae of the ER and enlarged swollen mitochondria are also usually evident to varying degrees in degenerating or anoxic tumor cells. Other degenerative changes that in their early stages may be confused with specific organelle alterations in viable tumor cells include condensed mitochondria with dilated compartments; vesiculation and vacuolization of the cytoplasm; the appearance of numerous autophagosomes; the formation of myelin figures (irregular, concentric, electron-dense phospholipid, or lipoprotein membranes); degranulation of the RER; blebs and discontinuities of the plasmalemma and organelle membranes; and the appearance of various metabolic inclusions (Ghadially, 1975; Trump et al., 1978).

As shown elsewhere in this monograph, there are cellular changes that reflect the altered state of viable neoplastic cells and are conspicuous in certain nosologic entities. Careful evaluation of the substructure of the neoplastic cells usually helps in determining whether an alteration of a specific structure or organelle is real or an artifact.

Cited References

Ghadially, F.N.: *Ultrastructural Pathology of the Cell.* A text and atlas of physiological and pathological alterations in cell fine structure. Butterworths, London, 1975.

Searle, J., Larson, T.A., Abbott, P.J., Harmon, B., and Kerr, J.F.R.: An electron-microscope study of the mode of cell death induced by cancer-chemotherapeutic agents in populations of proliferating normal and neoplastic cells. *J Pathol 116: 129–138, 1975.*

Trump, B.F., Jesudason, M.L., and Jones, R.T.: Ultrastructural features of diseased cells. In *Diagnostic Electron Microscopy* (vol. 1) B.F. Trump and R.T. Jones, Eds. John Wiley & Sons, New York, 1978, pp. 1–88.

Appendix C. Ultrastructural Tumor Diagnosis—Quick Reference Table

The following table may be used for quick identification of neoplasms by their ultrastructural features. General categories of neoplasms are marked with an asterisk. As stressed in the text, single fine structural features often are not diagnostic of a tumor *per se*. Naturally, interpretation should be made in a logical gross and clinical setting. A number of primitive or pleuripotential neoplasms and blastomas that have a varied nondiagnostic submicroscopic appearance, e.g., hemangiopericytoma and pulmonary blastoma, are not listed, but are discussed in the text. It must be emphasized that the more anaplastic tumors in each category may not have diagnostic ultrastructural markers. Numbers in parentheses refer to text pages on which the listed ultrastructural attributes are discussed in more detail, with cited references.

Tumor	Helpful Ultrastructural Features
Acinar Cell Carcinoma* (salivary glands, pancreas, etc.)	Zymogen granules, stacked cisternae of RER, Golgi, microvilli, junctional complex, cell junctions, basal lamina (29, 47)
Adenocarcinomas*	Lumens, intracellular lumens, microvilli, mucigen granules, glycogen, prominent Golgi, intermediate filaments (juxtanuclear), interdigitating cell membranes, cell junctions, rare cilia, basal lamina (44, 49)
Intestinal type	Rigid microvilli with prominent core microfilaments, glycocalyx, junctional complex, mucigen granules (104)
Adenoid Cystic Carcinoma	Reduplicated basal lamina (pseudocysts), true lumens with microvilli, junctional complex, intermediate filaments, myoepithelial cells (variable), intercellular mucus (91, 120)
Adrenocortical Tumors*	Mitochondria with tubulovesicular cristae (most prominent in tumors composed of zona fasciculata cells; not found in zona glomerulosa tumors—aldosterone-secreting tumors), SER, stacked cisternae of RER, lipofuscin, lipid, occasional primitive cell junctions, thin basal lamina (21, 30, 33)
Alveolar Cell Carcinoma (lung)	Lamellar inclusion body, microvilli, cell junctions, thin basal lamina (65)
Alveolar Soft Part Sarcoma	Inclusions that resemble mucigen and/or neurosecretory-type granules, rhomboid crystals (one-third of cases), organoid pattern (56, 62)
Apudomas—Neuroendocrine Tumors (eight tumors included in this category are listed separately) Carcinoid tumors Islet cell tumors Medullary thyroid carcinoma Pituitary adenomas	Neurosecretory-type granules (pleomorphic in midgut, pancreatic, ovarian, and testicular carcinoids), microfilaments, cell junctions, basal lamina (47)
Astrocytic Tumors	Prominent intermediate (glial) filaments that may form dense bundles (Rosenthal fibers) (86)
Brenner Tumor (ovary)	Epithelial cell nests surrounded by basal lamina, cell junctions, interdigitating plasma membranes, occasional lumens, cilia, microvilli (107, 112)

Tumor	Helpful Ultrastructural Features
Bronchiolar Carcinoma	Most consist of Clara cells (apical electron-dense secretory granules). Goblet cell types (mucigen granules). Nonciliated nonsecretory cells (short apical microvilli) and rare foci of neoplastic granular pneumocytes (lamellar inclusion body) are evident in mixed cell types (66, 107)
Cartilaginous Tumors* Chondroma Chondroblastoma Chondrosarcoma	Scalloped cell surface, RER, glycogen, lipid, intermediate filaments (higher-grade neoplasms). Cells may lie in electron-lucent lacunae (60, 95, 147)
Choroid Plexus Papilloma	Long tortuous microvilli, junctional complex, rare cilia, occasional blepharoplast, basal lamina (105, 107, 113)
Chordoma	Mitochondria–RER complexes, glycogen, vacuoles, primitive cell junctions (42, 115)
Clear Cell Carcinomas* (e.g., kidney, vagina)	Abundant glycogen and/or lipid (both are found in renal clear cell carcinomas), lumen, microvilli, junctional complex. Basal lamina may be reduplicated (58)
Dermatofibrosarcoma Protuberans	Nuclear membrane protrusions (satellite nuclei), deep nuclear indentations, long attenuated cell processes, rare foci of basal lamina (10)
Embryonal Carcinoma	Small lumens with microvilli, junctional complex, primitive cell junctions, Golgi, large nucleoli, basal lamina
Eosinophilic Granuloma	Langerhans granules—no cell junctions (64)
Ependymoma	Blepharoplasts (ciliary basal bodies), rare cilia, microvilli, primitive cell junctions, basal lamina, lumens and junctional complex if well differentiated (rosettes) (107, 112, 128)
Epithelioid Sarcoma	Variable appearance; desmosomes and primitive cell junctions (some cases), interdigitating cell membranes, intermediate filaments (96, 116, 155)
Ewing's Sarcoma	Prominent pools of cytoplasmic glycogen, rare primitive cell junctions, sparse organelles (58, 116)
Fibromatoses* Dupuytren's contracture Ledderhose's disease Infantile digital myofibroblastoma	Myofibroblasts and fibroblasts, well developed RER. Subplasmalemmal parallel bundles of actin myofilaments with fusiform dense bodies (90)

Tumor	**Helpful Ultrastructural Features**
Fibrosarcoma	Prominent branching cisternae of RER, myofibroblast component in low grade neoplasms, e.g., desmoid tumors. No cell junctions (30, 90)
Fibrous Histiocytoma (malignant)	Usually consist of a mixture of fibroblastic cells, myofibroblasts, and histiocytes. Branching cisternae of RER (often distended), lipid, lysosomes (4, 60)

Granular Cell Tumors*
  Granular cell ameloblastomas
  Congenital epulis
	Numerous secondary lysosomes (residual bodies and ceroid-lipofuscin), rare primitive cell junctions, basal lamina. Neural features (Schwann cell–axon complexes) in about 60% of cases (38)

Granulosa Cell Tumor	Cleaved nuclei, cystic intercellular spaces (Call-Exner bodies) delineated by an often reduplicated basal lamina, lipid, mitochondria may possess tubular cristae, SER, microfilaments, primitive cell junctions (33, 112)
Hepatocellular Carcinoma	Prominent SER, RER, mitochondria, alpha glycogen particles, lipid (30, 33)
Hepatoma—Focal Nodular Hyperplasia	Pseudocrystalline mitochondrial inclusions in addition to other organelles and inclusions found in hepatocytes (see above) (23, 60)
Hilus Cell Tumor (ovary)	SER, lipofuscin, Reinke's crystals (33, 60, 62)

Histiocytic Neoplasms*
  Malignant histiocytosis
  Histiocytic lymphoma (true)
	Prominent Golgi (in nuclear hof), lysosomes, lipid, bean-shaped nuclei, ruffled cell borders, phagocytosis (1, 38, 60)

Insulinoma	Neurosecretory-type granules with paracrystalline core separated from the limiting membrane by a clear space (55)
Interstitial (Leydig) Cell Tumor	Prominent SER, SER whorls, lysosomes, lipid droplets, rare Reinke crystals, some mitochondria with tubulovesicular cristae (22, 33, 60)
Juxtaglomerular Cell Neoplasms	Pleomorphic mature neurosecretory-type granules and rhomboid protogranules (55)
Leukemia Acute promonocytic (monocytic)	High nucleocytoplasmic ratio, large nucleolus, prominent Golgi, scattered small dense granules (more prominent in monocytic leukemias) (38)

Tumor	Helpful Ultrastructural Features
Acute myelomonocytic	Spectrum of monocytic and granulocytic cells (common bone marrow precursors). Promonocytes (see above) and granulocytes (see below)
Acute promyelocytic (granulocytic)	Auer bodies, primary, secondary and tertiary granules, primitive blast cells, dispersed or clumped chromatin, bilobed nuclei (63)
Eosinophilic	Charcot-Leyden crystals, membrane-limited inclusions with crystalline core (63)
Hairy cell	Ribosome–lamella complexes, numerous surface microvilli (hairy cell) (41)
Lymphoblastic (prolymphocytic)	Convoluted nuclei, marginated chromatin, small nucleoli; or round nuclei with dispersed chromatin, small nucleoli. The scanty cytoplasm contains free ribosomes (12)
Chronic lymphocytic	Cells resemble mature lymphocytes—uniform nucleus, clumped and marginated chromatin; small nucleolus. Some cases contain rectangular proteinaceous crystals in RER (63)
Liposarcoma	Small or large lipid droplets, glycogen, lipofuscin (60)
Lobular Carcinoma (infiltrating, breast)	Intracellular lumens, microvilli, primitive cell junctions, small desmosomes (99)
Luteoma	Prominent SER, mitochondria with tubulovesicular cristae, short stacks of RER, lipid, tight junctions (22, 33)
Lymphomas Hodgkin's disease, Reed-Sternberg cell	No cell junctions or basal lamina Cells resemble huge transformed lymphocytes or histiocytes. Large convoluted or hypersegmented nuclei, dispersed chromatin, large nucleoli (often centrally located), polysomes, RER, lipid droplets, lysosomes (17)
Lymphoblastic	Convoluted (T or null cell) type—convoluted nuclei, marginated chromatin, small nucleoli, prominent Golgi and polysomes. Nonconvoluted (T or null cell) type—round nuclei, finely dispersed chromatin, small nucleoli, scanty cytoplasm with few organelles (12)

Tumor	**Helpful Ultrastructural Features**
Lymphocytic—poorly differentiated	Nodular—small or medium sized B cells with cleaved, noncleaved or irregular nuclei, clumped chromatin, and scattered large transformed lymphocytes (large round nuclei, dispersed chromatin, large nucleoli, abundant polysomes).
	Diffuse—B and occasional T cell types (convoluted nuclei). The cells are generally smaller and less pleomorphic than those comprising histiocytic lymphomas (11)
Histiocytic (reticulum cell sarcoma)	A heterogeneous group of large B cell (rarely T or null cell) lymphomas with the fine structural features of transformed lymphocytes. Large noncleaved cells—round or irregular nuclei, moderately dispersed chromatin, multiple often marginated nucleoli, prominent polysome rosettes. Large cleaved cells—cleaved and convoluted nuclei; clumped, marginated or dispersed chromatin; multiple medium or large nucleoli; polysomes and ribosomes (13, 33)
Plasmacytoid	Lymphoid cells with fairly prominent stacked RER cisternae (29)
Undifferentiated	Burkitt's type—small noncleaved B cell lymphoma. Round nuclei with one or more short surface indentations or nuclear pockets, partially clumped and marginated chromatin, multiple small nucleoli, prominent polysome rosettes, and scattered lipid droplets in the scanty cytoplasm. (17)
	Non-Burkitt's—Cells and nuclei more pleomorphic, not diagnostic by EM
Malignant Melanoma	Premelanosomes and melanosomes (74, 131)
Meningothelial Meningioma	Entangled cell processes joined by numerous desmosomes; intermediate filaments (95, 112, 125)
Merkel Cell Tumor	Round cells, high nucleocytoplasmic ratio, small neurosecretory-type granules prominent in ectoplasm (50, 137)
Mesothelioma (epithelial) Adenomatoid tumor	Long tortuous microvilli, desmosomes, primitive cell junctions, basal lamina (104, 112)

Mixed Tumors* (pleomorphic adenoma)
    Salivary glands
    Chondroid syringoma
	Ductular epithelial cell component—lumens, microvilli, junctional complex, cytokeratin filaments, intermediate filaments.
	Myoepithelial cell component—nonspecific microfilaments, occasional clusters of perinuclear cytokeratin filaments, desmosomes, basal lamina, spindle cell and chondroid metaplasia (91)

Tumor	Helpful Ultrastructural Features
Mycosis Fungoides–Sézary Syndrome	Cerebriform nuclei, sparse cytoplasm, no cell junctions (T lymphocytes) (7)
Neuroblastoma Esthesioneuroblastoma	Small neurosecretory granules usually located within neuritic processes, round nuclei, small nucleoli, microtubules, neurofilaments, cell junctions (50, 78, 85)
Neurofibroma	Perineurial-like cells—long thin cell processes, pinocytotic vesicles, primitive cell junctions, external lamina. Schwann cell—axon complexes scattered throughout tumor (95, 122, 163)
Nevi* (melanocytic)	Uniform round cells, dispersed chromatin, scattered premelanosomes and melanosomes, microfilaments, occasional external lamina (72)
Blue nevus	Spindle-shaped cells containing large numbers of predominantly mature melanosomes (74)
Oat Cell Carcinoma (carcinoid type)	Spindle-shaped cells containing scattered, small neurosecretory-type granules, primitive cell junctions (50, 140)

Oncocytic Neoplasms*
  Hürthle cell tumor
  Oncocytoma
  Warthin's tumor
	Markedly abundant mitochondria with stacked lamelliform cristae that lack matrix granules. Intercellular junctions, lumens (microvilli) (23)

Osteogenic Sarcoma Parosteal	Osteoblasts—fibroblastic cells with often dilated RER cisternae, osteoid (dense collagen), hydroxyapetite crystals (30) Also contain neoplastic (?) myofibroblasts (90)
Ovarian Serous Cystic Tumors	Benign—columnar epithelial cells, some ciliated; scattered apical mucigen granules. Malignant—pleomorphic nuclei, large nucleoli, ciliated cells only evident in low-grade neoplasms; secretory granules rarely noted (47, 107)
Paragangliomas*	Chief cells—neurosecretory-type granules, desmosomes, Golgi. These cells may be enveloped by thin sustentacular cell processes (50)
Parathyroid Adenomas Chief cell type	Prominent organelles—Golgi, RER (whorls also noted), ribosomes, annulate lamellae, lysosomes, lipid, organelle complexes, interdigitating cell membranes, cell junctions (34, 95)
Clear cell type	Chief cells containing large amounts of cytoplasmic glycogen (60)

Tumor	Helpful Ultrastructural Features
Oxyphil cell type	Characterized by abundant mitochondria; when densely packed with lamelliform cristae, oncocytic adenomas (26)
Pheochromocytoma	Neurosecretory granules with distinct halo. The norepinephrine-containing granules with eccentrically positioned dense cores are particularly prominent in the extraadrenal tumors (55)
Plasmacytoma—Myeloma	Prominent RER and Golgi apparatus (29)
Primitive Neuroectodermal Tumor	Dispersed chromatin, dendritic processes that may contain neurofilaments and microtubules, primitive cell junctions; neurosecretory-type granules are rarely found (113)
Prostatic Carcinoma	Secondary lysosomes, mucigen granules, lumens (microvilli), junctional complex and primitive cell junctions (38)
Pulmonary Tumorlet	A spindle-cell variant of pulmonary carcinoid tumor—neurosecretory-type granules (50)
Retinoblastoma	Rosettes (Flexner-Wintersteiner), intercellular junctions, lumen, cilia (107, 115)
Rhabdomyosarcoma Rhabdomyoma	Actin (6-nm) filaments and myosin (15-nm) fibrils in parallel arrays closely associated with Z discs and linear ribosomes, sarcomeres, glycogen, primitive cell junctions, external lamina (79, 116, 144)
Schwannoma (benign)	Complexly entangled long cell processes, pseudomesaxon formation, intermediate filaments, microtubules, rare primitive cell junctions, external lamina, long-spacing collagen (77, 78, 95, 115, 122)
Schwannoma—Malignant Peripheral Nerve Sheath Tumors*	Long broad cytoplasmic processes, RER, microtubules, intermediate filaments, rare pseudomesaxon formation, primitive cell junctions, fragmented external lamina, long-spacing collagen, metaplastic changes, e.g., rhabdomyoblasts. (77, 82, 115)
Sertoli-Leydig Cell Tumor (arrhenoblastoma, androblastoma)	Well differentiated—ductular structures composed of Sertoli cells (lumens, interdigitating lateral cell membranes, basal lamina, cell junctions, Charcot-Bottcher crystalloids). (22, 62) Intermediate differentiation—biphasic pattern; Leydig cells more prominent (SER, Reinke crystals, lipid, lipofuscin) (22, 33, 60)

Tumor	Helpful Ultrastructural Features
Seminoma—Dysgerminoma	Round nuclei, elongated and twisted nucleolar strands (nucleolonema), glycogen, rare primitive cell junctions (18, 134)

Smooth Muscle Tumors*
  Leiomyoma
  Leiomyoblastoma
  Leiomyosarcoma
  Glomus tumor
	Actin microfilaments with interspersed fusiform dense bodies, plasmalemmal attachment plaques, pinocytotic vesicles, intermediate filaments, rare primitive cell junctions, external lamina (82, 116)

Squamous cell (epidermoid) Carcinoma—Squamous Metaplasia*	Cytokeratin filaments (tonofilaments), filopodia (fingerlike cell processes), well-developed desmosomes, primitive cell junctions (87, 108)
Sugar Tumor (lung)	Prominent free and membrane-bound glycogen (lysosomes), interdigitating cell membranes, cell junctions, basal lamina (60)
Synovial Sarcoma	Densely packed spindle cells, poorly developed RER, small lumens (microvilli), prominent tight junctions. Glandular areas—lumens, microvilli, junctional complex, basal lamina (116)
Thecoma	Ovarian stromal cell tumor composed of plump lipid-laden cells. Distinguished from ovarian fibromas consisting of fusiform fibroblastlike cells with prominent RER (60)
Thymoma	Cytokeratin filaments (tonofilaments), desmosomes, elongated cell processes, primitive cell junctions, occasional cells bounded by external lamina (85, 112)
Thyroid Tumors* (papillary and follicular)	Both papillary and follicular carcinomas consist of cells containing prominent electron-dense pleomorphic secondary lysosomes, some of which resemble neurosecretory-type granules. Lumens containing electron-dense colloid, microvilli, basal lamina, cell junctions (38)

Vascular Tumors* (endothelial cell origin)
  Hemangioma
  Hemangioendothelioma
  Angiosarcoma
  Lymphangiosarcoma
	Neoplastic endothelial cells forming vascular spaces. Weibel-Palade bodies, bundles of intermediate filaments, tight junctions and primitive cell junctions, pinocytotic vesicles, basal lamina. Intermediate filaments are particularly prominent in hemangioendotheliomas of bone. Lymphangiosarcoma—no basal lamina (66, 116)

Wilms' Tumor	Lumen, microvilli, junctional complex, primitive cell junctions, basal lamina, poorly differentiated spindle-shaped stromal cells, metaplastic changes, e.g., rhabdomyoblasts (4, 82)

References

1. Able, M.E., and Lee, J.C.: Ultrastructure of a Sertoli-cell adenoma of the testis.
   Cancer 23: 481–486, 1969.
2. Abt, A.B., and Carter, S.L.: Goblet cell carcinoid of the appendix.
   Arch Pathol Lab Med 100: 301–306, 1976.
3. Adelstein, R.S., Conti, M.A., Johnson, G., Pastan, I., and Pollard, T.D.: Isolation and characterization of myosin from cloned mouse fibroblasts.
   Proc Natl Acad Sci USA 69: 3693–3697, 1972.
4. Afzelius, B.A., Eliasson, R., Johnson, O., and Lindholmer, C.: Lack of dynein arms in immotile human spermatozoa.
   J Cell Biol 66: 225–232, 1975.
5. Ahearn, M.J., Trujillo, J.M., Cork, A., Fowler, A., and Hart, J.S.: The association of nuclear blebs with aneuploidy in human acute leukemia.
   Cancer Res 34: 2887–2896, 1974.
6. Ahmed, A.: *Atlas of the Ultrastructure of Human Breast Diseases.* Churchill Livingston, New York, 1978, pp. 58–64; 98–101.
7. Akhtar, M., Gosalbez, T., and Young, I.: Ultrastructural study of androgen-producing adrenocortical adenoma.
   Cancer 34: 322–327, 1974.
8. Albrecht-Buehler, G., and Bushnell, A.: The ultrastructure of primary cilia in quiescent 3T3 cells.
   Exp Cell Res 126: 427–437, 1980.
9. Alguacil-Garcia, A., Unni, K.K., and Goellner, J.R.: Malignant giant cell tumor of soft parts. An ultrastructural study of four cases.
   Cancer 40: 244–253, 1977.
10. Alguacil-Garcia, A., Unni, K.K., and Goellner, J.R.: Histogenesis of dermatofibrosarcoma protuberans. An ultrastructural study.
    Am J Clin Pathol 69: 427–434, 1978.
11. Alguacil-Garcia, A., Unni, K.K., and Goellner, J.R.: Malignant fibrous histiocytoma. An ultrastructural study of six cases.
    Am J Clin Pathol 69: 121–129, 1978.
12. Alguicil-Garcia, A., Unni, K.K., Goellner, J.R., and Winkelmann, R.K.: Atypical fibroxanthoma of the skin. An ultrastructural study of two cases.
    Cancer 40: 1471–1480, 1977.
13. Alroy, J., Pauli, B.U., Hayden, J.E., and Gould, V.E.: Intracytoplasmic lumina in bladder carcinomas.
    Hum Pathol 10: 549–555, 1979.
14. Alroy, J., Pauli, B.U., and Weinstein, R.S.: Correlation between numbers of desmosomes and the aggressiveness of transitional cell carcinoma in human urinary bladder.
    Cancer 47: 104–112, 1981.
15. Alroy, J., Pauli, B.U., Weinstein, R.S., and Merk, F.B.: Association of asymmetric unit membrane plaques formation in the urinary bladder of adult humans with therapeutic radiation.
    Experientia (Basel) 33: 1645–1647, 1977.
16. Altenähr, E., and Seifert, G.: Ultrastruktureller Vergleich menschlicher Epithelkörperchen bei sekundären Hyperparathyreoidismus und primärem Adenom.
    Virchows Arch (Pathol Anat) 353: 60–86, 1971.
17. Amin, H.K., Okagaki, T., and Richart, R.M.: Classification of fibroma and thecoma of the ovary. An ultra-structural study.
    Cancer 27: 438–446, 1971.
18. Anagnostou, D., Parker, J.W., Taylor, C.R., Tindle, B.H., and Lukes, R.J.: Lacunar cells of nodular sclerosing Hodgkin's disease. An ultrastructural and immunohistologic study.
    Cancer 39: 1032–1043, 1977.
19. Anderson, R.G.W.: The three-dimensional structure of the basal body from the Rhesus monkey oviduct.
    J Cell Biol 54: 246–265, 1972.
20. Andrew, A.: Further evidence that enterchromaffin cells are not derived from the neural crest.
    J Embryol Exp Morphol 31: 589–598, 1974.
21. Anteunis, A., Audebert, A.A., Krulik, M., Debray, J., and Robineaux, R.: Acute eosinophilic leukemia. An ultrastructural study.
    Virchows Archiv (Cell Pathol) 27: 237–248, 1978.
22. Aparisi, T., Arborgh, B., and Ericsson, J.L.E.: Studies on the fine structure of osteoblastoma with notes on the localization of nonspecific acid and alkaline phosphatase.
    Cancer 41: 1811–1822, 1978.
23. Archer, D.F., Salazar, H., Maroon, J.C., and Hough, L.J.: Prolactin-secreting pituitary adenomas: serum and tissue prolactin levels with ultrastructural correlation.
    Am J Obstet Gynecol 137: 646–652, 1980.
24. Archer, F., and Omar, M.: Pink cell (oncocytic) metaplasia in a fibro-adenoma of the human breast: Electron-microscope observations.
    J Pathol 99: 119–124, 1969.
25. Archer, G.T., and Blackwood, A.: Formation of Charcot-Leyden crystals in human eosinophils and basophils and study of the composition of isolated crystals.
    J Exp Med 122: 173–180, 1965.
26. Askin, F.B., and Kahn, C.: The cellular origin of pulmonary surfactant.
    Lab Invest 25: 260–268, 1971.
27. Azar, H.A.: Significance of the Reed-Sternberg cell.
    Hum Pathol 6: 479–484, 1975.
28. Azar, H.A.: The hematopoietic system. In: *Diagnostic Electron Microscopy*, Vol. 2. B.F. Trump and R.T. Jones (eds.). John Wiley & Sons, New York, 1979, pp. 126–140.
29. Azar, H.A., Jaffe, E.S., Berard, C.W., et al.: Diffuse large cell lymphomas. Correlation of morphologic features with functional markers.
    Cancer 46: 1428–1441, 1980.
30. Balázs, M.: Comparative electron-microscopic studies of benign hepatoma and icterus in patients on oral contraceptives.
    Virchows Arch (Pathol Anat) 381: 97–108, 1978.
31. Barajas, L., Bennett, C.M., Connor, G., and Lindstrom, R.R.: Structure of a juxtaglomerular cell tumor: The presence of a neural component. A light and electron microscopic study.
    Lab Invest 37: 357–368, 1977.
32. Barland, P., Novikoff, A.B., and Hamerman, D.: Electron microscopy of the human synovial membrane.
    J Cell Biol 14: 207–220, 1962.
33. Barr, R.J., Wuerker, R.B., and Graham, J.H.: Ultrastructure of atypical fibroxanthoma.
    Cancer 40: 736–743, 1977.

34. Basset, F., and Turiaf, J.: Identification par le microscopie electronique de particles de nature probablement viviale dans les lesions granulomateuses d'une histiocytosis-X pulmonaire.
CR Acad Sci (*Paris*) *261: 3701–3703, 1965.*

35. Battifora, H.: Hemangiopericytoma: Ultrastructural study of five cases.
Cancer 31: 1418–1432, 1973.

36. Battifora, H.: Intracytoplasmic lumina in breast carcinoma. A helpful histopathologic feature.
Arch Pathol 99: 614–617, 1975.

37. Battifora, H., Sun, T-T., Bahu, R.M., and Rao, S.: The use of antikeratin antiserum as a diagnostic tool: Thymoma versus lymphoma.
Hum Pathol 11: 635–641, 1980.

38. Bauserman, S.C., Hardman, J.M., Schochet, S.S., and Earle, K.M.: Pituitary oncocytoma. Indispensible role of electron microscopy in its identification.
Arch Pathol Lab Med 102: 456–459, 1978.

39. Beals, T.F., Pierce, B., and Schroeder, C.F.: The ultrastructure of human testicular tumors. 1. Interstitial cell tumors.
J Urol 93: 64–73, 1965.

40. Becker, N.H., and Soifer, I. Benign clear cell tumor ("sugar tumor") of the lung.
Cancer 27: 712–719, 1971.

41. Bedrossian, C.W.M., Weilbaecher, D.G., Bentinck, D.C., and Greenberg, D.S.: Ultrastructure of human bronchioloalveolar cell carcinoma.
Cancer 36: 1399–1413, 1975.

42. Bencosme, S.A., Raymond, M.J., Ross, R.C., et al.: A histochemical and ultrastructural study of human breast carcinomas with a view to their classification by cell of origin.
Exp Mol Pathol 31: 236–247, 1979.

43. Bennett, G.S., Fellini, S.A., Croop, J.M., et al.: Differences among 100Å filament subunits from different cell types.
Proc Natl Acad Sci USA 75: 4364–4368, 1978.

44. Berard, C.W., and Dorfman, R.F.: Histopathology of malignant lymphomas.
Clin Haematol 3: 39–76, 1974.

45. Berard, C.W., O'Conor, G.T., Thomas, L.B., and Torlani, H.: Histopathological definition of Burkitt's tumor.
Bull WHO 40: 601–607, 1969.

46. Berendsen, P.B., Smith, E.B., Abell, M.R., and Jaffe, R.B.: Fine structure of Leydig cells from an arrhenoblastoma of the ovary.
Am J Obstet Gynecol 103: 192–199, 1969.

47. Bernhard, W., and Granboulan, N.: The fine structure of the cancer cell nucleus.
Exp Cell Res Suppl 9: 19–53, 1963.

48. Bhawan, J.: Melanocytic nevi. A review.
J Cutan Pathol 6: 153–169, 1979.

49. Bhawan, J.: Amelanotic melanoma or poorly differentiated melanoma?
J Cutan Pathol 7: 55–56, 1980.

50. Bhawan, J., Bacchetta, C., Joris, I., and Majno, G.: A myofibroblastic tumor. Infantile digital fibroma (recurrent digital fibrous tumor of childhood).
Am J Pathol 94: 19–37, 1979.

51. Bhawan, J., Chang, W.H., and Edelstein, L.M.: Cellular blue nevus. An ultrastructural study.
J Cutan Pathol 7: 109–122, 1980.

52. Birbeck, M.S.C.: Electron microscopy of melanocytes: The fine structure of hair bulb melanosomes.
Ann NY Acad Sci 100: 540–547, 1963.

53. Birbeck, M.S., Breathnach, A.S., and Everall, J.D.: An electron microscopic study of basal melanocytes and high-level clear cells (Langerhan's cells) in vitiligo.
J Invest Dermatol 37: 51–64, 1961.

54. Bjersing, L., and Cajander, S.: Ultrastructure of gonadoblastoma and disgerminoma (seminoma) in a patient with XY gonadal dysgenesis.
Cancer 40: 1127–1136, 1977.

55. Black, W.C.: Enterochromaffin cell types and corresponding carcinoid tumors.
Lab Invest 19: 473–486, 1968.

56. Blaustein, A.: Calcitonin secreting struma-carcinoid tumor of the ovary.
Human Pathol 10: 222–228, 1979.

57. Blaustein, A., and Lee, H.: Surface cells of the ovary and pelvic peritoneum: a histochemical and ultrastructural comparison.
Gynecol Oncol 8: 34–43, 1979.

58. Bloodworth, J.M.B., Horvath, E., and Kovacs, K.: Fine structural pathology of the endocrine system. In: *Diagnostic Electron Microscopy*, Vol. 3. B.F. Trump and R.T. Jones (eds.). John Wiley & Sons, New York, 1980, pp. 359–527.

59. Bloom, W., and Fawcett, D.W.: *A Textbook of Histology*, 10th ed. W.B. Saunders, Philadelphia, 1975.

60. Bloustein, P.A., Silverberg, S.G., and Waddell, W.R.: Epithelioid sarcoma. Case report with ultrastructural review, histogenetic discussion, and chemotherapeutic data.
Cancer 38: 2390–2400, 1976.

61. Böcker, W., Dralle, H., Koch, G., de Heer, K., and Hagemann, J.: Immunohistochemical and electron microscope analysis of adenomas of the thyroid gland. II. Adenomas with specific cytological differentiation.
Virchows Arch (Pathol Anat) 380: 205–220, 1978.

62. Böcker, W., and Stegner, H.E.: Mixed müllerian tumor of the uterus. Ultrastructural studies on the differentiation of rhabdomyoblasts.
Virchows Arch (Pathol Anat) 3: 337–349, 1975.

63. Boesel, C.P., Suhan, J.P., and Bradel, E.J.: Ultrastructure of primitive neuroectodermal neoplasms of the central nervous system.
Cancer 42: 194–201, 1978.

64. Boesel, C.P., Suhan, J.P., and Sayers, M.P.: Melanotic medulloblastoma. Report of a case with ultrastructural findings.
J Neuropathol Exp Neurol 37: 531–543, 1978.

65. Bois, R.M.: The organization of the contractile apparatus of vertebrate smooth muscle.
Anat Rec 177: 61–78, 1973.

66. Bolen, J.W., and Thorning, D.: Benign lipoblastoma and myxoid liposarcoma. A comparative light- and electron-microscopic study.
Am J Surg Pathol 4: 163–174, 1980.

67. Bolen, J.W., and Thorning, D.: Mesotheliomas. A light- and electron-microscopical study concerning histogenetic relationships between the epithelial and the mesenchymal variants.
Am J Surg Pathol 4: 451–464, 1980.

68. Bonikos, D.S., Bensch, K.G., and Kempson, R.L.: The contribution of electron microscopy to the differential diagnosis of tumors.
Beitr Pathol 158: 417–444, 1976.

69. Bonikos, D.S., Hendrickson, M., and Bensch, K.G.: Pulmonary alveolar cell carcinoma. Fine structural and in vito study of a case and critical review of this entity.
Am J Surg Pathol 1: 93–108, 1977.

70. Boquist, L.: Annulate lamellae in human parathyroid adenoma.
    Virchows Arch Abt B Zellpathol 6: 234–246, 1970.
71. Boram, L.H., Erlandson, R.A., and Hajdu, S.I.: Mesodermal mixed tumor of the uterus. A cytologic, histologic, and electron microscopic correlation.
    Cancer 30: 1295–1306, 1972.
72. Bordi, C., and Bussolati, G.: Immunofluorescence, histochemical and ultrastructural studies for the detection of multiple endocrine polypeptide tumors of the pancreas.
    Virchows Archiv (Cell Pathol) 17: 13–27, 1974.
73. Bordi, C., and Tardini, A.: Electron microscopy of islet cell tumors. In: *Progress in Surgical Pathology*, Vol. 1. C.M. Fenoglio and M. Wolff (eds.). Masson, New York, 1980, pp. 135–155.
74. Boucheix, C., Diebold, J., Bernadou, A., et al.: Lymphoblastic lymphoma/leukemia with convoluted nuclei.
    Cancer 45: 1569–1577, 1980.
75. Bouteille, M., Kalifat, S.R., and Delarue, J.: Ultrastructural variations of nuclear bodies in human diseases.
    J Ultrastruct Res 19: 474–486, 1967.
76. Brandes, D., Kirchheim, D., and Scott, W.W.: Ultrastructure of human prostate: Normal and neoplastic.
    Lab Invest 13: 1541–1560, 1964.
77. Bransilver, B.R., Ferenczy, A., and Richart, R.M.: Brenner tumors and Walthard cell nests.
    Arch Pathol 98: 76–86, 1974.
78. Braun-Falco, O., Schmoeckel, C., and Hübner, G.: Zur Histogenese des Sarcoma idiopathicum multiplex haemorrhagicum (Morbus Kaposi). Eine histochemische und elektronenmikroskopische Studie.
    Virchows Arch (Pathol Anat) 369: 215–227, 1976.
79. Bretholz, A., and Steiner, H.: Les insulomes. Intérêt d'un diagnostic morpholigique précis.
    Virchows Arch (Pathol Anat) 359: 49–66, 1973.
80. Breton-Gorius, J., and Houssay, D.: Auer bodies in acute promyelocytic leukemia. Demonstration of their fine structure and peroxidase localization.
    Lab Invest 28: 135–141, 1973.
81. Bretscher, A., and Weber, K.: Fimbrin, a new microfilament-associated protein present in microvilli and other cell surface structures.
    J Cell Biol 86: 335–340, 1980.
82. Bretscher, A., and Weber, K.: Villin is a major protein of the microvillus cytoskeleton which binds both G and F actin in a calcium-dependent manner.
    Cell 20: 839–847, 1980.
83. Brown, W.J., Barajas, L., Waisman, J., and De Quattro, V.: Ultrastructure and biochemical correlates of adrenal and extra-adrenal pheochromocytoma.
    Cancer 29: 744–759, 1972.
84. Brownlee, T. R., and Murad, T.M.: Ultrastructure of mycosis fungoides.
    Cancer 26: 686–698, 1970.
85. Brunning, R.D., and Parkin, J.: Ribosome–lamella complexes in neoplastic hematopoietic cells.
    Am J Pathol 79: 565–578, 1975.
86. Buffa, R., Capella, C., Fontana, P., Usellini, L. and Solcia, E.: Types of endocrine cells in the human colon and rectum.
    Cell Tissue Res 192: 227–240, 1978.
87. Burns, R.E., Soloff, B.L., Hanna, C., and Buxton, D.F.: Nuclear pockets associated with the nucleolus in normal and neoplastic cells.
    Cancer Res 31: 159–165, 1971.
88. Burns, W.A., Matthews, M.J., Hamosh, M., et al.: Lipase-secreting acinar cell carcinoma of the pancreas with polyarthropathy. A light and electron microscopic, histochemical, and biochemical study.
    Cancer 33: 1002–1009, 1974.
89. Buss, D.H., Marshall, R.B., Holleman, I.L., and Myers, R.T.: Malignant lymphoma of the thyroid gland with plasma cell differentiation (plasmacytoma).
    Cancer 46: 2671–2675, 1980.
90. Camins, M.B., Cravioto, H.M., Epstein, F., and Ransohoff, J.: Medulloblastoma: An ultrastructural study— Evidence for astrocytic and neuronal differentiation.
    Neurosurgery 6: 398–411, 1980.
91. Campbell, W.G.: Ultrastructure of pneumocystis in human lung—Life cycle in human pneumocystosis.
    Arch Pathol 93: 312–324, 1972.
92. Cancilla, P. A., Lahey, M.E., and Carnes, W.H.: Cutaneous lesions of Letterer-Siwe disease. Electron microscopic study.
    Cancer 20: 1986–1991, 1967.
93. Cantrell, B.B., Cubilla, A.L., Erlandson, R.A., Fortner, J., and Fitzgerald, P.J.: Acinar cell cystadenocarcinoma of human pancreas.
    Cancer 47: 410–416, 1981.
94. Capella, C., Bordi, C., Monga, G., et al.: Multiple endocrine cell types in thyroid medullary carcinoma. Evidence for calcitonin, somatostatin, ACTH, 5HT, and small granule cells.
    Virchows Arch (Pathol Anat) 377: 111–128, 1978.
95. Capella, C., Gabrielli, M., Polak, J.M., et al.: Ultrastructural and histological study of 11 bronchial carcinoids. Evidence for different types.
    Virchows Arch (Pathol Anat) 381: 313–329, 1979.
96. Capella, C., Solcia, E., Frigerio, B., et al.: The endocrine cells of the pancreas and related tumors. Ultrastructural study and classification.
    Virchows Arch (Pathol Anat) 373: 327–352, 1977.
97. Capella, C., Usellini, L., Frigerio, B., et al.: Argyrophil pituitary tumors showing TSH cells or small granule cells.
    Virchows Arch (Pathol Anat) 381: 295–312, 1979.
98. Carstens, P.H.B.: Ultrastructure of granular cell myoblastoma.
    Acta Pathol Microbiol Scand (A) 78: 685–694, 1970.
99. Carstens, P.H.B.: Ultrastructure of human fibroadenoma.
    Arch Pathol 98: 23–32, 1974.
100. Carstens, P.H.B., and Schrodt, G.R.: Ultrastructure of sclerosing hemangioma.
    Am J Pathol 77: 377–386, 1974.
101. Carter, L.P., Beggs, J., and Waggener, J.D.: Ultrastructure of three choroid plexus papillomas.
    Cancer 30: 1130–1136, 1972.
102. Castleman, B., and Roth, S.I.: Tumors of the parathyroid glands. In: *Atlas of Tumor Pathology*, 2nd ser., fasc. 14. Armed Forces Institute of Pathology, Washington, D.C., 1978.
103. Cebelin, M.S.: Melanocytic bronchial carcinoid tumor.
    Cancer 46: 1843–1848, 1980.
104. Cervós-Navarro, J., and Vazquez, J.J.: An electron microscopic study of meningiomas.
    Acta Neuropathol (Berl) 13: 301–323, 1969.
105. Chang, V., Aikawa, M., and Druet, R.: Uterine leiomyoblastoma. Ultrastructural and cytological studies.
    Cancer 39: 1563–1569, 1977.

106. Chaudhry, A.P., Haar, J.G., Koul, A., and Nickerson, P.A.: A nonfunctioning paraganglioma of vagus nerve. An ultrastructural study.
Cancer 43: 1689–1701, 1979.

107. Chaudhry, A.P., Haar, J.G., Koul, A., and Nickerson, P.A.: Olfactory neuroblastoma (esthesioneuroblastoma). A light and ultrastructural study of two cases.
Cancer 44: 564–579, 1979.

108. Chaudhry, A.P., Montes, M., and Cohn, G.A.: Ultrastructure of cerebellar hemangioblastoma.
Cancer 42: 1834–1850, 1978.

109. Chaudhry, A.P., Satchidanand, S.K., Gaeta, J.F., et al.: Light and ultrastructural studies of renal oncocytic adenoma.
Urology 14: 392–396, 1979.

110. Chejfec, G., and Gould, V.E.: Malignant gastric neuroendocrinomas. Ultrastructural and biochemical characterization of their secretory activity.
Hum Pathol 8: 433–440, 1977.

111. Christ, M.I., and Ozzello, L.: Myogenous origin of a granular cell tumor of the urinary bladder.
Am J Clin Pathol 56: 736–749, 1971.

112. Churg, A., Johnston, W.H., and Stulbarg, M.: Small cell squamous and mixed small cell squamous-small cell anaplastic carcinomas of the lung.
Am J Surg Pathol 4: 255–263, 1980.

113. Churg, A.M., and Kahn, L.B.: Myofibroblasts and related cells in malignant fibrous and fibrohistiocytic tumors.
Hum Pathol 8: 205–218, 1977.

114. Churg, A., and Ringus, J.: Ultrastructural observations on the histogenesis of alveolar rhabdomyosarcoma.
Cancer 41: 1355–1361, 1978.

115. Cinti, S., Osculati, F., and LoCascio, V.: Submicroscopic aspects of the chief cells in a case of parathyroid adenoma.
J Submicrosc Cytol 12: 293–300, 1980.

116. Clark, W. H., and Bretton, R.: A comparative fine structural study of melanogenesis in normal human epidermal melanocytes and in certain human malignant melanoma cells. In: *The Skin.* E.B. Helwig and F.K. Mostofi (eds.). International Academy of Pathology Monograph 10. Williams & Wilkins, Baltimore, 1971, pp. 197–214.

117. Clark, W.H., Jr., Goldman, L.I., and Mastrgelo, M.J. (eds.): *Human Malignant Melanoma.* Clinical Oncology Monographs. Grune & Stratton, New York, 1979.

118. Conforti, A., Medolago-Albani, L., and Alessio, L.: Ultrastructural changes in human leukemic cell nuclei.
Virchows Archiv (Cell Pathol) 22: 143–149, 1976.

119. Conley, F.K., Rubinstein, L.J., and Spence, A.M.: Studies on experimental malignant nerve sheath tumors maintained in tissue and organ culture systems.
Acta Neuropathol 34: 293–310, 1976.

120. Conley, J., Lattes, R., and Orr, W.: Desmoplastic malignant melanoma (a rare variant of spindle cell melanoma).
Cancer 28: 914–936, 1971.

121. Cooper, P.H., and Goodman, D.M.: Multilayering of the capillary basal lamina in the granular cell tumor. A marker of cellular injury.
Hum Pathol 5: 327–338, 1974.

122. Cooper, P.H., and Warkel, R.L.: Ultrastructure of the goblet cell type of adenocarcinoid of the appendix.
Cancer 42: 2687–2695, 1978.

123. Copeland, D.D., Bell, S.N., and Shelburne, J.D.: Hemidesmosome-like intercellular specializations in human meningiomas.
Cancer 41: 2242–2249, 1978.

124. Cornog, J.L., Jr.: Gastric leiomyoblastoma. A clinical and ultrastructural study.
Cancer 34: 711–719, 1974.

125. Cravioto, H., and Lockwood, R.: Long-spacing fibrous collagen in human acoustic nerve tumors. In vivo and in vitro observations.
J Ultrastruct Res 24: 70–85, 1968.

126. Creutzfeldt, W. Endocrine tumors of the pancreas: Clinical, chemical and morphologic findings. In: *The Pancreas.* P.J. Fitzgerald and A.B. Morrison (eds.). Williams & Wilkins, Baltimore, 1980, pp. 208–230.

127. Creutzfeldt, W., Arnold, R., Creutzfeldt, C., and Track, N.S.: Pathomorphologic, biochemical, and diagnostic aspects of gastrinomas (Zollinger-Ellison syndrome).
Hum Pathol 6: 47–76, 1975.

128. Creutzfeldt, W., Arnold, R., Creutzfeldt, C., et al.: Biochemical and morphological investigations of 30 human insulinomas. Correlations between the tumor content of insulin and the histological and ultrastructural appearance.
Diabetologia 9: 217–231, 1973.

129. Crissman, J.D., and Rosenblatt, A.: Acinous cell carcinoma of the larynx.
Arch Pathol Lab Med 102: 233–236, 1978.

130. Crissman, J.D., Wirman, J.A., and Harris, A.: Malignant myoepithelioma of the parotid gland.
Cancer 40: 3042–3049, 1977.

131. Cristina, M.L., Lehy, T., Zeitoun, P., and Dufougeray, F.: Fine structural classification and comparative distribution of endocrine cells in normal human large intestine.
Gastroenterology 75: 20–28, 1978.

132. Cubilla, A.L., and Woodruff, J.M.: Primary carcinoid tumor of the breast. A report of eight patients.
Am J Surg Pathol 1: 283–292, 1977.

133. Curran, R.C., and McCann, B.G.: The ultrastructure of benign pigmented naevi and melanocarcinomas in man.
J Pathol 119: 135–146, 1976.

134. Cutler, L.S., and Krutchkoff, D.: An ultrastructural study of eosinophilic granuloma: The Langerhans cell—Its role in histogenesis and diagnosis.
Oral Surg Med Pathol 44: 246–252, 1977.

135. Dahl, E.: The fine structure of nuclear inclusions.
J Anat 106: 255–262, 1970.

136. Damjanov, I., Niejadlik, D.C., Rabuffo, J.V., and Donadio, J.A.: Cribriform and sclerosing seminoma devoid of lymphoid infiltrates.
Arch Pathol Lab Med 104: 527–530, 1980.

137. David, H.: Physiologische und pathologische Modifikationen der submikroskopischen Kernstruktur. I. Das Karyoplasma Kerneinschlüsse.
Z Mikr-anat Forsch 71: 412–456, 1964.

138. Davison, P.F., Hong, B-S., and Cooke, P.: Classes of distinguishable 10 nm cytoplasmic filaments.
Exp Cell Res 109: 471–474, 1977.

139. Dehner, L.P., Sibley, R.K., Sauk, J.J., et al.: Malignant melanotic neuroectodermal tumor of infancy. A clinical, pathologic, ultrastructural and tissue culture study.
Cancer 43: 1389–1410, 1979.

140. DeRobertis, E.D.P., and DeRobertis, E.M.F., Jr.: *Cell and Molecular Biology,* 7th ed. Saunders College, Philadelphia, 1980, pp. 187–197.

141. DeWolf-Peeters, C., Marien, K., Mebis, J., and Desmet, V.: A cutaneous APUDoma or Merkel cell tumor? A morphologically recognizable tumor with a biological and

histological malignant aspect in contrast with its clinical behavior.
Cancer 46: 1810–1816, 1980.

142. Dickersin, G.R., Welch, W.R., Erlandson, R., and Robboy, S.J.: Ultrastructure of 16 cases of clear cell adenocarcinoma of the vagina and cervix in young women.
Cancer 45: 1615–1624, 1980.

143. Dische, F.E., Darby, A.J., and Howard, E.R.: Malignant synovioma: Electron microscopical findings in three patients and review of the literature.
J Pathol 124: 149–155, 1978.

144. Dorfman, R.F.: Diagnosis of Burkitt's tumor in the United States.
Cancer 21: 563–574, 1968.

145. Doyle, L.E., Lynn, J.A., Panopio, I.T., and Crass, G.: Ultrastructure of the chondroid regions of benign mixed tumor of salivary gland.
Cancer 22: 225–233, 1968.

146. Dubin, H.V., Creehand, E.P., and Headington, J.T.: Lymphangiosarcoma and congenital lymphedema of the extremities.
Arch Dermatol 110: 608–614, 1974.

147. Dustin, P.: *Microtubules.* Springer-Verlag, New York, 1978.

148. Dustin, P.: Microtubules.
Sci Am 243: 66–76, 1980.

149. Ehrenreich, J.H., Bergeron, J.J.M., Siekevitz, P., and Palade, G.E.: Golgi fractions prepared from rat liver homogenates.
J Cell Biol 59: 45–72, 1973.

150. Eimoto, T.: Ultrastructure of an infantile hemangiopericytoma.
Cancer 40: 2161–2170, 1977.

151. Ekfors, T.O., Kalimo, H., Rantakakko, V., Latvala, M., and Parvinen, M.: Alveolar soft part sarcoma. A report of two cases with some histochemical and ultrastructural observations.
Cancer 43: 1672–1677, 1979.

152. El-Hashimi, W.: Charcot-Leyden crystals. Formation from primate and lack of formation from nonprimate eosinophils.
Am J Pathol 65: 311–324, 1971.

153. Elliott, R.L., and Arhelger, R.B.: Fine structure of parathyroid adenomas. With special reference to annulate lamellae and septate desmosomes.
Arch Pathol 81: 200–212, 1966.

154. Eng, L.F., Vanderhaegen, J.J., Bignami, A., and Gerstl, B.: An acidic protein isolated from fibrous astrocytes.
Brain Res 28: 351–354, 1971.

155. Enzinger, F.M.: Epithelioid sarcoma. A sarcoma simulating a granuloma or a carcinoma.
Cancer 26: 1029–1041, 1970.

156. Ericsson, J.L.E., Seljelid, R., and Orrenius, S.: Comparative light and electron microscopic observations of the cytoplasmic matrix in renal carcinomas.
Virchows Arch (Pathol Anat) 341: 204–223, 1966.

157. Erlandson, R.A.: Electron microscopy of human tumors: A short review.
Clin Bull (MSKCC) 3: 14–19, 1973.

158. Erlandson, R.A.: Nuclear envelope changes in human tumor cells.
Anat Rec 81: 353, 1975. (Abst.)

159. Erlandson, R.A., and Huvos, A.G.: Chondrosarcoma. A light and electron microscopic study.
Cancer 34: 1642–1652, 1974.

160. Erlandson, R.A., and Melamed, M.R.: The subclassification of peripheral lung adenocarcinoma in man.
Proc Electron Microsc Soc Am 37: 224–225, 1979.

161. Erlandson, R.A., and Tandler, B.: Ultrastructure of acinic cell carcinoma of the parotid gland.
Arch Pathol 93: 130–140, 1972.

162. Erlandson, R.A., Tandler, B., Lieberman, P.H., and Higinbotham, N.L.: Ultrastructure of human chordoma.
Cancer Res 28: 2115–2125, 1968.

163. Erlandson, R.A., and Woodruff, J.M.: Peripheral nerve sheath tumors. An electron microscopic study of 43 cases.
Cancer (In press.)

164. Eto, T., Kumamamoto, K., Kawasaki, T., et al.: Ultrastructural types of cell in adrenal cortical adenoma with primary aldosteronism.
J Pathol 128: 1–6, 1979.

165. Farmer, P.M.: Electron microscopy in the diagnosis of pituitary tumors.
Ann Clin Lab Sci 9: 275–288, 1979.

166. Farquhar, M.G., and Palade, G.E.: Junctional complexes in various epithelia.
J Cell Biol 17: 375–309, 1963.

167. Fawcett, D.W.: Surface specializations of absorbing cells.
J Histochem Cytochem 13: 75–91, 1965.

168. Fawcett, D.W.: On the occurrence of a fibrous lamina on the inner aspect of the nuclear envelope in certain cells of vertebrates.
Am J Anat 119: 129–145, 1966.

169. Fawcett, D.W., and Burgos, M.H.: Studies on the fine structure of the mammalian testis. II. The human interstitial cells.
Am J Anat 107: 245–269, 1960.

170. Fawcett, D.W., and Porter, K.R.: A study of the fine structure of ciliated epithelia.
J Morphol 94: 221–281, 1954.

171. Fechner, R.E., and Bentinck, B.R.: Ultrastructure of bronchial oncocytoma.
Cancer 31: 1451–1457, 1973.

172. Fechner, R.E., Bentinck, B.R., and Askew, J.B., Jr.: Acinic cell tumor of the lung. A histologic and ultrastructural study.
Cancer 29: 501–508, 1972.

173. Feldman, P.S.: A comparative study including ultrastructure of intramuscular myxoma and myxoid liposarcoma.
Cancer 43: 512–525, 1979.

174. Feldman, P.S., Horvath, E., and Kovacs, K.: Ultrastructure of three Hürthle cell tumors of the thyroid.
Cancer 30: 1279–1285, 1972.

175. Feldman, P.S., Horvath, E., and Kovacs, K.: An ultrastructural study of seven cardiac myxomas.
Cancer 40: 2216–2232, 1977.

176. Feldman, P.S., Sheidman, D., and Kaplan, C.: Ultrastructure of infantile hemangioendothelioma of the liver.
Cancer 42: 521–527, 1978.

177. Fenoglio, C.M.: Overview article: Ultrastructural features of the common epithelial tumors of the ovary.
Ultrastruct Pathol 1: 419–444, 1980.

178. Fenoglio, C.M., Castadot, M-J., Ferenczy, A., Cottral, G.A., and Richart, R.M.: Serous tumors of the ovary. I. Ultrastructural and histochemical studies on the epithelium of the benign serous neoplasms, serous cystadenoma and serous cystadenofibroma.
Gynecol Oncol 5: 203–218, 1977.

179. Feremans, W.W., Neve, P., and Caudron, M.: IgM

lambda cytoplasmic crystals in three cases of immuno-cytoma: A clinical, cytochemical, and ultrastructural study.
J Clin Pathol 31: 250–258, 1978.

180. Ferenczy, A.: The ultrastructural morphology of gynecologic neoplasms.
Cancer 38: 463–468, 1976.

181. Ferenczy, A.: Recent advances in endometrial neoplasia.
Exp Mol Pathol 31: 226–235, 1979.

182. Ferenczy, A., and Richart, R.M.: Gynecology. In: *Diagnostic Electron Microscopy*, Vol. 2. B.F. Trump and R.T. Jones (eds.). John Wiley & Sons, New York, 1979, pp. 269–308.

183. Ferenczy, A., Richart, R.M., and Okagaki, T.: A comparative ultrastructural study of leiomyosarcoma, cellular leiomyoma, and leiomyoma of the uterus.
Cancer 28: 1004–1018, 1971.

184. Ferenczy, A., Talens, M., Zoghby, M., and Hussain, S.: Ultrastructural studies on the morphogenesis of psammoma bodies in ovarian serous neoplasia.
Cancer 39: 2451–2459, 1977.

185. Fernandez, B.B., and Hernandez, F.J.: Poorly differentiated synovial sarcoma. A light and electron microscopic study.
Arch Pathol Lab Med 100: 221–223, 1976.

186. Fisher, E.R., Palekar, A., and Paulson, J.D.: Comparative histopathologic, histochemical, electron microscopic and tissue culture studies of bronchial carcinoids and oat cell carcinomas of lung.
Am J Clin Pathol 69: 165–172, 1978.

187. Fitzpatrick, T.B., Quevedo, W.C. Jr., Szabo, G., and Selji, M.: Biology of the melanin pigmentary system. In: *Dermatology in General Medicine*. T.B. Fitzpatrick, K.A. Arndt, W.H. Clarke, A.Z. Eisen, E.J. Van Scott, and J.H. Vaughan (eds.). McGraw-Hill, New York, 1971, pp. 117–146.

188. Florentin, I.: The immunoblast.
Biomedicine 22: 457–460, 1975.

189. Foa, C., and Aubert, C.: Ultrastructural comparison between cultured and tumor cells of human malignant melanoma.
Cancer Res 37: 3957–3963, 1977.

190. Fox, B., Bull, T.B., and Arden, G.B.: Variations of human nasal cilia including abnormalities found in retinitis pigmentosa.
J Clin Pathol 33: 327–335, 1980.

191. Franke, W.W., Schmid, E., Freudenstein, C., et al.: Intermediate-sized filaments of the prekeratin type in myoepithelial cells.
J Cell Biol 84: 633–654, 1980.

192. Franke, W.W., Schmid, E., Osborn, M., and Weber, K.: Intermediate-sized filaments of human endothelial cells.
J Cell Biol 81: 570–580, 1979.

193. Friede, R.L., and Pollak, A.: The cytogenetic basis for classifying ependymomas.
J Neuropathol Exp Neurol 37: 103–118, 1978.

194. Fu, Y-S., Chen, A.T.L., Kay, S., and Young, H.F.: Is subependymoma (subependymal glomerate astrocytoma) an astrocytoma or ependymoma? A comparative ultrastructural and tissue culture study.
Cancer 34: 1992–2008, 1974.

195. Fu, Y-S., Gabbiani, G., Kaye, G.I., and Lattes, R.: Malignant soft tissue tumors of probable histiocytic origin (malignant fibrous histiocytoma): General considerations and electron microscopic and tissue culture studies.
Cancer 35: 176–198, 1975.

196. Fu, Y-S., and Kay, S.: Congenital mesoblastic nephroma and its recurrence.
Arch Pathol 96: 66–70, 1973.

197. Fulker, M.J., Cooper, E.H., and Tanaka, T.: Proliferation and ultrastructure of papillary transitional cell carcinoma of the human bladder.
Cancer 27: 71–82, 1971.

198. Fung, C.H., Lo, J.W., Yonan, T.N., et al.: Pulmonary blastoma. An ultrastructural study with a brief review of literature and a discussion of pathogenesis.
Cancer 39: 153–163, 1977.

199. Gabbiani, G., Csank-Brassert, J., Schneeberger, J-C., et al.: Contractile proteins in human cancer cells. Immunofluorescent and electron microscopic study.
Am J Pathol 83: 457–474, 1976.

200. Gabbiani, G., Kaye, G.I., Lattes, R., and Majno, G.: Synovial sarcoma. Electron microscopic study of a typical case.
Cancer 28: 1031–1039, 1971.

201. Gabbiani, G., and Majno, G.: Dupuytren's contracture: Fibroblast contraction? An ultrastructural study.
Am J Pathol 66: 131–145, 1972.

202. Gabbiani, G., Ryan, G.B., and Majno, G.: Presence of modified fibroblasts in granulation tissue and their possible role in wound contraction.
Experientia 27: 549–550, 1971.

203. Gullivan, M.V.E., Chun, B., Rowden, G., and Lack, E.E.: Laryngeal paraganglioma. Case report with ultrastructural analysis and literature review.
Am J Surg Pathol 3: 85–92, 1979.

204. Garancis, J.C., Tang, T., Panares, R., and Jurevics, I.: Hepatic adenoma. Biochemical and electron microscopic study.
Cancer 24: 560–568, 1969.

205. Garcia-Buñuel, R., and Brandes, D.: Luteoma of pregnancy: Ultrastructural features.
Hum Pathol 7: 205–214, 1976.

206. Genton, C.Y.: Some observations on the fine structure of human granulosa cell tumors.
Virchows Arch (Pathol Anat) 387: 353–369, 1980.

207. Ghadially, F.N.: *Ultrastructural Pathology of the Cell.* (A text and atlas of physiological and pathological alterations in cell fine structure.) Butterworths, London, 1975.

208. Ghadially, F.N.: *Diagnostic Electron Microscopy of Tumors.* Butterworths, London, 1980.

209. Ghadially, F.N.: Overview article: The articular territory of the reticuloendothelial system.
Ultrastruct Pathol 1: 249–264, 1980.

210. Ghadially, F.N., and Mehta, P.N.: Ultrastructure of osteogenic sarcoma.
Cancer 25: 1457–1467, 1970.

211. Gillespie, J.J.: The ultrastructural diagnosis of diffuse large-cell ("histiocytic") lymphoma. Fine structural study of 30 cases.
Am J Surg Pathol 2: 9–20, 1978.

212. Gillespie, J.J., Luger, A.M., and Callaway, L.A.: Peripheral spindled carcinoid tumor: A review of its ultrastructure, differential diagnosis, and biologic behavior.
Hum Pathol 10: 601–606, 1979.

213. Glenner, G.G.: Amyloid deposits and amyloidosis. The β-fibrilloses.
N Engl J Med 302: 1283–1292; 1333–1343, 1980.

214. Glick, A.D.: Acute leukemia: Electron microscope diagnosis.
Semin Oncol 3: 229–241, 1976.

215. Glick, A.D., Leech, J.H., Flexner, J.M., and Collins, R.D.: Ultrastructural study of Reed-Sternberg cells. Comparison with transformed lymphocytes and histiocytes. *Am J Pathol 85: 195–208, 1976.*

216. Glick, A.D., Leech, J.H., Waldron, J.A., et al.: Malignant lymphomas of follicular center cell origin in man. II. Ultrastructural and cytochemical studies. *J Natl Cancer Inst 54: 23–36, 1975.*

217. Goellner, J.R., and Soule, E.H.: Desmoid tumors. An ultrastructural study of eight cases. *Human Pathol 11: 43–50, 1980.*

218. Goldman, J.E., Schaumburg, H.H., and Norton, W.T.: Isolation and characterization of glial filaments from human brain. *J Cell Biol 78: 426–440, 1978.*

219. Gondos, B.: Ultrastructure of a metastatic granulosa-theca cell tumor. *Cancer 24: 954–959, 1969.*

220. Gondos, B.: Electron microscopic study of papillary serous tumors of the ovary. *Cancer 27: 1455–1464, 1971.*

221. Gonzalez-Crussi, F., and Black-Schaffer, S.: Rhabdomyosarcoma of infancy and childhood. *Am J Surg Pathol 3: 157–171, 1979.*

222. Goodman, T.F., and Abele, D.C.: Multiple glomus tumors. A clinical and electron microscopic study. *Arch Dermatol 103: 11–23, 1971.*

223. Gould, V.E.: Neuroendocrinomas: APUD-cell system neoplasms and their aberrant secretory activities. In: *Pathology Annual*, Vol. 12. S.C. Sommers (ed.). Appleton-Century-Crofts, New York, 1977, pp. 33–62.

224. Gould, V.E., and Chejfec, G.: Ultrastructural and biochemical analysis of "undifferentiated" pulmonary carcinomas. *Hum Pathol 9: 377–384, 1978.*

225. Granger, B.L., and Lazarides, E.: Desmin and vimentin coexist at the periphery of the myofibril Z disc. *Cell 18: 1053–1063, 1979.*

226. Granger, B.L., and Lazarides, E.: Synemin: A new high molecular weight protein associated with desmin and vimentin filaments in muscle. *Cell 22: 727–738, 1980.*

227. Gray, G.F. Jr., Gonzales-Licea, A., Hartmann, W.H., and Woods, A.C.: Angiosarcoma in lymphedema: An unusual case of Stewart-Treves syndrome. *Bull Hopkins Hosp 119: 117–128, 1966.*

228. Greenberg, D.S., Smith, M.N., and Spjut, H.J.: Bronchioloalveolar carcinoma—Cell of origin. *Am J Clin Pathol 63: 153–167, 1975.*

229. Greider, M.H., Rosai, J., and McGuigan, J.E.: The human pancreatic islet cells and their tumors. II. Ulcerogenic and diarrheogenic tumors. *Cancer 33: 1423–1443, 1974.*

230. Grimley, P.M., and Glenner, G.G.: Histology and ultrastructure of carotid body paragangliomas. Comparison with the normal gland. *Cancer 20: 1473–1488, 1967.*

231. Gyorkey, F., Min, K-W., Krisko, I., and Gyorkey, P.: The usefulness of electron microscopy in the diagnosis of human tumors. *Hum Pathol 6: 421–441, 1975.*

232. Hage, E.: Histochemistry and fine structure of bronchial carcinoid tumors. *Virchows Arch (Pathol Anat) 361: 121–128, 1973.*

233. Hahn, M.J., Dawson, R., Esterly, J.A., and Joseph, D.J.: Hemangiopericytoma. An ultrastructural study. *Cancer 31: 255–261, 1973.*

234. Hajdu, S.I., Erlandson, R.A., and Paglia, M.A.: Light and electron microscopic studies of a gastric leiomyoblastoma. *Arch Pathol 93: 36–41, 1972.*

235. Hamperl, H.: Benign and malignant oncocytoma. *Cancer 15: 1019–1025, 1962.*

236. Hamperl, H.: The myothelia (myoepithelial cells). Normal state; regressive changes; hyperplasia; tumors. *Curr Top Pathol 53: 160–220, 1970.*

237. Hanaoka, H., and Friedman, B.: Paired cisternae in human tumor cells. *J Ultrastruct Res 32: 323–333, 1970.*

238. Harris, M., and Balgobin, B.: Pure Sertoli cell tumor of the ovary: Report of a case with ultrastructural observations. *Histopathology 2: 449–459, 1978.*

239. Hart, M.N., and Earle, K.M.: Primitive neuroectodermal tumors of the brain in children. *Cancer 32: 890–897, 1973.*

240. Hashimoto, K., Brownstein, M.H., and Jakobiec, F.A.: Dermatofibrosarcoma protuberans. A tumor with perineurial and endoneurial cell features. *Arch Dermatol 110: 874–885, 1974.*

241. Hassan, M.O., Khan, M.A., and Kruse, T.V.: Apocrine cystadenoma. An ultrastructural study. *Arch Dermatol 115: 194–200, 1979.*

242. Hassan, M.O., and Olaizola, M.Y.: Ultrastructural observations on gynecomastia. *Arch Pathol Lab Med 103: 624–630, 1979.*

243. Hasumi, K., Sakamoto, G., Sugano, H., Kasuga, T., and Masubuchi, K.: Primary malignant melanoma of the vagina. Study of four autopsy cases with ultrastructural findings. *Cancer 42: 2675–2686, 1978.*

244. Hattori, S., Matsuda, M., Tateishi, R., Nishihara, H., and Horai, T.: Oat-cell carcinoma of the lung. Clinical and morphological studies in relation to its histogenesis. *Cancer 30: 1014–1024, 1972.*

245. Hazard, J.B.: The C cells (parafollicular cells) of the thyroid gland and medullary thyroid carcinoma. A review. *Am J Pathol 88: 214–249, 1977.*

246. Heitz, P.U., and Wegmann, W.: Identification of neoplastic paneth cells in an adenocarcinoma of the stomach using lysozyme as a marker, and electron microscopy. *Virchows Arch (Pathol Anat) 386: 107–116, 1980.*

247. Herman, I.M., and Pollard, T.D.: Electron microscopic localization of cytoplasmic myosin with ferritin-labeled antibodies. *J Cell Biol 88: 346–351, 1981.*

248. Hernandez, F.J.: Malignant blue nevus. A light and electron microscopic study. *Arch Dermatol 107: 741–744, 1973.*

249. Hernandez, F.J.: Primary leiomyosarcoma of the aorta. *Am J Surg Pathol 3: 251–256, 1979.*

250. Herndon, R.M., Rubinstein, L.J., Freeman, J.M., and Mathieson, G.: Light and electron microscopic observations on Rosenthal fibers in Alexander's disease and in multiple sclerosis. *J Neuropathol Exp Neurol 29: 524–551, 1970.*

251. Herrera, G.A., Crofts, J.L., and Roberts, C.R.: Neurosecretory granule-like structures in lymphomas. *Hum Pathol 11: 449–457, 1980.*

252. Hickey, W.F., and Seiler, M.W.: Ultrastructural markers of colonic adenocarcinoma.

Cancer 47: 140–145, 1981.

253. Hicks, R.M.: The function of the Golgi complex in transitional epithelium. Synthesis of the thick cell membrane.
J Cell Biol 30: 623–644, 1966.

254. Hirano, A., Ghatak, N.R., and Zimmerman, H.M.: The fine structure of ependymoblastoma.
J Neuropathol Exp Neurol 32: 144–152, 1973.

255. Hoch, W.S., Patchefsky, A.S., Takeda, M., and Gordon, G.: Benign clear cell tumor of the lung. An ultrastructural study.
Cancer 33: 1328–1336, 1974.

256. Holstein, A.F., and Körner, F.: Light and electron microscopical analysis of cell types in human seminoma.
Virchows Arch (Pathol Anat) 363: 97–112, 1974.

257. Horie, A., Kotoo, Y., and Hayashi, I.: Ultrastructural comparison of hepatoblastoma and hepatocellular carcinoma.
Cancer 44: 2184–2193, 1979.

258. Horie, A., Yano, Y., Kotoo, Y., and Miwa, A.: Morphogenesis of pancreatoblastoma, infantile carcinoma of the pancreas. Report of two cases.
Cancer 39: 247–254, 1977.

259. Horoupian, D.S., Kerson, L.A., Saiontz, H., and Valsamis, M.: Paraganglioma of cauda equina. Clinicopathologic and ultrastructural studies of an unusual case.
Cancer 33: 1337–1348, 1974.

260. Horvath, E., and Kovacs, K.: Morphogenesis and significance of fibrous bodies in human pituitary adenomas,
Virchows Archiv (Cell Pathol) 27: 69–78, 1978.

261. Horvath, E., Kovacs, K., Singer, W., Ezrin, C., and Kerenyi, N.A.: Acidophil stem cell adenoma of the human pituitary.
Arch Pathol Lab Med 101: 594–599, 1977.

262. Hoshino, M.: "Polysome-lamellae complex" in the adenoma cells of the human adrenal cortex.
J Ultrastruct Res 27: 205–215, 1969.

263. Hoshino, M., and Yamamoto, L.: Ultrastructure of adenoid cystic carcinoma.
Cancer 25: 186–198, 1970.

264. Hubbard, B.D., and Lazarides, E.: Copurification of actin and desmin from chicken smooth muscle and their copolymerization in vitro to intermediate filaments.
J Cell Biol 80: 166–182, 1979.

265. Hübner, G., Klein, H.J., Kleinsasser, O., and Schiefer, H.G.: Role of myoepithelial cells in the development of salivary gland tumors.
Cancer 27: 1255–1261, 1971.

266. Huhn, D., and Meister, P.: Malignant histiocytosis. Morphologic and cytochemical findings.
Cancer 42: 1341–1349, 1978.

267. Hull, B.E., and Staehelin, A.L.: The terminal web. A reevaluation of its structure and function.
J Cell Biol 81: 67–82, 1979.

268. Hunter, J.A.A., Zaynoun, S., Paterson, W.D., et al.: Cellular fine structure in the invasive nodules of different histogenetic types of malignant melanoma.
Br J Dermatol 98: 255–272, 1978.

269. Huvos, A.G., Marcove, R.C., Erlandson, R.A., and Mike, V.: Chondroblastoma of bone. A clinicopathologic and electron microscopic study.
Cancer 29: 760–771, 1972.

270. Ishida, T., Okagaki, T., Tagatz, G.E., Jacobson, M.E., and Doe, R.P.: Lipid cell tumor of the ovary: An ultrastructural study.
Cancer 40: 234–243, 1977.

271. Ito, S.: Structure and function of the glycocalyx.
Fed Proc 28: 12–25, 1969.

272. Jacob, J., Ludgate, C.M., Forde, J., and Tulloch, W.S.: Recent observations on the ultrastructure of human urothelium.
Cell Tissue Res 193: 543–560, 1978.

273. Jamiesen, J.P., and Palade, G.E.: Intracellular transport of secretory proteins in the pancreatic exocrine cell. I, II.
J Cell Biol 34: 577–615, 1967.

274. Janssen, M., and Johnston, W.H.: Anaplastic seminoma of the testis. Ultrastructural analysis of three cases.
Cancer 41: 538–544, 1978.

275. Jao, W., Vazquez, L.T., Keh, P.C., and Gould, V.E.: Myoepithelial differentiation and basal lamina deposition in fibroadenoma and adenosis of the breast.
J Pathol 126: 107–122, 1978.

276. Jimbow, K., Oikawa, O., Sugiyama, S., and Takeuchi, T.: Comparison of eumelanogenesis and pheomelanogenesis in retinal and follicular melanocytes; role of vesiculoglobular bodies in melanosome differentiation.
J Invest Dermatol 73: 278–284, 1979.

277. Jimbow, K., Quevedo, W.C., Fitzpatrick, T.B., and Szabo, G.: Some aspects of melanin biology: 1950–1975.
J Invest Dermatol 67: 72–89, 1976.

278. Jimbow, K., Szabo, G., and Fitzpatrick, T.B.: Ultrastructure of giant pigment granules (macromelanosomes) in the cutaneous pigmented macules of neurofibromatosis.
J Invest Dermatol 61: 300–309, 1973.

279. Johns, M.E., Regezi, J.A., and Batsakis, J.G.: Oncocytic neoplasms of salivary glands: An ultrastructural study.
Laryngoscope 87: 862–871, 1977.

280. Johnson, L., Diamond, D., and Jolly, G.: Ultrastructure of fallopian tube carcinoma.
Cancer 42: 1291–1297, 1978.

281. Johnson, W.W., Coburn, T.P., Pratt, C.B., et al.: Ultrastructure of malignant histiocytoma arising in the acromion.
Hum Pathol 9: 199–209, 1978.

282. Julian Garvin, A., Pratt-Thomas, H.R., Spector, M., Spicer, S.S., and Williamson, H.O.: Gonadoblastoma: Histologic, ultrastructural and histochemical observations in five cases.
Am J Obstet Gynecol 125: 459–471, 1976.

283. Kahn, L.B., and Schoub, L.: Myoepithelioma of the palate. Histochemical and ultrastructural observations.
Arch Pathol 95: 209–212, 1973.

284. Kalderon, A.E., and Tucci, J.R.: Ultrastructure of a human chorionic gonadotropin- and adrenocorticotropin-responsive functioning Sertoli-Leydig cell tumor (type 1).
Lab Invest 29: 81–89, 1973.

285. Kamperdijk, E.W.A., Raaymaker, E.M., de Leeuw, J.H.S., and Hoefsmit, E.Ch.M.: Lymph node macrophages and reticulum cells in the immune response. I. The primary response to parathyroid vaccine.
Cell Tissue Res 192: 1–23, 1978.

286. Kanabe, S., Watanabe, I., and Lotuaco, L.: Multiple granular-cell tumors of the ascending colon: Microscopic study.
Dis Colon Rectum 21: 322–328, 1978.

287. Kaneko, H., Yanaihara, N., Ito, S., et al: Somatostatinoma of the duodenum.
Cancer 44: 2273–2279, 1979.

288. Kano, K-i., Sato, S., and Hama, H.: Adrenal adenomata causing primary aldosteronism. An ultrastructural study of twenty-five cases.
Virchows Arch (Pathol Anat) 384: 93–102, 1979.

289. Kanwar, Y.S., and Manaligod, J.R.: Glomus tumor of the stomach. An ultrastructural study.
Arch Pathol 99: 392–397, 1975.

290. Katayama, I., and Schneider, G.B.: Further ultrastructural characterization of hairy cells of leukemic reticuloendotheliosis.
Am J Pathol 86: 163–182, 1977.

291. Katayama, I., Uehara, H., Gleser, R.A., and Weintraub, L.: The value of electron microscopy in the diagnosis of Burkitt's lymphoma.
Am J Clin Pathol 61: 540–548, 1974.

292. Kawanami, O., Ferrans, V.J., Fulmer, J.O., and Crystal, R.G.: Nuclear inclusions in alveolar epithelium of patients with fibrotic lung disorders.
Am J Pathol 94: 301–322, 1979.

293. Kay, S.: Hyperplasia and neoplasia of the adrenal gland. In: *Pathology Annual*, Vol. 11. S.C. Sommers (ed.). Appleton-Century-Crofts, New York, 1976, pp. 103–139.

294. Kay, S., Elzay, R.P., and Willson, M.A.: Ultrastructural observations on a gingival granular cell tumor (congenital epulis).
Cancer 27: 674–680, 1971.

295. Kay, S., Fu, Y-S, Koontz, W.W., and Chen, A.T.L.: Interstitial-cell tumor of the testis. Tissue culture and ultrastructural studies.
Am J Clin Pathol 63: 366–376, 1975.

296. Kay, S., and Schatzki, P.F.: Ultrastructure of a benign liver cell adenoma.
Cancer 28: 755–762, 1971.

297. Kay, S., and Schatzki, P.F.: Ultrastructure of acinic cell carcinoma of the parotid salivary gland.
Cancer 29: 235–244, 1972.

298. Kay, S., and Schatzki, P.F.: Ultrastructural observations of a chordoma arising in the clivus.
Hum Pathol 3: 403–413, 1972.

299. Kay, S., Still, W.J.S., and Borochovitz, D.: Sclerosing hemangioma of the lung: An endothelial or epithelial neoplasm.
Hum Pathol 8: 468–474, 1977.

300. Kay, S., and Terz, J.J.: Ultrastructural observations on a follicular carcinoma of the thyroid gland.
Am J Clin Pathol 65: 328–336, 1976.

301. Kelly, R.E., and Rice, R.V.: Localization of myosin filaments in smooth muscle.
J Cell Biol 37: 104–116, 1968.

302. Kempson, R.L.: Ultrastructure of ovarian stromal cell tumors. Sertoli-Leydig cell tumor and lipid cell tumor.
Arch Pathol 86: 492–507, 1968.

303. Kermarec, J., and Varim, J-P.: Etude microscopie et ultrastructurale d'un tumeur de Stewart-Treves.
Arch Anat Pathol 23: 193–198, 1975.

304. Kern, H.F., and Ferner, H.: Die Feinstruktur des exocrinen Pankreasgewebes von Menschen.
Z Zellforsch 133: 322–343, 1971.

305. Kessel, R.G.: Fine structure of annulate lamellae.
J Cell Biol 36: 658–663, 1968.

306. Kimula, Y.: A histochemical and ultrastructural study of adenocarcinoma of the lung.
Am J Surg Pathol 2: 253–264, 1978.

307. Kindblom, L-G., and Säve-Söderbergh, J.: The ultrastructure of liposarcoma. A study of 10 cases.
Acta Pathol Microbiol Scand (A) 87: 109–121, 1979.

308. Klein, M.J., and Valensi, Q.J.: Proximal tubular adenomas of the kidney with so-called oncocytic features.
Cancer 38: 906–914, 1976.

309. Kleinman, G.M., Liszczak, T., Tarlov, E., and Richardson, E.P., Jr.: Microcystic variant of meningioma. A light-microscopic and ultrastructural study.
Am J Surg Pathol 4: 383–389, 1980.

310. Klemi, P.J., and Nevalainen, T.J.: Ultrastructure of the benign and borderline Brenner tumors.
Acta Pathol Microbiol Scand (A) 85: 826–838, 1977.

311. Klemi, P.J., and Nevalainen, T.J.: Ultrastructural and histochemical observations on serous ovarian cystadenomas.
Acta Pathol Microbiol Scand (A) 86: 303–312, 1978.

312. Klima, M., Spjut, H.J., and Seybold, W.D.: Diffuse malignant mesothelioma.
Am J Clin Pathol 65: 583–600, 1976.

313. Kline, K.T., Damjanov, I., Moriber Katz, S., and Schmidek, H.: Pineoblastoma: An electron microscopic study.
Cancer 44: 1692–1699, 1979.

314. Klug, H.: Über Kenanomalien bei malignen Melanomen des Menschen.
Zentralbl Allg Pathol 116: 316–324, 1972.

315. Klug, H., and Gunther, W.: Ultrastructural differences in human malignant melanomata.
Br J Dermatol 86: 395–407, 1972.

316. Koide, O., Watanabe, Y., and Sato, K.: A pathological survey of intracranial germinoma and pinealoma in Japan.
Cancer 45: 2119–2130, 1980.

317. Konrad, K., Wolff, K., and Hönigsmann, H.: The giant melanosome: A model of deranged melanosome-morphogenesis.
J Ultrastruct Res 48: 102–123, 1974.

318. Koppersmith, D.L., Powers, J.M., and Hennigar, G.R.: Angiomatoid neuroblastoma with cytoplasmic glycogen. A case report and histogenetic considerations.
Cancer 45: 553–560, 1980.

319. Korényi-Both., Lapis, K., and Gallai, M.: Uber die Feinstruktur des undifferenzierten, adulten, pleomorphen Rhabdomyosarkoms.
Beitr Pathol Anat 138: 96–108, 1968.

320. Koss, L.G.: The asymmetric unit membranes of the epithelium of the urinary bladder of the rat. An electron microscopic study of a mechanism of epithelial maturation and function.
Lab Invest 21: 154–168, 1969.

321. Koss, L.G.: Some ultrastructural aspects of experimental and human carcinoma of the bladder.
Cancer Res 37: 2824–2835, 1977.

322. Koss, L.G., Brannan, C.D., and Ashikari, R.: Histologic and ultrastructural features of adenoid cystic carcinoma of the breast.
Cancer 26: 1271–1279, 1970.

323. Koss, L.G., Rothschild, E.O., Fleisher, M., and Francis, J.E.: Masculinizing tumor of the ovary, apparently with adrenocortical activity. A histologic, ultrastructural and biochemical study.
Cancer 23: 1245–1258, 1969.

324. Kovacs, K.K., and Horvath, E.: Pituitary "chromophobe" adenoma composed of oncocytes. A light and electron microscopic study.
Arch Pathol 95: 235–239, 1973.

325. Kovacs, K., Horvath, E., and Ezrin, C.: Pituitary adenomas. In: *Pathology Annual*, Vol. 12. S.C. Sommers (ed.). Appleton-Century-Crofts, New York, 1977, pp.

341–382.

326. Kovacs, K., Horvath, E., and Murray, T.M.: Large-clear cell adenoma of the parathyroid gland associated with primary hyperparathyroidism. A light and electron microscopic study.
J Submicrosc Cytol 9: 323–328, 1977.

327. Kovacs, K., Horvath, E., Ryan, N., and Ezrin, C.: Null cell adenoma of the human pituitary.
Virchows Arch (Pathol Anat) 387: 165–174, 1980.

328. Kuhn, C.: Fine structure of bronchiolo-alveolar cell carcinoma.
Cancer 30: 1107–1118, 1972.

329. Kumar, P., Kumar, S., Marsden, H.B., Lynch, P.G., and Earnshaw, E.: Weibel-Palade bodies in endothelial cells as a marker for angiogenesis in brain tumors.
Cancer Res 40: 2010–2019, 1980.

330. Kurki, P., Linder, E., Virtanen, I., and Stenman, S.: Human smooth muscle autoantibodies reacting with intermediate (100Å) filaments.
Nature 268: 240–241, 1977.

331. Labaze, J.J., Moscovic, E.A., Pham, T.D., and Azar, H.A.: Histological and ultrastructural findings in a case of the Sézary syndrome.
J Clin Pathol 25: 312–319, 1972.

332. Labrecque, P.G., Hu, C-H., and Winkelmann, R.K.: On the nature of desmoplastic melanoma.
Cancer 38: 1205–1213, 1976.

333. Lack, E.E., Cubilla, A.L., and Woodruff, J.M.: Paragangliomas of the head and neck region. A pathologic study of tumors from 71 patients.
Hum Pathol 10: 191–218, 1979.

334. Lack, E.E., Stillinger, R.A., Colvin, D.B., Groves, R.M., and Burnette, D.G.: Aortico-pulmonary paraganglioma. Report of a case with ultrastructural study and review of the literature.
Cancer 43: 269–278, 1979.

335. Lagacé, R., Bouchard, H-Ls., Delage, C., and Seemeyer, T.A.: Desmoplastic fibroma of bone. An ultrastructural study.
Am J Surg Pathol 3: 423–430, 1979.

336. Lagios, M.D., Friedlander, L.M., Wallerstein, R.O., and Bohannon, R.A.: Atypical azurophilic crystals in chronic lymphocytic leukemia.
Am J Clin Pathol 62: 342–349, 1974.

337. Landolt, A.M., and Oswald, U.W.: Histology and ultrastructure of an oncocyte adenoma of the human pituitary.
Cancer 31: 1099–1105, 1973.

338. Lane, B.P., and Rhodin, J.A.G.: Cellular interrelationships and electrical activity in two types of smooth muscle.
J Ultrastruct Res 10: 470–488, 1964.

339. Larsson, L-I.: Endocrine pancreatic tumors.
Hum Pathol 9: 401–416, 1978.

340. Lazarides, E.: Actin, α-actinin, and tropomyosin interactions in the structural organization of actin filaments in nonmuscle cells.
J Cell Biol 68: 202–219, 1976.

341. Lazarides, E.: Intermediate filaments as mechanical integrators of cellular space.
Nature 283: 249–256, 1980.

342. Lazarides, E., and Revel, J.P.: The molecular basis of cell movement.
Sci Am 240: 100–113, 1979.

343. Lazarus, S.S., and Trombetta, L.D.: Ultrastructural identification of a benign perineurial cell tumor.
Cancer 41: 1823–1829, 1978.

344. Leak, L.V., and Burke, J.F.: Fine structure of the lymphatic capillary and the adjoining connective tissue area.
Am J Anat 118: 785–807, 1966.

345. Leifer, C., Miller, A.S., Putong, P.B., and Harwick, R.D.: Myoepithelioma of the parotid gland.
Arch Pathol 98: 312–319, 1974.

346. Levine, A.M., Reddick, R., and Triche, T.: Intracellular collagen fibrils in human sarcomas.
Lab Invest 39: 531–540, 1978.

347. Levine, G.D.: Primary thymic seminoma—A neoplasm ultrastructurally similar to testicular seminoma and distinct from epithelial thymoma.
Cancer 31: 729–741, 1973.

348. Levine, G.D., and Bensch, K.G.: Chondroblastoma—The nature of the basic cell. A study by means of histochemistry, tissue culture, electron microscopy, and autoradiography.
Cancer 29: 1546–1562, 1972.

349. Levine, G.D., and Dorfman, R.F.: Nodular lymphoma: An ultrastructural study of its relationship to germinal centers and a correlation of light and electron microscopic findings.
Cancer 35: 148–164, 1975.

350. Levison, D.A., and Semple, P. d'A.: Primary cardiac Kaposi's sarcoma.
Thorax 31: 595–600, 1976.

351. Lewis, P.D., and Van Noorden, S.: "Nonfunctioning" pituitary tumors. A light and electron microscopical study.
Arch Pathol 97: 178–182, 1974.

352. Li, C.L., Chen, E.C., Huang, D.P., and Ho, H.C.: Intracytoplasmic desmosomes in tumor cells.
Cell Biol Int Rep 4: 593–597, 1980.

353. Lieberman, P.H., Foote, F.W., Stewart, F.W., and Berg, J.W.: Alveolar soft-part sarcoma.
J Am Med Assoc 198: 1047–1051, 1966.

354. Lieberman, P.H., Jones, C.R., Dargeon, H.W.K., and Begg, C.F.: A reappraisal of eosinophilic granuloma of bone, Hand-Schüller-Christian syndrome and Letterer-Siwe syndrome.
Medicine 48: 375–400, 1969.

355. Lieberman, P.H., Jones, C.R., and Filippa, D.A.: Langerhans cell (eosinophilic) granulomatosis.
J Invest Dermatol 75: 71–72, 1980.

356. Liebow, A.A.: Bronchiolo-alveolar carcinoma.
Adv Intern Med 10: 329–358, 1960.

357. Like, A.A., and Orci, L.: Embryogenesis of the human pancreatic islets: A light and electron microscopic study.
Diabetes 21 (Suppl 2): 511–534, 1972.

358. Limacher, J., Delage, C., and Lagacé, R.: Malignant fibrous histiocytoma. Clinicopathologic and ultrastructural study of 12 cases.
Am J Surg Pathol 2: 265–274, 1978.

359. Limas, C., and Tio, F.O.: Meningeal melanocytoma ("melanocytic meningioma"). Its melanocytic origin as revealed by electron microscopy.
Cancer 30: 1286–1294, 1972.

360. Llombart-Bosch, A., Blache, R., and Peydro-Olaya, A.: Ultrastructural study of 28 cases of Ewing's sarcoma: Typical and atypical forms.
Cancer 41: 1362–1373, 1978.

361. Lokich, J., Anderson, N., Rossini, A., et al.: Pancreatic alpha cell tumors: Case report and review of the literature.
Cancer 45: 2675–2683, 1980.

362. Lombardi, L., Carbone, A., Pilotti, S., and Rilke, F.: Malignant histiocytosis: A histological and ultrastructural study of lymph nodes in six cases. *Histopathology 2: 315–328, 1978.*

363. Long, J.A., and Jones, A.L.: Observations on the fine structure of the adrenal cortex of man. *Lab Invest 17: 355–370, 1967.*

364. Lopez, O.A., Silvers, D.N., and Helwig, E.B.: Cutaneous meningiomas—A clinicopathologic study. *Cancer 34: 728–744, 1974.*

365. Lukes, R.J., and Collins, R.D.: Immunologic characterization of human malignant lymphomas. *Cancer 34: 1488–1503, 1974.*

366. Lukes, R.J., Craver, L.F., Hall, T.C., and Rappaport, H.: Report of the nomenclature committee. Symposium on obstacles to the control of Hodgkin's disease. *Cancer Res 26: 1311, 1966.*

367. Lunda, M.A., MacKay, B., and Gamez-Araujo, J.: Myoepithelioma of the palate: Report of a case with histochemical and electron microscopic observations. *Cancer 32: 1429–1435, 1973.*

368. Luse, S.A.: Electron microscopic studies of brain tumors. *Neurology (Minneap) 10: 881–905, 1960.*

369. Lutzner, M.A., Emerit, I., Durepaire, R., et al.: Cytogenetic, cytophotometric, and ultrastructural study of large cerebriform cells of the Sézary syndrome and description of a small cell variant. *J Natl Cancer Inst 50: 1145–1162, 1973.*

370. Lutzner, M.A., Hobbs, J.W., and Horvath, P.: Ultrastructure of abnormal cells in Sézary syndrome, mycosis fungoides, and parapsoriasis en plaque. *Arch Dermatol 103: 375–386, 1971.*

371. Lutzner, M.A., and Jordan, H.W.: The ultrastructure of an abnormal cell in Sézary syndrome. *Blood 31: 719–726, 1968.*

372. Ma, M.H., and Blackburn, C.R.B.: Fine structure of primary liver tumors and tumor-bearing livers in man. *Cancer Res 33: 1766–1774, 1973.*

373. Macartney, J.C., Trevithick, M.A., Kricka, L., and Curran, R.C.: Identification of myosin in human epithelial cancers with immunofluorescence. *Lab Invest 41: 437–445, 1979.*

374. MacAulay, M.A., Welicky, I., and Schulz, R.A.: Ultrastructure of a biosynthetically active granulosa cell tumor. *Lab Invest 17: 562–570, 1967.*

375. Mackay, B., Bennington, J.L., and Skoglund, R.W.: The adenomatoid tumor: Fine structural evidence for mesothelial origin. *Cancer 27: 109–115, 1971.*

376. Mackay, B., Luna, M.A., and Butler, J.J.: Adult neuroblastoma. Electron microscopic observations in nine cases. *Cancer 37: 1334–1351, 1976.*

377. Mackay, B., and Osborne, B.M.: The contribution of electron microscopy to the diagnosis of tumors. *Pathobiol Annu 8: 359–405, 1978.*

378. Mackay, B., Osborne, B.M., and Wilson, R.A.: Ultrastructure of lung neoplasms. In: *Diagnosis and Treatment of Lung Carcinoma.* (M. J. Straus ed.). Grune & Stratton, New York, 1977, pp. 71–84.

379. Magalhães, M.C.: A new crystal-containing cell in human adrenal cortex. *J Cell Biol 55: 126–133, 1972.*

380. Mahoney, J.P., and Alexander, R.W.: Ewing's sarcoma. A light and electron-microscopic study of 21 cases.

Am J Surg Pathol 2: 283–298, 1978.

381. Mahoney, J.P., and Alexander, R.W.: Primary histiocytic lymphoma of bone. A light and ultrastructural study of four cases. *Am J Surg Pathol 4: 149–161, 1980.*

382. Mahoney, J.P., Ballinger, W.E., and Alexander, R.W.: So-called extraskeletal Ewing's sarcoma. Report of a case with ultrastructural analysis. *Am J Clin Pathol 70: 926–931, 1978.*

383. Mahoney, J.P., Saffos, R.O., and Rhatigan, R.M.: Follicular adenoacanthoma of the thyroid gland. *Histopathology 4: 547–557, 1980.*

384. Majno, G., Gabbiani, G., Hirschel, B.J., Ryan, G.B., and Statkov, P.R.: Contraction of granulation tissue in vitro: Similarity with smooth muscle. *Science 173: 548–549, 1971.*

385. Maldonaldo, J.E., Brown, A.L., Bayrd, E.D., and Pease, G.: Ultrastructure of myeloma cell. *Cancer 19: 1613–1627, 1966.*

386. Mandard, A.M., Herlin, P., Chasle, J., et al.: Cutaneous pseudosarcomas. Electron microscopic study of three tumors. *J Submicrosc Cytol 10: 441–456, 1978.*

387. Mandybur, T.I.: Melanotic nerve sheath tumors. *J Neurosurg 41: 187–192, 1974.*

388. Mao, P., Nakao, K., and Angrist, L.: Human prostatic carcinoma: An electron microscopic study. *Cancer Res 26: 955–973, 1966.*

389. Marcus, P.B., Martin, J.H., Green, R.H., and Krause, M.A.: Glycocalyceal bodies and microvillous core rootlets: Their value in tumor typing. *Arch Pathol Lab Med 103: 89–92, 1979.*

390. Marinozzi, V., Derenzini, M., Nardi, F., and Gallo, P.: Mitochondrial inclusions in human cancer of the gastrointestinal tract. *Cancer Res 37: 1556–1563, 1977.*

391. Markesbery, W.R., Brooks, W.H., Milsow, L., and Mortara, R.H.: Ultrastructural study of the pineal germinoma in vivo and in vitro. *Cancer 37: 327–337, 1976.*

392. Markesbery, W.R., and Challa, V.R.: Electron microscopic findings in primitive neuroectodermal tumors of the cerebrum. *Cancer 44: 141–147, 1979.*

393. Matsudaira, P.T., and Burgess, D.R.: Identification and organization of the components in the isolated microvillus cytoskeleton. *J Cell Biol 83: 667–673, 1979.*

394. Matsusaka, T., Watanabe, H., and Enjoji, M.: Anaplastic carcinoma of the esophagus: Report of three cases and their histogenetic consideration. *Cancer 37: 1352–1358, 1976.*

395. Matsuyama, M., Inoue, T., Ariyoshi, Y., et al.: Argyrophil cell carcinoma of the uterine cervix with ectopic production of ACTH, β-MSH, serotonin, histamine, and amylase. *Cancer 44: 1813–1823, 1979.*

396. Mazanec, K.: Présence de la "zonula nucleum limitans" dans quelques cellules humaines. *J Microscopie 6: 1027–1032, 1967.*

397. Mazur, M.T., and Askin, F.B.: Endolymphatic stromal myosis. Unique presentation and ultrastructural study. *Cancer 42: 2661–2667, 1978.*

398. Mazur, M.T., and Katzenstein, A-L. A.: Metastatic melanoma: The spectrum of ultrastructural morphology. *Ultrastruct Pathol 1: 337–356, 1980.*

399. Mazur, M.T., and Kraus, F.T.: Histogenesis of morphologic variations in tumors of the uterine wall. *Am J Surg Pathol 4: 59–74, 1980.*

400. McDowell, E.M., Barrett, L.A., Harris, C.C., and Trump, B.F.: Abnormal cilia in human bronchial epithelium. *Arch Pathol Lab Med 100: 429–436, 1976.*

401. McDowell, E.M., Barrett, L.A., and Trump, B.F.: Observations on small granule cells in adult human bronchial epithelium and in carcinoid and oat cell tumors. *Lab Invest 34: 202–206, 1976.*

402. McGregor, D.H., Lotuaco, L.G., Rao, M.S., and Chu, L.H.: Functioning oxyphil adenoma of parathyroid gland. An ultrastructural and biochemical study. *Am J Pathol 92: 691–712, 1978.*

403. McNutt, N.S., Hershberg, R.A., and Weinstein, R.S.: Further observation on the occurrence of nexuses in benign and malignant human cervical epithelium. *J Cell Biol 51: 805–825, 1971.*

404. Melicow, M.M.: The urothelium: A battleground for oncogenesis. *J Urol 120: 43–47, 1978.*

405. Mennemeyer, R.P., Hammar, S.P., Tytus, J.S., et al.: Melanotic schwannoma. Clinical and ultrastructural studies of three cases with evidence of intracellular melanin synthesis. *Am J Surg Pathol 3: 3–10, 1979.*

406. Merkow, L.P., Burt, R.C., Hayeslip, D.W., et al.: A cellular and malignant blue nevus: A light and electron microscopic study. *Cancer 24: 888–896, 1969.*

407. Merkow, L.P., Slifkin, M., Acevedo, H.F., Pardo, M., and Greenberg, W.V.: Ultrastructure of an interstitial (hilar) cell tumor of the ovary. *Obstet Gynecol 37: 845–859, 1971.*

408. Merrick, T.A., Erlandson, R.A., and Hajdu, S.I.: Lymphangiosarcoma of a congenitally lymphedematous arm. *Arch Pathol 91: 365–371, 1971.*

409. Meyer, C.J.L.M., van Leeuwen, A.W.F.M., van der Loo, E.M., van de Putte, L.B.A., and van Vloten, W.A.: Cerebriform (Sézary like) mononuclear cells in healthy individuals: A morphologically distinct population of T cells. *Virchows Archiv (Cell Pathol) 25: 95–104, 1977.*

410. Michel, R.P., Case, B.W., and Moinuddin, M.: Immunoblastic lymphosarcoma. A light, immunofluorescence, and electron microscopic study. *Cancer 43: 224–236, 1979.*

411. Mickelson, M.R., Brown, G.A., Maynard, J.A., Cooper, R.R., and Bonfiglio, M.: Synovial sarcoma. An electron microscopic study of monophasic and biphasic forms. *Cancer 45: 2109–2118, 1980.*

412. Mierau, G.W., and Favara, B.E.: Rhabdomyosarcoma in children: Ultrastructural study of 31 cases. *Cancer 46: 2035–2040, 1980.*

413. Miller, A.S., Leifer, C., Chen, S-Y., and Harwick, R.D.: Oral granular-cell tumors. Report of twenty-five cases with electron microscopy. *Oral Surg Med Pathol 44: 227–239, 1977.*

414. Miller, F., de Harven, E., and Palade, G.E.: The structure of eosinophilic leukocyte granules in rodents and in man. *J Cell Biol 31: 349–362, 1966.*

415. Miller, R., Kreutner, A., and Kurtz, S.M.: Malignant inflammatory histiocytoma (inflammatory fibrous histiocytoma). Report of a patient with four lesions. *Cancer 45: 179–187, 1980.*

416. Minor, R.R.: Collagen metabolism. A comparison of diseases of collagen and diseases affecting collagen. *Am J Pathol 98: 226–280, 1980.*

417. Mintzis, M.M., and Silvers, D.N.: Ultrastructural study of superficial spreading melanoma and benign simulants. *Cancer 42: 502–511, 1978.*

418. Mishima, Y.: Macromolecular changes in pigmentary disorders. *Arch Dermatol 91: 519–557, 1965.*

419. Mishima, Y.: Melanotic tumors. In: *Ultrastructure of Normal and Abnormal Skin.* A.S. Zelickson (ed.). Lea & Febiger, Philadelphia, 1967, pp. 388–424.

420. Mitschke, H., Saeger, W., and Breustedt, H-J.: Feminizing adrenocortical tumor. Histological and ultrastructural study. *Virchows Arch (Pathol Anat) 377: 301–309, 1978.*

421. Mollo, F., Canese, M.G., and Stramignoni, A.: Nuclear sheets in epithelial and connective tissue cells. *Nature 221: 869–870, 1969.*

422. Mollo, F., and Stramignoni, A.: Nuclear projections in blood and lymph node cells of human leukaemias and Hodgkin's disease and in lymphocytes cultured with phytohaemagglutinin. *Br J Cancer 21: 519–523, 1967.*

423. Moore, J.H., Crum, C.P., Chandler, J.G., and Feldman, P.S.: Benign cystic mesothelioma. *Cancer 45: 2395–2399, 1980.*

424. Morales, A.R., Fine, G., and Horn, R.C., Jr.: Rhabdomyosarcoma: An ultrastructural appraisal. In: *Pathology Annual,* Vol. 7. S.C. Sommers (ed.). Appleton-Century-Crofts, New York, 1972, pp. 81–106.

425. Morales, A.R., Fine, G., Horn, R.C., and Watson, J.H.L.: Langerhans cells in a localized lesion of the eosinophilic granuloma type. *Lab Invest 20: 412–423, 1969.*

426. Morales, A.R., Fine, G., Pardo, V.J., and Horn, R.C., Jr.: The ultrastructure of smooth muscle tumors with a consideration of the possible relationship of glomangiomas, hemangiopericytomas, and cardiac myxomas. In: *Pathology Annual,* Vol. 10. S.C. Sommers (ed.). Appleton-Century-Crofts, New York, 1975, pp. 65–92.

427. More, I.A.R., Jackson, A.M., and MacSween, R.N.M.: Renin-secreting tumor associated with hypertension. *Cancer 34: 2093–2102, 1974.*

428. Mottaz, J.H., and Zelickson, A.S.: Electron microscope observations of Kaposi's sarcoma. *Acta Dermatol Venerol 46: 195–200, 1966.*

429. Moxey, P.C., and Trier, J.S.: Endocrine cells in the human fetal small intestine. *Cell Tissue Res 183: 33–50, 1977.*

430. Mughal, S., and Filipe, M.I.: Ultrastructural study of the normal mucosa-adenoma-cancer sequence in the development of familial polyposis coli. *J Natl Cancer Inst 60: 753–768, 1978.*

431. Mullins, J.D.: A pigmented differentiating neuroblastoma. A light and ultrastructural study. *Cancer 46: 522–528, 1980.*

432. Mullins, J.D., Newman, R.K., and Coltman, C.A.: Primary oat cell carcinoma of the larynx. A case report and review of the literature. *Cancer 43: 711–717, 1979.*

433. Murad, T.M., Mancini, R., and George, J.: Ultrastructure of a virilizing ovarian Sertoli-Leydig cell tumor with familial incidence. *Cancer 31: 1440–1450, 1973.*

434. Murphy, G.F., Pilch, B.Z., Dickersin, G.R., Goodman,

M.L., and Nadol, J.B., Jr.: Carcinoid tumor of the middle ear.
Am J Clin Pathol 73: 816–822, 1980.

435. Nabarra, B., Sonsino, E., and Andrianarison, I.: Ultrastructure of a polysome–lamellae complex in a human paraganglioma.
Am J Pathol 86: 523–532, 1977.

436. Nagai, T.: Electron microscopic studies of pigmented nevi.
Jpn J Dermatol 78: 390–408, 1968.

437. Nagano, T., and Ohtsuki, I.: Reinvestigation of the fine structure of Reinke's crystal in the human testicular interstitial cell.
J Cell Biol 51: 148–161, 1971.

438. Napolitano, L., Kyle, R., and Fisher, E.R.: Ultrastructure of meningiomas and the derivation and nature of their cellular components.
Cancer 17: 233–241, 1964.

439. Nathwani, B.N.: A critical analysis of the classifications of non-Hodgkin's lymphomas.
Cancer 44: 347–384, 1979.

440. Nathwani, B.N., Kim, H., and Rappaport, H.: Malignant lymphoma, lymphoblastic.
Cancer 38: 964–983, 1976.

441. Navarrete, A.R., and Smith, M.: Ultrastructure of granular cell ameloblastoma.
Cancer 27: 948–955, 1971.

442. Navas Palacios, J.J.: Malignant melanotic neuroectodermal tumor. Light and electron microscopic study.
Cancer 46: 529–536, 1980.

443. Nevalainen, T.J., and Linna, M.I.: Ultrastructure of gastric leiomyosarcoma.
Virchows Arch (Pathol Anat) 379: 25–33, 1978.

444. Nezelof, C., Basset, F., and Rousseau, M.F.: Histiocytosis X. Histogenetic arguments for a Langerhans cell origin.
Biomedicine 18: 365–371, 1973.

445. Nilsson, O.: Studies on the ultrastructure of the human parathyroid glands in various pathological conditions.
Acta Pathol Microbiol Scand (A) Suppl 263, 1977.

446. Novikoff, A.B., and Novikoff, P.M.: Cytochemical contributions to differentiating GERL from the Golgi apparatus.
Histochem J 9: 525–551, 1977.

447. Nunez-Alonso, C., and Battifora, H.A.: Plexiform tumors of the uterus. Ultrastructural study.
Cancer 44: 1707–1714, 1979.

448. Nunez-Alonso, C., Gashti, E.N., and Christ, M.L.: Maxillofacial synovial sarcoma. Light- and electron-microscopic study of two cases.
Am J Surg Pathol 3: 23–30, 1979.

449. O'Conor, G.T., Tralka, T.S., Henson, E., and Vogel, C.L.: Ultrastructural survey of primary liver cell carcinomas from Uganda.
J Natl Cancer Inst 48: 587–603, 1972.

450. O'Hare, M.J., Monaghan, P., and Neville, A.M.: The pathology of adrenocortical neoplasia: A correlated structural and functional approach to the diagnosis of malignant disease.
Hum Pathol 10: 137–154, 1979.

451. O'Neal, L.W., Kipnis, D.M., Luse, S.A., Lacy, P.E., and Jarett, L.: Secretion of various endocrine substances by ACTH-secreting tumors—gastrin, melanotropin, norepinephrine, serotonin, parathormone, vasopressin, glucagon.
Cancer 21: 1219–1232, 1968.

452. Ohtani, H., and Sasano, N.: Myofibroblasts and myoepithelial cells in human breast carcinoma. An ultra-

structural study.
Virchows Arch (Pathol Anat) 385: 247–261, 1980.

453. Olufemi Williams, A., and Ajayi, O.O.: Ultrastructure of Wilms' tumor (nephroblastoma).
Exp Mol Pathol 24: 35–47, 1976.

454. Palutke, M., Patt, D.J., Weise, R., et al.: T cell leukemia-lymphoma in young adults.
Am J Clin Pathol 68: 429–439, 1977.

455. Papadaki, L., and Beilby, J.O.W.: Ovarian cystadenofibroma: A consideration of the role of estrogen in its pathogenesis.
Am J Obstet Gynecol 212: 501–512, 1975.

456. Parker, J.B., Marcus, P.B., and Martin, J.H.: Spinal melanotic clear-cell sarcoma. A light and electron microscopic study.
Cancer 46: 718–724, 1980.

457. Patchefsky, A.S., Gordon, G., Harrier, W.V., and Hoch, W.S.: Carcinoid tumor of the pancreas. Ultrastructural observations of a lymph node metastasis and comparison with bronchial carcinoid.
Cancer 33: 1349–1354, 1974.

458. Patchefsky, A.S., Soriano, R., and Kostianovsky, M.: Epithelial sarcoma. Ultrastructural similarity to nodular synovitis.
Cancer 39: 143–152, 1977.

459. Pearse, A.G.: Common cytochemical and ultrastructural characteristics of cells producing polypeptide hormones (the APUD series) and their relevance to thyroid and ultimobranchial C cells and calcitonin.
Proc R Soc Lond (Biol) 170: 71–80, 1968.

460. Pearse, A.G.E.: The APUD cell concept and its implications in pathology. In: *Pathology Annual*, Vol. 9. S.C. Sommers (ed.). Appleton-Century-Crofts, New York, 1974, pp. 27–41.

461. Pearse, A.G.E., and Polak, J.M.: Endocrine tumors of neural crest origin—neurolophomas, apudomas and the APUD concept.
Med Biol 52: 3–18, 1974.

462. Pearse, A.G.E., and Polak, J.M.: The diffuse neuroendocrine system and the APUD concept. In: *Gut Hormones*, S.R. Bloom (ed.). Churchill Livingstone, 1978, pp. 33–39.

463. Pearse, A.G.E., Polak, J.M., and Heath, C.M.: Polypeptide hormone production by "carcinoid" apudomas and their relevant cytochemistry.
Virchows Archiv (Cell Pathol) 16: 95–109, 1974.

464. Phillips, G., and Mukherjee, T.M.: A juxtaglomerular cell tumor: Light and electron microscopic studies of a renin-secreting kidney tumor containing both juxtaglomerular cells and mast cells.
Pathology 4: 193–204, 1972.

465. Pierce, G.B.: Ultrastructure of human testicular tumors.
Cancer 19: 1963–1983, 1966.

466. Pieslor, P.C., Orenstein, J.M., Hogan, D.L., and Breslow, A.: Ultrastructure of myofibroblasts and decidualized cells in leiomyomatosis peritonealis disseminata.
Am J Clin Pathol 72: 875–882, 1979.

467. Pinkus, G.S., and Said, J.W.: Characterization of non-Hodgkin's lymphomas using multiple cell markers. Immunologic, morphologic, and cytochemical studies of 72 cases.
Am J Pathol 94: 349–380, 1979.

468. Pinkus, G.S., Said, J.W., and Hargreaves, H.: Malignant lymphoma, T-cell type. A distinct morphologic variant with large multilobated nuclei, with a report of four cases.

Am J Clin Pathol 72: 540–550, 1979.

469. Pollak, A., and Friede, R.L.: Fine structure of medulloepithelioma.
J Neuropathol Exp Neurol 36: 712–725, 1977.

470. Pollard, T.D., and Weihing, R.R.: Cytoplasmic actin and myosin and cell movement. In: *CRC Critical Review of Biochemistry*, Vol. 2. G.D. Fassman (ed.). Chemical Rubber Company, Cleveland, 1974, pp. 1–65.

471. Popoff, N.A., and Ellsworth, R.M.: The fine structure of retinoblastoma. In vivo and in vitro observations.
Lab Invest 25: 389–402, 1971.

472. Popoff, N.A., Malinin, T.I., and Rosomoff, H.L.: Fine structure of intracranial hemangiopericytoma and angiomatous meningioma.
Cancer 34: 1187–1197, 1974.

473. Porter, K.R., Kenyon, K., and Badenhausen, S.: Specializations of the unit membrane.
Protoplasma 63: 262–274, 1967.

474. Prota, G.: Recent advances in the chemistry of melanogenesis in mammals.
J Invest Dermatol 75: 122–127, 1980.

475. Rambaud, J-C., Galian, A., Scotto, J., et al.: Pancreatic cholera (W.D.H.A. syndrome). Histochemical and ultrastructural studies.
Virchows Arch (Pathol Anat) 367: 35–45, 1975.

476. Ramsey, H.J.: Fibrous long-spacing collagen in tumors of the nervous system.
J Neuropathol Exp Neurol 24: 40–48, 1965.

477. Ramsey, H.J.: Ultrastructure of a pineal tumor.
Cancer 18: 1014–1025, 1965.

478. Ramzy, I., and Bos, C.: Sertoli cell tumors of ovary. Light microscopic and ultrastructural study with histogenetic considerations.
Cancer 38: 2447–2456, 1976.

479. Ranchod, M.: The histogenesis and development of pulmonary tumorlets.
Cancer 39: 1135–1145, 1977.

480. Ranchod, M., Kempson, R.L., and Dorgeloh, J.R.: Strumal carcinoid of the ovary.
Cancer 37: 1913–1922, 1976.

481. Rao, U., Cheng, A., and Dibolkar, M.S.: Extraosseous osteogenic sarcoma. Clinicopathological study of eight cases and review of literature.
Cancer 41: 1488–1496, 1978.

482. Rausch, E., Kaiserling, E., and Goos, M.: Langerhans cells and interdigitating reticulum cells in the thymus-dependent region in human dermatopathic lymphadenitis.
Virchows Archiv (Cell Pathol) 25: 327–343, 1977.

483. Reddick, R.L., Michelitch, H. J., Levine, A.M., and Triche, T.J.: Osteogenic sarcoma. A study of the ultrastructure.
Cancer 45: 64–71, 1980.

484. Reddick, R.L., Michelitch, H., and Triche, T.J.: Malignant soft tissue tumors (malignant fibrous histiocytoma, pleomorphic liposarcoma, and pleomorphic rhabdomyosarcoma): An electron microscopic study.
Hum Pathol 10: 327–343, 1979.

485. Reddick, R.L., Popovsky, M.A., Fantone, J.C., and Michelitch, H.J.: Parosteal osteogenic sarcoma. Ultrastructural observations in three cases.
Hum Pathol 11: 373–380, 1980.

486. Regezi, J.A., Hayward, J.R., and Pickens, T.N.: Superficial melanomas of oral mucous membranes.
Oral Surg Med Pathol 45: 730–740, 1978.

487. Reyes, J.W., Shinozuka, H., Garry, P., and Putong, P.B.: A light and electron microscopic study of a hemangiopericytoma of the prostate with local extension.
Cancer 40: 1122–1126, 1977.

488. Rhodin, J.A.G.: Ultrastructure of mammalian venous capillaries, venules, and small collecting veins.
J Ultrastruct Res 25: 452–500, 1968.

489. Rhodin, J.A.G.: *Histology: A Text and Atlas.* Oxford University Press, New York, 1974.

490. Ridolfi, R.L., Lieberman, P.H., Erlandson, R.A., and Moore, O.S.: Schneiderian papillomas: A clinicopathologic study of 30 cases.
Am J Surg Pathol 1: 43–53, 1977.

491. Rilke, F., Pilotti, S., Carbone, A., and Lombardi, L.: Morphology of lymphatic cells and of their derived tumours.
J Clin Pathol 31: 1009–1056, 1978.

492. Risdall, R.J., Sibley, R.K., McKenna, R.W., Brunning, R.D., and Dehner, L.P.: Malignant histiocytosis. A light- and electron-microscopic and histochemical study.
Am J Surg Pathol 4: 439–450, 1980.

493. Robert, F., and Hardy, J.: Prolactin-secreting adenomas. A light and electron microscopical study.
Arch Pathol 99: 625–633, 1975.

494. Roberts, D.K., Marshall, R.B., and Wharton, J.T.: Ultrastructure of ovarian tumors. I. Papillary serous cystadenocarcinoma.
Cancer 25: 947–958, 1970.

495. Roberts, K.: Cytoplasmic microtubules and their functions.
Prog Biophys Mol Biol 28: 371–420, 1974.

496. Rodriguez, E.M., and Caorsi, I.: A second look at the ultrastructure of the Langerhans cell of the human epidermis.
J Ultrastruct Res 65: 279–295, 1978.

497. Romansky, S.G., Crocker, D.W., and Shaw, K.N.F.: Ultrastructural studies on neuroblastoma. Evaluation of cytodifferentiation and correlation of morphology and biochemical and survival data.
Cancer 42: 2392–2398, 1978.

498. Rosai, J., and Levine, G.D.: Tumors of thymus. In: *Atlas of Tumor Pathology*, 2nd ser., fasc. 13. Armed Forces Institute of Pathology, Washington, D.C., 1976, pp. 108–130.

499. Rosai, J., Levine, G., Weber, W.R., and Higa, E.: Carcinoid tumors and oat cell carcinomas of the thymus. In: *Pathology Annual*, Vol. 11. S.C. Sommers (ed.). Appleton-Century-Crofts, New York, 1976, pp. 201–226.

500. Rosai, J., Summer, H.W., Kostianovsky, M., and Perez-Mesa, C.: Angiosarcoma of the skin. A clinicopathologic and fine structural study.
Hum Pathol 7: 83–109, 1976.

501. Rosner, M.C., and Golomb, H.M.: Ribosome–lamella complex in hairy cell leukemia. Ultrastructure and distribution.
Lab Invest 42: 236—247, 1980.

502. Ross, R., and Greenlee, T.K.: Electron microscopy: Attachment sites between connective tissue cells.
Science 153: 997–999, 1966.

503. Roth, J.A., Enzinger, F.M., and Tannenbaum, M.: Synovial sarcoma of the neck: A followup study of 24 cases.
Cancer 35: 1243–1253, 1975.

504. Roth, L.M.: Fine structure of the Brenner tumor.
Cancer 27: 1482–1488, 1971.

505. Roth, L.M., Nicholos, T.R., and Ehrlich, C.E.: Juvenile granulosa cell tumor. A clinicopathologic study of three cases with ultrastructural observations.
Cancer 44: 2194–2205, 1979.

506. Rubinstein, L.J.: Tumors of the central nervous system. In: *Atlas of Tumor Pathology*, 2nd ser., fasc. 6. Armed Forces Institute of Pathology, Washington, D.C., 1972, pp. 104–115; pp. 257–262.

507. Rubinstein, L.J., Herman, M.M., and Hanbery, J.W.: The relationship between differentiating medulloblastoma and dedifferentiating diffuse cerebellar astrocytoma. Light, electron microscopic, tissue, and organ culture observations. *Cancer 33: 675–690, 1974.*

508. Ryan, G.B., Cliff, W.J., Gabbiani, G., et al.: Myofibroblasts in human granulation tissue. *Hum Pathol 5: 55–67, 1974.*

509. Ryder, D.R., Horvath, E., and Kovacs, K.: Fine structural features of secretion in adenomas of human pituitary gland. *Arch Pathol Lab Med 104: 518–522, 1980.*

510. Sacchi, T.B., Bartolini, G., Biliotti, G., and Allara, E.: Behavior of the intercalated ducts of the pancreas in patients with functioning insulinomas. *J Submicrosc Cytol 11: 243–248, 1979.*

511. Said, J.W., Hargreaves, H.K., and Pinkus, G.S.: Non-Hodgkin's lymphomas: An ultrastructural study correlating morphology with immunologic cell type. *Cancer 44: 504–528, 1979.*

512. Said, J.W., and Pinkus, G.S.: Immunoblastic sarcoma of the T cell type. An ultrastructural study of five cases. *Am J Pathol 101: 515–526, 1980.*

513. Salazar, H., Merkow, L.P., Walter, W.S., and Pardo, M.: Human ovarian neoplasms: Light and electron microscopic correlations. II. The clear cell tumor. *Obstet Gynecol 44: 551–563, 1974.*

514. Salazar, H., and Totten, R.S.: Leiomyoblastoma of the stomach. An ultrastructural study. *Cancer 25: 176–185, 1970.*

515. Santiago, H., Feinerman, L.K., and Lattes, R.: Epithelioid sarcoma. A clinical and pathologic study of nine cases. *Hum Pathol 3: 133–147, 1972.*

516. Santos-Briz, A., Terron, J., Sastre, R., Romero, L., and Valle, A.: Oncocytoma of the lung. *Cancer 40: 1330–1336, 1977.*

517. Sasadaira, H., Kameya, T., Shimosato, Y., Baba, K., and Amemya, R.: Immunohistochemical identification of actomyosin-containing (myoepithelial) cells in nonneoplastic and neoplastic tissues. *Acta Pathol Jpn 28: 345–355, 1978.*

518. Schachenmayr, W., and Friede, R.L.: The origin of subdural neomembranes. I. Fine structure of the dura-arachnoid interface in man. *Am J Pathol 92: 53–68, 1978.*

519. Schajowicz, F., Cabrini, R.L., Simes, R.J., and Klein-Szanto, A.J.P.: Ultrastructure of chondrosarcoma. *Clin Orthopaed 100: 378–386, 1974.*

520. Schechter, J.: Electron microscopic studies of human pituitary tumors. I. Chromophobic adenomas. *Am J Anat 138: 371–386, 1973.*

521. Schechter, J.: Electron microscopic studies of human pituitary tumors. II. Acidophilic adenomas. *Am J Anat 138: 387–400, 1973.*

522. Schmid, K.O., Auböck, L. and Albegger, K.: Endocrine-amphicrine enteric carcinoma of the nasal mucosa. *Virchows Arch (Pathol Anat) 383: 329–343, 1979.*

523. Schochet, S.S., McCormick, W.F., and Halmi, N.S.: Acidophil adenomas with intracytoplasmic filamentous aggregates. A light and electron microscopic study. *Arch Pathol 94: 16–22, 1972.*

524. Schulz, A., Maerker, R., and Delling, G.: Ultrastructural study of tumor cell differentiation in osteosarcoma of jaw bones. *J Oral Pathol 7: 69–84, 1978.*

525. Scott, R.E., and Horn, R.G.: Ultrastructural aspects of neutrophil granulocyte development in humans. *Lab Invest 23: 202–215, 1970.*

526. Scully, R.E.: Tumors of the ovary and maldeveloped gonads. In *Atlas of Tumor Pathology.* 2nd ser., fasc 16. Armed Forces Institute of Pathology, Washington, D.C., 1979.

527. Seemayer, T.A., Schürch, W., Lagacé, R., and Tremblay, G.: Myofibroblasts in the stroma of invasive and metastatic carcinoma. A possible host response to neoplasia. *Am J Surg Pathol 3: 525–533, 1979.*

528. Seman, G., and Gallager, H.S.: Intramitochondrial rodlike inclusions in human breast tumors. *Anat Rec 194: 267–272, 1979.*

529. Serratoni, F.T., and Robboy, S.J.: Ultrastructure of primary and metastatic ovarian carcinoids: Analysis of 11 cases. *Cancer 36: 157–160, 1975.*

530. Shabtai, F., Lewinski, U.H., Har-Zahav, L., et al.: A hypodiploid clone and its duplicate in acute lymphoblastic leukemia. *Am J Clin Pathol 72: 1018–1024, 1979.*

531. Shamoto, M.: Langerhans cell granule in Letterer-Siwe disease. An electron microscopic study. *Cancer 26: 1102–1108, 1970.*

532. Shamoto, M., Kaplan, C., and Katoh, A.K.: Langerhans cell granules in human hyperplastic lymph nodes. *Arch Pathol 92: 46–52, 1971.*

533. Shaw, M.T.: Monocytic leukemias. *Hum Pathol 11: 215–227, 1980.*

534. Shelley, W.B., and Juhlin, L.: The Langerhans cell: Its origin, nature, and function. *Acta Dermatovener (Stockh) Suppl 79: 7–22, 1978.*

535. Shen, S.C., and Yunis, E.J.: A study of the cellularity and ultrastructure of congenital mesoblastic nephroma. *Cancer 45: 306–314, 1980.*

536. Shin, W-Y., Aftalion, B., Hotchkiss, E., Schenkman, R., and Berkman, J.: Ultrastructure of a primary fibrosarcoma of the human thyroid gland. *Cancer 44: 584–591, 1979.*

537. Shipkey, F.H., Lieberman, P.H., Foote, F.W., and Stewart, F.W.: Ultrastructure of alveolar soft part sarcoma. *Cancer 17: 821–830, 1964.*

538. Sibley, R.K., Rosai, J., Foucar, E., Dehner, L.P., and Bosl, G.: Neuroendocrine (Merkel cell) carcinoma of the skin. A histologic and ultrastructural study of two cases. *Am J Surg Pathol 4: 211–221, 1980.*

539. Sidhu, G.S.: The endodermal origin of digestive and respiratory tract APUD cells. *Am J Pathol 96: 5–20, 1979.*

540. Sidhu, G.S., Feiner, H., and Flotte, T.J.: Merkel cell neoplasms. Histology, electron microscopy, biology, and histogenesis. *Am J Dermatopathol 2: 101–119, 1980.*

541. Sidhu, G.S., and Forrester, E.M.: Acinic cell carcinoma: Long term survival after pulmonary metastases. Light and electron microscopic study. *Cancer 40: 756–765, 1977.*

542. Silverberg, S.G., Kay, S., and Koss, L.G.: Postmastectomy lymphangiosarcoma: Ultrastructural observa-

tions.
Cancer 27: 100–108, 1971.

543. Smetana, K., Gyorkey, F., Gyorkey, P., and Busch, H.: Ultrastructural studies on human myeloma plasmacytes.
Cancer Res 33: 2300–2309, 1973.

544. Smith, G.F., and O'Hara, P.T.: Structure of nuclear pockets in human leukocytes.
J Ultrastruct Res 21: 415–423, 1968.

545. Smith, H.S., Riggs, J.L., and Mosesson, M.W.: Production of fibronectin by human epithelial cells in culture.
Cancer Res 39: 4138–4144, 1979.

546. Smith, T.W., and Bhawan, J.: Tactile-like structures in neurofibromas.
Acta Neuropathol 50: 233–236, 1980.

547. Sobel, H.J., Marquet, E., Avrin, E., and Schwarz, R.: Granular cell myoblastoma. An electron microscopic and cytochemical study illustrating the genesis of granules and aging of myoblastoma cells.
Am J Pathol 65: 59–78, 1971.

548. Sobel, H.J., Marquet, E., and Schwarz, R.: Is schwannoma related to granular cell myoblastoma?
Arch Pathol 95: 396–401, 1973.

549. Sobel, H.J., Schwarz, R., and Marquet, E.: Nonviral nuclear inclusions. I. Cytoplasmic invaginations.
Arch Pathol 87: 179–192, 1969.

550. Sohval, A.R., Churg, J., Suzuki, Y., Katz, N., and Gabrilove, J.L.: Electron microscopy of a feminizing Leydig cell tumor of the testis.
Hum Pathol 8: 621–634, 1977.

551. Soifer, D.: The biology of cytoplasmic microtubules.
Ann NY Acad Sci 253: 1–848, 1975.

552. Solcia, E. Polak, J.M., Pearse, A.G.E., et al.: Lausanne 1977 classification of gastroenteropancreatic endocrine cells. In: *Gut Hormones*, S.R. Bloom (ed.), Churchill Livingstone, New York, 1978, pp. 40–48.

553. Spence, A.M., and Rubinstein, L.J.: Cerebellar capillary hemangioblastoma: Its histogenesis studied by organ culture and electron microscopy.
Cancer 35: 326–341, 1975.

554. Staehelin, L.A.: Structure and function of intercellular junctions.
Int Rev Cytol 39: 191–283, 1974.

555. Stahl, R.E., and Sidhu, G.S.: Primary carcinoid of the kidney. Light and electron microscopic study.
Cancer 44: 1345–1349, 1979.

556. Stahlberger, R., and Friede, R.L.: Fine structure of myomedulloblastoma.
Acta Neuropathol 37: 43–48, 1977.

557. Stefani, S., Chandra, S., Schrek, R., Tonaki, H., and Knospe, W.H.: Endoplasmic reticulum-associated structures in lymphocytes from patients with chronic lymphocytic leukemia.
Blood 50: 125–139, 1977.

558. Steiner, G.C.: Ultrastructure of osteoid osteoma.
Hum Pathol 7: 309–325, 1976.

559. Steiner, G.C.: Ultrastructure of osteoblastoma.
Cancer 39: 2127–2136, 1977.

560. Steiner, G.C.: Ultrastructure of benign cartilagenous tumors of intraosseous origin.
Hum Pathol 10: 71–86, 1979.

561. Steiner, G.C., and Dorfman, H.D.: Ultrastructure of hemangioendothelial sarcoma of bone.
Cancer 29: 122–135, 1972.

562. Steiner, G.C., Ghosh, L., and Dorfman, H.D.: Ultrastructure of giant cell tumors of bone.
Hum Pathol 3: 569–586, 1972.

563. Stenman, S. and Vaheri, A.: Distribution of a major connective tissue protein, fibronectin, in normal human tissues.
J Exp Med 147: 1054–1064, 1978.

564. Stiller, D., and Katenkamp, D.: Cellular features in desmoid fibromatosis and well-differentiated fibrosarcomas. An electron microscopic study.
Virchows Arch (Pathol Anat) 369: 155–164, 1975.

565. Stingl, G.: New aspects of Langerhans' cell function. (Review.)
Int J Dermatol 19: 189–213, 1980.

566. Stromeyer, F.W., Haggitt, R.C., Nelson, J.F., and Hardman, J.M.: Myoepithelioma of minor salivary gland origin.
Arch Pathol 99: 242–245, 1975.

567. Sun, C.N., Bissada, N.K., White, H.J., and Redman, J.F.: Spectrum of ultrastructural patterns of renal cell adenocarcinoma.
Urology 9: 195–200, 1977.

568. Sun, C.N., and White, H.J.: Annulate lamellae in human tumor cells.
Tissue Cell 11: 139–146, 1979.

569. Sun, C.N., White, H.J., and Thompson, B.W.: Oncocytoma (mitochondrioma) of the parotid gland. An electron microscopic study.
Arch Pathol 99: 208–214, 1975.

570. Suzuki, H., and Matsuyama, M.: Ultrastructure of functioning beta cell tumors of the pancreatic islets.
Cancer 28: 1302–1313, 1971.

571. Talerman, A., Gratama, S., Miranda, S., and Okagaki, T.: Primary carcinoid tumor of the testis. Case report, ultrastructure and review of the literature.
Cancer 42: 2696–2706, 1978.

572. Tandler, B.: Ultrastructure of adenoid cystic carcinoma of salivary gland origin.
Lab Invest 24: 504–512, 1971.

573. Tandler, B., Denning, C. R., Mandel, I.D., and Kutscher, A.H.: Ultrastructure of human labial salivary glands. II. Intranuclear inclusions in the acinar secretory cells.
Z Zellforsch 94: 555–564, 1969.

574. Tandler, B., Denning, C.R., Mandel, I.D., and Kutscher, A.H.: Ultrastructure of human labial salivary glands. III. Myoepithelium and ducts.
J Morphol 130: 227–245, 1970.

575. Tandler, B., and Hoppel, C.L.: Mitochondria. In *Ultrastructure of Cells and Organisms*. M. Locke, ser. ed. Academic Press, New York, 1972.

576. Tandler, B., Hutter, R.V.P., and Erlandson, R.A.: Ultrastructure of oncocytoma of the parotid gland.
Lab Invest 23: 567–580, 1970.

577. Tandler, B., and Rossi, E.P.: Granular cell ameloblastoma: Electron microscopic observations.
J Oral Pathol 6: 401–412, 1977.

578. Tandler, B., and Shipkey, F.H.: Ultrastructure of Warthin's tumor. I. Mitochondria.
J Ultrastruct Res 11: 292–305, 1964.

579. Tandler, B., and Shipkey, F.H.: Ultrastructure of Warthin's tumor. II. Crystalloids.
J Ultrastruct Res 11: 306–314, 1964.

580. Tang, C-K., and Toker, C.: Trabecular carcinoma of the skin. An ultrastructural study.
Cancer 42: 2311–2321, 1978.

581. Tani, E., Ikeda, K., Yamagata, S., Nishivira, M., and Higoshi, N.: Specialized junctional complexes in human meningiomas.
Acta Neuropathol 28: 305–315, 1974.

582. Tani, E., Kawamura, Y., Ametani, T., et al.: Immuno-

cytochemistry of acidophil granules of human pituitary.
Arch Neurol 20: 634–643, 1969.

583. Tani, E., Takeuchi, J., Ishijima, Y., et al.: Elongated nuclear sheet and intranuclear myelin figure of human medulloblastoma.
Cancer Res 31: 2120–2129, 1971.

584. Tannenbaum, M.: Ultrastructural pathology of the adrenal medullary tumors. In: *Pathology Annual*, Vol. 5. S.C. Sommers (ed.). Appleton-Century-Crofts, New York, 1970, pp. 145–171.

585. Tannenbaum, M.: Ultrastructural pathology of the adrenal cortex. In: *Pathology Annual*, Vol. 8. S.C. Sommers (ed.). Appleton-Century-Crofts, New York, 1973, pp. 109–156.

586. Tasso, F., and Sarles, H.: Cellules canalaires et oncocytes dans le pancréas humain.
Ann Anat Pathol (Paris) 18: 277–300, 1973.

587. Tateishi, R., Taniguchi, K., Horai, T., et al.: Argyrophil cell carcinoma (Apudoma) of the esophagus. A histopathologic entity.
Virchows Arch (Pathol Anat) 371: 283–294, 1976.

588. Tavassoli, F.A., and Norris, H.J.: Secretory carcinoma of the breast.
Cancer 45: 2404–2413, 1980.

589. Tavassoli, F.A., and Norris, H.J.: Sertoli tumors of the ovary. A clinicopathologic study of 28 cases with ultrastructural observations.
Cancer 46: 2281–2297, 1980.

590. Taxy, J.B.: Electron microscopy in the diagnosis of neuroblastoma.
Arch Pathol Lab Med 104: 355–360, 1980.

591. Taxy, J.B., and Battifora, H.: Malignant fibrous histiocytoma. An electron microscopic study.
Cancer 40: 254–267, 1977.

592. Taxy, J.B., Battifora, H., and Oyasu, R.: Adenomatoid tumors: A light microscopic, histochemical, and ultrastructural study.
Cancer 34: 306–316, 1974.

593. Taxy, J.B., Ettinger, D.S., and Wharam, M.D.: Primary small cell carcinoma of the skin.
Cancer 46: 2308–2311, 1980.

594. Taxy, J.B., and Gray, S.R.: Cellular angiomas of infancy. An ultrastructural study of two cases.
Cancer 43: 2322–2331, 1979.

595. Taxy, J.B., and Hildvegi, D.F.: Olfactory neuroblastoma. An ultrastructural study.
Cancer 39: 131–138, 1977.

596. Thiele, J., Reale, E., and Georgii, A.: Elektronenmikroskopische Befunde an Epithelkörperadenomen unterschiedlicher endokriner Aktivität.
Virchows Arch Abt B Zellpathol 12: 168–188, 1973.

597. Timpl, R., Rohde, H., Robey, P.G., et al.: Laminin–A glycoprotein from basement membranes.
J Biol Chem 254: 9933–9937, 1979.

598. Tobon, H., and Price, H.M.: Lobular carcinoma in situ. Some ultrastructural observations.
Cancer 30: 1082–1091, 1972.

599. Toduyasu, K., Madden, S.C., and Zelois, L.J.: Fine structure alterations of interphase nuclei of lymphocytes stimulated to growth activity in vitro.
J Cell Biol 39: 630–660, 1968.

600. Tomec, R., Ahmed, I., Fu, Y.S., and Jaffe, S.: Malignant hemangioendothelioma (angiosarcoma) of the salivary gland. An ultrastructural study.
Cancer 43: 1664–1671, 1979.

601. Toshima, S., Moore, G.E., and Sandberg, A.A.: Ultra-structure of human melanoma in cell culture. Electron microscopic studies.
Cancer 21: 202–216, 1968.

602. Toth, J.: Benign human mammary myoepithelioma.
Virchows Arch (Pathol Anat) 374: 263–269, 1977.

603. Tremblay, G.: Stromal aspects of breast carcinoma.
Exp Mol Pathol 31: 248–260, 1979.

604. Tremblay, M.: Ultrastructure of Wilms' tumor and myogenesis.
J Pathol 105: 269–277, 1971.

605. Triche, T.J., and Ross, W.E.: Glycogen-containing neuroblastoma with clinical and histopathologic features of Ewing's sarcoma.
Cancer 41: 1425–1432, 1978.

606. Trier, J.S.: Studies on small intestinal crypt epithelium. I. The fine structure of the crypt epithelium of the proximal small intestines of fasting humans.
J Cell Biol 18: 599–620, 1963.

607. Trump, B.F., Jesudason, M.L., and Jones, R.T.: Ultrastructural features of diseased cells. In: *Diagnostic Electron Microscopy*, Vol. 1. B.F. Trump and R.T. Jones (eds.). John Wiley & Sons, New York, 1978, pp. 1–88.

608. Ts'o, M.O.M., Fine, D.S., and Zimmerman, L.E.: The Flexner-Wintersteiner rosettes in retinoblastoma.
Arch Pathol 88: 664–671, 1969.

609. Unni, K.K., and Soule, E.: Alveolar soft part sarcoma. An electron microscopic study.
Mayo Clin Proc 50: 591–598, 1975.

610. Usui, M., Ishii, S., Yamawaki, S., et al.: Malignant granular cell tumor of the radial nerve.
Cancer 39: 1547–1555, 1977.

611. Uzman, B.G., Saito, H., and Kasac, M.: Tubular arrays in the endoplasmic reticulum in human tumor cells.
Lab Invest 24: 492–498, 1971.

612. Valdez, V.A., Planas, A.T., Lopez, V.F., Goldberg, M., and Herra, N.E.: Adenocarcoma of uterus and ovary. A clinicopathologic study of two cases.
Cancer 43: 1439–1447, 1979.

613. Valensi, Q.J.: Desmoplastic malignant melanoma. A light and electron microscopic study of two cases.
Cancer 43: 1148–1155, 1979.

614. Valenta, L.J., Michel-Bechet, M., Mattson, J.C., and Singer, F.R.: Microfollicular thyroid carcinoma with amyloid rich stroma, resembling the medullary carcinoma of the thyroid (MCT).
Cancer 39: 1573–1586, 1977.

615. Valenta, L.J., Michel-Bechet, M., Warshaw, J.B., and Maloof, F.: Human thyroid tumors composed of mitochondrion-rich cells: Electron microscopic and biochemical findings.
J Clin Endocrinol Metab 39: 719–733, 1974.

616. Valente, M., Pennelli, N., Segato, P. Bevilacqua, L., and Thiene, G.: Androgen producing adrenocortical carcinoma. A histological and ultrastructural study of two cases.
Virchows Arch (Pathol Anat) 378: 91–103, 1978.

617. van Haelst, U.J.G.M.: General consideration on electron microscopy of tumors of soft tissues. In: *Progress in Surgical Pathology*, Vol. 2. C.M. Fenoglio and M. Wolff (eds.). Masson, New York, 1980, pp. 225–257.

618. Varela-Duran, J., Diaz-Flores, L., and Varela-Nunez, R.: Ultrastructure of chondroid syringoma. Role of the myoepithelial cell in the development of mixed tumor of the skin and soft tissues.
Cancer 44: 148–156, 1979.

619. Vasudev, K.S., and Harris, M.: A sarcoma of myofibroblasts. An ultrastructural study.

Arch Pathol Lab Med 102: 185–188, 1978.

620. Velasco, M.E., Dahl, D., Roessmann, U., and Gambetti, P.: Immunohistochemical localization of glial fibrillary acidic protein in human glial neoplasms.
Cancer 45: 484–494, 1980.

621. Venkatachalam, M.A., and Greally, J.G.: Fine structure of glomus tumor: Similarity of glomus cells to smooth muscle.
Cancer 23: 1176–1184, 1969.

622. Vernon, M.L., Fountain, L., Krebs, H.M., et al.: Birbeck granules (Langerhans cell granules) in human lymph nodes.
Am J Clin Pathol 60: 771–779, 1973.

623. Volmer, J., Pickartz, H., and Jautzke, G.: Vascular tumors in the region of the breast.
Virchows Arch (Pathol Anat) 385: 201–214, 1980.

624. Vracko, R.: Basal lamina scaffold—Anatomy and significance for maintenance of orderly tissue structure. A review.
Am J Pathol 77: 314–345, 1974.

625. Vuletin, J.C.: Myofibroblasts in parosteal osteogenic sarcoma.
Arch Pathol Lab Med 101: 272, 1977.

626. Wang, N-S.: Electron microscopy in the diagnosis of pleural mesotheliomas.
Cancer 31: 1046–1054, 1973.

627. Wang, N-S., Seemayer, T.A., Ahmed, M.N., and Morin, J.: Pulmonary leiomyosarcoma associated with arteriovenous fistula.
Arch Pathol 98: 100–105, 1974.

628. Wang, T-Y., Erlandson, R.A., Marcove, R.C., and Huvos, A.G.: Primary leiomyosarcoma of bone.
Arch Pathol Lab Med 104: 100–104, 1980.

629. Warner, T.F.C.S., and Seo, I.S.: Aggregates of cytofilaments as the cause of the appearance of hyaline tumor cells.
Ultrastruct Pathol 1: 395–401, 1980.

630. Warner, T.F.C.S., Seo, I.S., Madura, J.A., Polak, J.M., and Pearse, A.G.E.: Pancreatic-polypeptide-producing apudoma of the liver.
Cancer 46: 1146–1151, 1980.

631. Watanabe, S., Berard, C.W., and Triche, T.: Annulate Lamellae in four cases of diffuse lymphocytic lymphoma.
J Natl Cancer Inst 58: 777–780, 1977.

632. Weibel, E.R., and Palade, G.E.: New cytoplasmic components in arterial endothelia.
J Cell Biol 23: 101–112, 1964.

633. Weinstein, R.S., Merk, F.B., and Alroy, J.: The structure and function of intercellular junctions in cancer.
Adv Cancer Res 23: 23–89, 1976.

634. Weiser, G.: Neurofibrom und Perineuralzelle. Elektronenoptische Untersuchung an 9 Neurofibromen.
Virchows Arch (Pathol Anat) 379: 73–83, 1978.

635. Weiser, G.: Granularzelltumor (granuläres neurom Feyrter) und Schwannsche phagen. Electronenoptische Untersuchung von 3 Fällen.
Virchows Arch (Pathol Anat) 380: 49–57, 1978.

636. Welsh, R.A., Bray, D.M., Shipkey, F.H., and Meyer, A.T.: Histogenesis of alveolar soft part sarcoma.
Cancer 29: 191–204, 1972.

637. Welsh, R.A., and Meyer, A.T.: Intracellular collagen fibers—In human mesenchymal tumors and inflammatory states.
Arch Pathol 84: 354–362, 1967.

638. Weston, J.A.: The migration and differentiation of neural crest cells.
Adv Morphogen 8: 41–115, 1970.

639. White, D.K., Chen, S-Y., Hartman, K.S., Miller, A.S., and Gomez, L.F.: Central granular-cell tumor of the jaws (the so-called granular-cell ameloblastic fibroma).
Oral Surg Med Pathol 45: 396–405, 1978.

640. Wigger, H.J., Salazar, G.H., and Blanc, W.A.: Extraskeletal Ewing sarcoma. An ultrastructural study.
Arch Pathol Lab Med 101: 446–449, 1977.

641. Williams, E.D., and Sandler, M.: The classification of carcinoid tumors.
Lancet 1: 238–239, 1963.

642. Wills, E.J.: Crystalline structures in the mitochondria of normal human liver parenchymal cells.
J Cell Biol 24: 511–514, 1965.

643. Wirman, J.A.: Nodular fasciitis, a lesion of myofibroblasts. An ultrastructural study.
Cancer 38: 2378–2389, 1976.

644. Wolff, M., Santiago, H., and Duby, M.M.: Delayed distant metastasis from a subcutaneous sacrococcygeal ependymoma. Case report, with tissue culture, ultrastructural observations, and a review of the literature.
Cancer 30: 1046–1067, 1972.

645. Wolin, S.L., and Kucherlapati, R.S.: Expression of microtubule networks in normal cells, transformed cells, and their hybrids.
J Cell Biol 82: 76–85, 1979.

646. Wolosewick, J.J., and Porter, K.R.: Microtrabecular lattice of the cytoplasmic ground substance. Artifact or reality.
J Cell Biol 82: 114–139, 1979.

647. Woodruff, J.M., Chernik, N.L., Smith, M.C., Millett, W.B., and Foote, F.W.: Peripheral nerve tumors with rhabdomyosarcomatous differentiation (malignant "Triton" tumors).
Cancer 32: 426–439, 1973.

648. Yagishita, S., Itoh, Y., Chiba, Y., and Fujino, H.: Primary rhabdomyosarcoma of the cerebrum. An ultrastructural study.
Acta Neuropathol 45: 111–115, 1979.

649. Yokoyama, M, Okada, K., Tokue, A., Takayasu, H., and Yamada, R.: Ultrastructural and biochemical study of neuroblastoma and ganglioneuroblastoma.
Invest Urol 9: 156–164, 1971.

650. Yu, G.S.M., Rendler, S., Herskowitz, A., and Molnar, J.J.: Renal oncocytoma. Report of five cases and review of literature.
Cancer 45: 1010–1018, 1980.

651. Yunis, E.J., Agostini, R.M., Walpusk, J.A., and Hubbard, J.D.: Glycogen in neuroblastomas. A light- and electron-microscopic study of 40 cases.
Am J Surg Pathol 3: 313–323, 1979.

652. Zampighi, G., Corless, J.M., and Robertson, J.D.: On gap junction structure.
J Cell Biol 86: 190–198, 1980.

653. Zimmerman, L.E., Font, R.L., and Andersen, S.R.: Rhabdomyosarcomatous differentiation in malignant intraocular medulloepithelioma.
Cancer 30: 817–835, 1972.

654. Zucker-Franklin, D.: Virus-like particles in the lymphocyte of a patient with chronic lymphocytic leukemia.
Blood 21: 509–512, 1963.

Index

Acinar cell tumors
    bronchial, 152
    pancreas, 29, 47
    parotid, 29, 47
Actin, 78, 83
    and microvilli, 99
Adenocarcinoid tumors, 49
Adenocarcinoma, 99–104
    anaplastic lung, 8, 103
    duct cell, 45
    and intracellular lumen, 99–104
    of lung, 18, 104
    mucin-producing, 45
    papillary, 118
    serous, 152
    sigmoid colon, 2, 45
Adenoid cystic carcinoma and basal lamina, 120, 121
Adenoma
    adrenocortical, 22
    benign hepatic, 60
    black, 22
    Hürthle cell, 36
    oxyphilic parathyroid, 24, 26
    parathyroid, 34, 36, 96, 98
    pleomorphic, 91, 92, 93, 119
Adenomatoid tumors, 105, 112
Adenomyoepitheliomas, 91
Adenosarcoma (uterus), 107
Adenosis, florid sclerosing, 91
Adolescents, round cell tumor, 146
Adrenal cortex, 23, 33
Adrenal gland tumors, 22, 33
Adrenocortical carcinoma, 29, 30, 33
Alpha-actinin, 79
Alpha glycogen, 58
Alveolar cell carcinoma, 65
Alveolar rhabdomyosarcoma, 79
Alveolar soft part sarcoma, 56, 62
Amelanotic melanoma, 4, 74, 76
Ameloblastoma, granular cell, 38
Amphicrine cell, 49
Anaplastic tumors, 4
Angiosarcoma, 67, 68, 69, 116
Angulate bodies in granular cell tumors, 38
Annulate lamellae, 33–35
Anterior mediastinal tumors, 6, 18, 137
Apoptosis, 160
APUD concept, 49
Apudoma, 49
Artifacts and TEM, 1, 160

Astrocytoma, malignant, 85
Auer bodies, 63
Autophagosomes, 160
Axoneme, 106

Basal lamina, 117–122, 130
    in neoplasms, 117
    myoepithelial cells, 91
    reduplication, 120
    and smooth muscles, 83
Basement membrane, 117
Benign hepatic adenoma, 60
Beta glycogen, 58
Birbeck body, 63–65
Black adenomata, 22
Blastema, 4
Blastoma, pulmonary, 4, 34
Blebs, nuclear, 10
Blepharoplasts, 107, 130
Blue nevi, 74
B lymphocytes, 12
    B-immunoblastic lymphoma, 16
    noncleaved, 17
Botryoid rhabdomyosarcoma, 79, 81
Breast
    adenocarcinoma, 99
    fibroadenoma, 91, 120
    infiltrating duct carcinoma, 102
    lobular carcinoma, 91
    myoepitheliomas, 93–94
Brenner tumor, 107, 112
Bronchiolar carcinoma, 65, 66
Brush border, 99
Burkitt's lymphoma, 17

Café-au-lait spots, 74
Carcinoid tumors, 50–54, 56
    bronchial, 143
    definition, 51
    and Kutschitzky-Masson cell, 56
Carcinoma
    acinic cell, 29, 46, 47, 152
    adenoid cystic, 91, 120
    adrenocortical, 30, 33
    alveolar cell, 65
    basal cell, 86
    bronchiolar, 66
    epidermoid, 87, 89, 110
    feminizing adrenocortical, 22
    hepatocellular, 30

infiltrating duct, 3, 88, 102, 121
  lobular in breast, 91, 92, 103
  medullary, 42, 50
  Merkel cell, 35, 50, 138, 139
  skin appendage origin, 155
  squamous cell, 8, 87–89
  trabecular, 139
Carotid body tumor, 51
Cartilaginous tumors, 95, 148
Cell junctions, 107–116
  gap junction, 109
  hemidesmosome, 109
  in neoplasms other than carcinomas and sarcomas, 111
  junctional complex, 108–109
  primitive, 111, 116
  in sarcoma, 115, 116
Cell surface, 95–116
  junctions, 107–116
  membrane specializations, 95–107
Central nervous system neoplasms, 112
Centriole, 106
Cerebriform nuclei, 7
Charcot-Böttcher crystalloids, 62
Charcot-Leyden crystals, 63
Chief cells in parathyroid adenoma, 60
Childhood sarcoma of undetermined histogenesis, 82, 146
Chondrosarcoma, 88, 89, 95
  and glycogen, 60
  mesenchymal, 148–150
Chordoma, 42, 43
Choroid plexus papilloma, 105, 113
Chromatin, 7, 13, 139
Chromosomes, 7, 10
Chrondoblastoma, 10
Chronic lymphocytic leukemia, 63
Cilia, 106–107, 130
Ciliated columnar epithelium, 105
Cisternae (RER), 29, 30, 42
Clara cells, 66
Clear cell carcinoma
  in female reproductive tract, 60, 120
  in kidney, 58
Clear cell sarcoma, spinal melanotic, 77
Cleaved nuclei, 7, 17
Collagen fibrils, 117, 122
Contractile cells, hybrid, 89–94
Conus medullaris, 131
Convoluted nuclei, 7, 13, 16, 17
Crystalline inclusions in cytoplasm, 60–63
Cushing's syndrome, 22
Cylindroma, dermal eccrine, 120, 122
Cystadenfibroma, 9, 107
Cystadenocarcinoma, papillary serous, 47, 106
Cystadenoma
  apocrine, 91, 94
  benign serous, 107
  ovarian serous, 47, 107, 112
Cystic Hyperplastic mastopathy, 91
Cytokeratin, 86, 87, 112
  and junctional complexes, 109
  and myoepithelial cells, 94

Cytoplasm, 21–94
  granularity and eosinophilia, 26
  inclusions, 42–77
  intracytoplasmic fibers, 77–94
  invaginations, 7
  organelles, 21–42
Cytosarcoma phyllodes, 82

Dark cells, 160
Deoxyribonucleoprotein, 7
Dermal eccrine cylindroma, 120, 122
Dermatofibrosarcoma protuberans, 10, 12
Desmin, 79, 85, 86
Desmoid tumors, 90
Desmoplastic malignant melanoma, 77
Desmosomes, 87, 112
  hemidesmosomes, 109–111
  and junctional complex, 109
  and myoepithelial cells, 91
Discoid (fusiform) vesicle, 98
DNA in nucleus, 7
Dynein arms, 106
Dysgerminoma, ovarian, 18, 137

Ectoblast, 49
Ectopic meningiomas, 126
Embryonal rhabdomyosarcoma, 5, 79–81
Endoplasmic reticulum, 26–33
  rough, 29–30
  smooth, 33
Endosecretory granules, 47
Endothelial cell
  junctions, 116
  and pinocytotic vesicles, 95
  tumors, 67
Enterochromaffin cells, 49, 56
Envelope, nuclear, 7
Eosinophilia
  and crystalline inclusions, 63
  and cytoplasmic granularity, 26
Eosinophilic granuloma, 64
Ependymoblastoma, 112
Ependymoma, 112–113, 130
  myxopapillary, 108, 131
Epidermoid carcinoma, 87–89, 110
Epithelioid sarcoma, 95, 96, 116, 155
Epulis, congenital, 38
Esthesioneuroblastoma, 50
Euchromatin, 7
Eumelanin, 71
Ewing's sarcoma, 5, 7, 58
  cell junctions, 116
  extraskeletal, 58, 60
  glycogen in, 58, 59
  and nucleoli, 17
Exocytosis and secretory granules, 44
External lamina, 117
Extracellular constituents, 117

Feminizing adrenocortical carcinoma, 22
Fibrillar nuclear body, 19

Fibroadenoma, breast, 91
  and basal lamina, 120
Fibroblasts and RER, 30
Fibroma
  desmoplastic, of bone, 90
  granular cell ameloblastic, 38
  infantile digital, 90
Fibromatoses, 90
Fibronectin, 117
Fibrosarcoma, 30
  and lipid, 60
  low-grade, 29
  myxoid, 120
Fibrous histiocytoma, 4, 60, 89
Fibrous lamina, 10
Fibroxanthoma, 60
Filopodia, 95
Filum terminale, 131
Fimbrin, 99
Flexner-Wintersteiner rosettes, 115
Focal nodular hyperplasia (liver), 23, 24
Foregut carcinoids, 51
Fusiform dense bodies, 83
  and myoepithelial cells, 91, 93

Gap junction (nexus), 109
Gastrinomas, 54
Gastroenteropancreatic cells, 52
Genome, 4
GERL (Golgi-Endoplasmic Reticulum-Lysosome), 35
Germ cell tumors, 112
Germinoma, pineal, 137
Giant cell tumor, 96
Giant mitochondria, 22
Glial fibrillary acidic protein, 86
Glial filaments, 85
Glioma, 18
Glomus tumors, 83
Glycocalyx, 99, 104
Glycogen, 42, 58-60
Glycosaminoglycans, 117
Goblet cells, 44
Golgi apparatus, 35
Granular cell carcinoma in kidney, 26
Granular cell tumors, 38, 40, 41
Granular nuclear body, 19
Granulation tissue, 90
Granulocytes, neoplastic, 63
Granulocytic sarcoma, 62-63
Granulosa cell tumors, 7
Granulosa-theca cell tumor, 33, 112, 113
Gynecomastia, 104

Hairy cell leukemia, 40, 41
Hand-Schuller-Christian disease, 64
Hemangioblastoma, cerebellar, 70
Hemangioendotheliomas, 67, 89, 116, 119
Hemangioma, 67
Hemangiomatosis, 67
Hemangiopericytoma, 69, 70, 116
Hemidesmosomes, 109-111

Hepatocellular carcinoma, 22, 33
Hepatomas, benign, 23, 33
Heterochromatin, 7
Hilus cell tumor, 33
Hindgut carcinoids, 53
Histiocytes, 1, 60
Histiocytosis
  malignant, 38
  -X, 64
Histogenesis and classification of tumors, 1
Hodgkin's disease, 6, 16, 17
Homer-Wright pseudorosettes, 113
Hormone production and apudoma, 55
Hürthle cell tumor, 26, 36
Hybrid cells, 4
  contractile, 89-94
Hyperplasia
  adenomatous, 23, 27
  focal nodular, 23, 24, 58
  sebaceous, 60

IgM lambda crystals, 63
Ileum, carcinoid tumor, 48, 56
Immunoblasts in lymphoma, 12, 16
  polysomes, 33
Immunocytoma and crystalline inclusions, 63
Immunofluorescence, indirect, 78
Inclusions in cytoplasm, 42-77
  crystalline inclusions, 60-63
  definition, 42
  glycogen and lipid, 58-60
  lamellar inclusion body, 65-66
  Langerhans granule, 63-65
  melanin, 71-77
  nuclear, 18-19
  secretory granules, 44-58
  Weibel-Palade body—vascular tumors, 66-71
Infantile digital fibroma, 90
Infiltrating duct carcinoma, 3, 88, 102, 121
Insulinoma, 54, 55
Interchromatin granules, 7
Intermediate filaments, 85-89
  in mesenchymal tumors, 89
Intermediate junction, 108
Interstitial (Leydig) cell tumors, 22, 33, 38
Intracytoplasmic fibers, 77-94
  fibrils, 89
  hybrid contractile cells, 89-94
  intermediate filament, 85-89
  microfilaments-myofilaments, 78-85
  microtrabecular system, 78
  microtubules, 77-78
Intracellular cilia, 106
Islet cell carcinoma, 48, 50

Jejunum, 100
Junctional complex, 108-109
Juxtaglomerular cell tumor, 55-56

Kaposi's sarcoma, 70, 116
Keratinocytes, neoplastic, 87

Keratosis, actinic, 110
Kidney
    clear cell carcinoma, 58, 59
    granular cell carcinoma, 26
    oncocytoma, 26
Kultschitzky-Masson cell, 56

Lacunar cell in Hodgkin's disease, 17
Lamellar cristae in mitochondria, 22
Lamellar inclusion body, 65–66
Laminin, 117
Langerhans cells, 63–65
Leiomyoblastoma, 83
Leiomyocyte, 82–85
    and pinocytotic vesicles, 95
Leiomyomas, 83, 84
Leiomyomatosis peritonealis disseminata, 90
Leiomyosarcoma, 11, 83, 84, 85
    and basal lamina, 117
Letterer-Siwe disease, 64
Leukemia
    acute promyelocytic, 63
    and basal lamina, 120
    chronic lymphocytic, 63
    hairy cell, 40, 41, 42
    myelomonocytic, 38, 39
    unclassifiable, 10, 13
Leydig (interstitial) cell tumors, 22, 33, 38
    and crystalline inclusions, 61, 62
Lipid, 58–60
    lipoid cell tumors, 33
Lipofuscin pigment, 38
Liposarcoma, 30, 60
    and lipid, 60
Liver, focal nodular hyperplasia, 23, 58
Lobular carcinoma in breast, 91, 103
Low-grade follicular carcinoma, 36
Lumen
    intracellular, 99–104
Lung
    adenocarcinoma, 18, 66, 103–104
    alveolar cell carcinoma, 65
    blastoma, 4, 34
    bronchiolar carcinoma, 65, 66
    carcinoid tumor, 51, 53, 143
    sugar tumor, 60
    tumorlet, 50
Luse bodies, 122
Luteoma, 22, 33, 164
Lymphangiosarcoma, 116
    postmastectomy, 70
Lymphocytes
    B, 12, 16, 17
    null, 13
    prolymphocytes, 13
    T, 13, 15, 16
    transformed, 16
Lymphomas, 10–17
    and basal lamina, 120
    non-Hodgkin's, 1

    B-immunoblastic, 16
    histiocytic type, 13, 14, 15
    lymphoblastic, 11, 12, 13, 14, 17–18, 95
    plasmacytoid, 29, 30
    poorly-differentiated lymphocytic, 9, 11, 12
    T-immunoblastic, 15, 16
    undifferentiated, Burkitt-type, 15, 17, 31
    well-differentiated lymphocytic, 11
    true histiocytic, 1, 37, 38
Lysosomes, 35–41
    and collagen, 122
    granular cell tumors, 38, 40, 41
    primary, 35
    secondary, 38

Macromelanosomes, 74
Malignant fibrous histiocytoma, 4, 60, 89
Marginal folds in endothelial cell tumors, 67
Medullary thyroid carcinoma, 50
Medulloblastoma (cerebellar), 10, 113
    melanotic, 77
Medulloepithelioma, 113
Melanin, 71–77
Melanocytes, 71
Melanocytic nevi, 72
    blue, 74
    compound, 72, 73
    intradermal, 72
    junctional, 72
Melanocytoma, meningeal, 77
Melanoma (malignant), 74–77
    amelanotic, 4, 74, 76, 134
    balloon cell, 71
    desmoplastic, 77
    and nuclear protrusions, 10
    pigmented, 74
    superficial spreading, 76
Melanophages, 74
Melanosomes, 21
    giant, 74
Membrane of cell, specialization, 95–107
    asymmetric (urothelium), 95, 98, 99
    cilia, 106–107
    interdigitating, 95, 155
    microvilli, 99–105
    pinocytotic vesicles, 95
    plasmalemmal configurations, 95
Meningothelial meningioma, 85, 95, 112
    ectopic, 126
Merkel cell carcinoma, 35, 50, 139
Meromyosin, 78
Mesodermal mixed tumor in uterus, 82
Mesothelial cells, 112
Mesothelioma, epithelial, 104, 112
Metaplasia, 4
    squamous, 152
Microfilaments, 78
    and microvilli, 99, 104
    and myoepithelial cells, 91, 94
    and myofilaments, 78

Microtrabecular system, 78
Microtubules, 21, 77–78
  -associated proteins, 77
Microvilli, 99–105
  configurations, 104, 105
Midgut carcinoids, 53, 56
Mitochondria, 21–26
  giant, 22
  in cells synthesizing steroid hormones, 21
  inclusions, 23
  oncocytic, 23, 25, 26
  and RER, 42
Mixed tumor (pleomorphic adenomas), 91, 93
Mucigen, 44
Mucin-producing adenocarcinoma, 45
Müllerian tumor (uterus), 82
Multilobated nuclei, 10
  in lymphoma, 13, 17
Multiple myeloma, 29
Multipotential cells, 4
Multivesicular bodies, 38
Mycosis fungoides, 7
Myelin figures, 160
Myeloma, plasma cell, 29
Myelomonocytic leukemia, 38, 39
Myoblast precursor cells, 82, 146
Myoepithelial cells, 90–94
  definition, 90
Myoepithelioma, 87, 93
Myofibrils, 79
Myofibroblast, 89–90, 94
  neoplastic, 90
Myofilaments, 78–85
Myosin, 78, 83
Myxoma, cardiac, 90

Necrosis, 160
Neoplasm, basal lamina in, 117
Neoplastic germ cells, immature, 34
Nephroblastoma (Wilms' tumor), 4
Nephroma, congenital mesoblastic, 90
Neural crest, 115
  and apudomas, 49
  and melanin, 71
Neurites, 113
Neuroblastoma, 5, 50
  nucleoli, 18
Neuroectodermal tumor of infancy, 5, 77
Neuroendocrine tumors, 47
Neuroendocrinomas, 49
Neuroepithelial tumor of skin, 139
Neurofibroma, 95
  and collagen, 122
  and pinocytotic vesicle, 95
Neurofilaments, 85
Neuromelanin, 71
Neurosecretory-type granules, 47–58, 139
Nevus cell, 72, 73
Nodular fasciitis, 90
Non-Hodgkin's lymphoma, 1, 6, 10–17, 33

Norepinephrine, 55
Nucleolonema, 7, 18, 136
Nucleolus, 7, 17–18, 136
Nucleoplasm, 7
Nucleus, 7–19
  configurations, 7–14
  envelope, 7
  inclusions, 18–19
  in malignant lymphoma, 11–12
  pockets, 10
  pore, 7
  projection, 10
  pseudoinclusions, 18
  satellite, 10, 17
  sheets, 10
Null lymphocytes, 13

Oat cell carcinoma, 50, 143
Oncocytes, 23, 25, 26
Oncocytoma, 26
Organelles in cytoplasm, 21–42
  annulate lamellae, 33–35
  complexes, 41, 42
  definition, 21
  endoplasmic reticulum and ribosomes, 26–33
  Golgi apparatus, 35
  lysosomes, 35–41
  mitochondria, 21–26
Osteogenic sarcoma, 30
Osteoid
  fibrils, 117
  -producing neoplasms, 30
Ovarian neoplasms
  adenosarcoma, 107
  Brenner, 107, 112
  carcinoid, 56
  cystic, 47, 107, 112
  Sertoli cell, 22, 62
  sex cord-stromal, 7, 22, 33, 62, 112
Oxyphilic parathyroid adenoma, 24, 26

Pancreas
  acinar cell tumor, 29, 47
  and Kultschitzky-Masson cell, 56
Pancreatic islet cells, 49, 50
Pancreatoblastoma, 4, 47
Paneth cells, 47
Papilloma
  benign, 10
  choroid plexus, 105, 107
  Schneiderian, 107
Paracrystalline inclusions, 23
Paraganglioma, 50
Parathyroid adenoma
  and annulate lamellae, 34
  and cell membrane, 95
  chief cell, 34, 60
  and glycogen, 60
  oxyphilic, 24, 26
Parosteal osteogenic sarcoma, 90

Parotid gland, acinic cell carcinoma, 29, 47
Perichromatin granules, 7
Pericyte, 70
  and pinocytotic vesicles, 95
Perineurial cells, 95
Peripheral nerve sheath tumor, 95, 120
  and collagen, 122
  melanotic, 77
Peroxisomes, 21
Phagosomes, 38
Pheochromocytomas, 50
  extradrenal, 55
Physaliferous cells, 115
Pineal germinoma, 137
Pineoblastoma, 107
Pinkus tactile hair disc, 139
Pinocytotic vesicles, 95
  and myoepithelial cells, 91
  and smooth muscles, 83
Pituitary gland tumors, 26, 50
Plasma cell myeloma, 29
Plasmacytoma, 28, 29
Plasmalemmal attachment plaques, 83
Plasmalemmal configurations, 95
Plexiform tumors of uterus, 83
Pneumocytes, 65
Pockets, nuclear, 10
Polysomes, 12, 16, 17
  definition, 26
  and ribosomes, 33
Poorly differentiated neoplastic cells, 7
Poorly differentiated tumors, 4
Pore, nuclear, 7
Premelanosomes, 21, 71, 74
Primitive cell junctions, 111, 116, 137, 146
Procollagen type IV, 117
Prohormone and apudomas, 54
Projections, nuclear, 10
Prolymphocytes, 13
Prostate gland
  carcinoma, 37
  secondary lysosome, 38
Pseudocrystalline inclusions, 23
Pseudoinclusion (nuclear), 18
Pseudopods, 95
Pseudorosettes, 113, 130
Pseudosarcoma, cutaneous, 90
Pulmonary blastoma, 4, 34
Pulmonary tumorlets, 50

Reduplication of basal lamina, 120
Reed-Sternberg cells, 17
Reinke crystals, 62
Renin, 55
RER (rough endoplasmic reticulum), 29–30, 42
Residual bodies and lysosomes, 38
Reticulin, 117
Reticulum cell sarcoma, 16
Retinoblastoma, 115
  and cilia, 107

Rhabdomyosarcoma, 79–82
  alveolar, 79
  and external lamina, 117
  botryoid, 79, 81
  embryonal, 79, 80, 81, 146
  pleomorphic, 79, 81
Rhomboid granules, 56, 62
Ribsome, 26–33
  definition, 26
  -lamella complexes, 41
RNA in nucleus, 7
Rosenthal fibers, 86
Rosettes (neural), 113, 115
Rough endoplasmic reticulum, 29–30, 42

Salivary glands, pleomorphic adenomas, 91
Sarcoma
  alveolar soft part, 56, 62
  childhood, 82, 146
  cell junctions, 115–116
  epithelioid, 95, 96, 116, 155
  Ewing's, 7, 17, 58, 59, 60, 116
  granulocytic, 62–63
  hemangioendothelial, 67, 89, 116, 119
  Kaposi's, 70, 116
  osteogenic, 30
  parosteal osteogenic, 90
  reticulum cell, 16
  spindle cell, 4
  synovial, 4, 116
Sarcomeres, 79
Satellite nuclei, 10, 17
Scalloped cell membrane (chondrocytes), 95
Schneiderian membrane, 106
  papilloma, 107
Schwannoma, 95, 120
  and collagen, 122
Scirrhous carcinoma of breast, 90
Sebaceous hyperplasia, 60
Secretory granules, 44–58
  mucigen, 44
  neurosecretory, 47–58
  zymogen, 44–47
Seminoma, 6
  mediastinal, 137
  testicle, 18, 137
Septate junctions, 108
SER (smooth endoplasmic reticulum), 33
Serous granules, 47
Sertoli cell tumors, 22
  and crystalline inclusions, 62
  Sertoli-Leydig cell tumors, 33, 112
Sex-cord stromal tumors, 22, 33, 62, 112
Sézary cells, 7
Sheets, nuclear, 10
Sigmoid colon, adenocarcinoma, 2, 45
Skeletin, 85
Smooth endoplasmic reticulum, 33
Smooth muscle tumors, 4, 82–85
Spindle cell tumors, 4, 106

Squamous cell carcinoma, 8, 87–89
Squamous metaplasia, 4, 152
Steroid hormones, 33
Stewart-Treves syndrome, 70
Sugar tumor, 60
Superficial spreading malignant melanoma, *76*
Synemin, 79, 86
Synovial sarcoma, 4, 116
Syringoma, chondroid, 93

Tables
    1-1, small round cell tumor, 5
    1-2, anterior mediastinal tumors, 6
    3-1, cells of anterior pituitary, 51
    3-2, gastroenteropancreatic system, 52
    3-3, intracytoplasmic fibers, 77
    4-1, cell junctions, 108
TEM—see Transmission electron microscopy
Terminal web region, 108
Thecoma, ovarian, 60
Thymoma, 6, 85, 112
Thymus-derived lymphocyte, 13
Thyroid gland
    Hürthle cell tumors, 26, 36
    oncocytoid adenomatous hyperplasia, 26
    secondary lysosome, 38
Tight junction, 108
T lymphocytes, 13
    T-immunoblastic lymphoma, 15, 16
Tonofilament, 85
Trabecular carcinoma of skin, 139
Transformed lymphocytes, 12
Transmembrane effusion, 44
Transmission electron microscopy
    procedure for evaluating human tumors, 1–6
    and tumor diagnosis, 125–156
Troponin, 79
Tropmyosin, 79
True histiocytic lymphoma, 1, 37, 38
Tubulins, 77, 106
Tubulovesicular cristae in mitochondria, 22
Tumor
    adenomatoid, 105, 112
    adrenal gland, 22, 30, 33
    anaplastic, 4
    anterior mediastinal, 6, 18, 137

cartilagenous, 95, 148
granular cell, 38, 40, 41
granulosa cell, 7, 33, 112
histiocytic, 60, 120
histogenesis and classification, 1
Hürthle cell, 26, 36
interstital cell, 38
Leydig cell, 22
and myofibroblasts, 89–90
Müllerian, 82
neuroendocrine, 47
oncocytic, 26
ovarian sex cord-stromal, 22, 33, 62, 112
primitive neuroectodermal, 113
Stertoli cell, 22, 62
small, round to oval cell, 4
smooth muscle, 4, 82–85
ultrastructural diagnosis, 160–168
vascular, 66–71
Warthin's, 26
Type 2 alveolar pneumocytes, 65
Tyrosinase, 71

Urethra, amelanotic malignant melanoma, 134
Urothelium, 95

Vagina, clear cell carcinoma, 60, 120
Vascular tumors, 66–71
Vesiculoglobular bodies, 74
Villin, 99
Vimentin, 79, 86, 89

Warthin's tumor, 26
    and crystalline inclusions, 62
Weibel-Palade body—Vascular Tumors, 66–71
Wilm's tumor, 4
    and rhabdomyoblasts, 82

Xanthoma, malignant fibrous, 30

Z discs, 79
Zona fasciculata, 22
Zona glomerulosa, 22
Zona reticularis, 22
Zonula adherens and occludens, 108
Zymogen, 44–47